Molecular Immunobiology of Self-Reactivity

IMMUNOLOGY SERIES

1. Mechanisms in Allergy: Reagin-Mediated Hypersensitivity
   Edited by Lawrence Goodfriend, Alec Sehon and Robert P. Orange
2. Immunopathology: Methods and Techniques
   Edited by Theodore P. Zacharia and Sidney S. Breese, Jr.
3. Immunity and Cancer in Man: An Introduction
   Edited by Arnold E. Reif
4. *Bordetella pertussis:* Immunological and Other Biological Activities
   J.J. Munoz and R.K. Bergman
5. The Lymphocyte: Structure and Function (in two parts)
   Edited by John J. Marchalonis
6. Immunology of Receptors
   Edited by B. Cinader
7. Immediate Hypersensitivity: Modern Concepts and Development
   Edited by Michael K. Bach
8. Theoretical Immunology
   Edited by George I. Bell, Alan S. Perelson, and George H. Pimbley, Jr.
9. Immunodiagnosis of Cancer (in two parts)
   Edited by Ronald B. Herberman and K. Robert McIntire
10. Immunologically Mediated Renal Diseases: Criteria for Diagnosis and Treatment
    Edited by Robert T. McCluskey and Giuseppe A. Andres
11. Clinical Immunotherapy
    Edited by Albert F. LoBuglio
12. Mechanisms of Immunity to Virus-Induced Tumors
    Edited by John W. Blasecki
13. Manual of Macrophage Methodology: Collection, Characterization, and Function
    Edited by Herbert B. Herscowitz, Howard T. Holden, Joseph A. Bellanti, and Abdul Ghaffar
14. Suppressor Cells in Human Disease
    Edited by James S. Goodwin
15. Immunological Aspects of Aging
    Edited by Diego Segre and Lester Smith
16. Cellular and Molecular Mechanisms of Immunologic Tolerance
    Edited by Tomáš Hraba and Milan Hašek

17. Immune Regulation: Evolution and Biological Significance
Edited by Laurens N. Ruben and M. Eric Gershwin

18. Tumor Immunity in Prognosis: The Role of Mononuclear Cell Infiltration
Edited by Stephen Haskill

19. Immunopharmacology and the Regulation of Leukocyte Function
Edited by David R. Webb

20. Pathogenesis and Immunology of Treponemal Infection
Edited by Ronald F. Schell and Daniel M. Musher

21. Macrophage-Mediated Antibody-Dependent Cellular Cytotoxicity
Edited by Hillel S. Koren

22. Molecular Immunology: A Textbook
Edited by M. Zouhair Atassi, Carel J. van Oss, and Darryl R. Absolom

23. Monoclonal Antibodies and Cancer
Edited by George L. Wright, Jr.

24. Stress, Immunity, and Aging
Edited by Edwin L. Cooper

25. Immune Modulation Agents and Their Mechanisms
Edited by Richard L. Fenichel and Michael A. Chirigos

26. Mononuclear Phagocyte Biology
Edited by Alvin Volkman

27. The Lactoperoxidase System: Chemistry and Biological Significance
Edited by Kenneth M. Pruitt and Jorma O. Tenovuo

28. Introduction to Medical Immunology
Edited by Gabriel Virella, Jean-Michel Goust, H. Hugh Fudenberg, and Christian C. Patrick

29. Handbook of Food Allergies
Edited by James C. Breneman

30. Human Hybridomas: Diagnostic and Therapeutic Applications
Edited by Anthony J. Strelkauskas

31. Aging and the Immune Response: Cellular and Humoral Aspects
Edited by Edmond A. Goidl

32. Complications of Organ Transplantation
Edited by Luis H. Toledo-Pereyra

33. Monoclonal Antibody Production Techniques and Applications
Edited by Lawrence B. Schook

34. Fundamentals of Receptor Molecular Biology
Donald F. H. Wallach

35. Recombinant Lymphokines and Their Receptors
Edited by Steven Gillis

36. Immunology of the Male Reproductive Organs
Edited by Pierluigi E. Bigazzi

37. The Lymphocyte: Structure and Function
Edited by John J. Marchalonis

38. Differentiation Antigens in Lymphohemopoietic Tissues
Edited by Masayuki Miyasaka and Zdenek Trnka

39. Cancer Diagnosis In Vitro Using Monoclonal Antibodies
Edited by Herbert Z. Kupchik

40. Biological Response Modifiers and Cancer Therapy
Edited by J. W. Chiao

41. Cellular Oncogene Activation
Edited by George Klein

42. Interferon and Nonviral Pathogens
Edited by Gerald I. Byrne and Jenifer Turco

43. Human Immunogenetics: Basic Principles and Clinical Relevance
Edited by Stephen D. Litwin, with David W. Scott, Lorraine Flaherty, Ralph A. Reisfeld, and Donald M. Marcus

44. AIDS: Pathogenesis and Treatment
Edited by Jay A. Levy

45. Cell Surface Antigen Thy-1: Immunology, Neurology, and Therapeutic Applications
Edited by Arnold E. Reif and Michael Schlesinger

46. Immune Mechanisms in Cutaneous Disease
Edited by David A. Norris

47. Immunology of Fungal Diseases
Edited by Edouard Kurstak

48. Adoptive Cellular Immunotherapy of Cancer
Edited by Henry C. Stevenson

49. Colony-Stimulating Factors: Molecular and Cellular Biology
Edited by T. Michael Dexter, John M. Garland, and Nydia G. Testa

50. Introduction to Medical Immunology, Second Edition
Edited by Gabriel Virella, Jean-Michel Goust, and H. Hugh Fudenberg

51. Tumor Suppressor Genes
Edited by George Klein

52. Organ-Specific Autoimmunity
Edited by Pierluigi E. Bigazzi, Georg Wick, and Konrad Wicher

53. Immunodiagnosis of Cancer: Second Edition
Edited by Ronald B. Herberman and Donald W. Mercer

54. Systemic Autoimmunity
Edited by Pierluigi E. Bigazzi and Morris Reichlin

55. Molecular Immunobiology of Self-Reactivity
Edited by Constantin A. Bona and Azad K. Kaushik

Additional Volumes in Preparation

Molecular Immunobiology of Self-Reactivity

edited by

Constantin A. Bona
Mount Sinai School of Medicine
New York, New York

Azad K. Kaushik
Ontario Veterinary College
University of Guelph
Guelph, Ontario, Canada

Marcel Dekker, Inc. New York • Basel • Hong Kong

Library of Congress Cataloging--in--Publication Data

Molecular immunobiology of self-reactivity/edited by Constantin A. Bona, Azad K. Kaushik.
p. cm. -- -- (Immunology)
Includes bibliographical references and index.
ISBN 0-8247-8553-3 (alk. paper)
1. Autoimmunity-- --Molecular aspects. I. Bona, Constantin A. II. Kaushik, Azad K. III. Series: Immunology (Marcel Dekker, Inc.)
[DNLM: 1. Autoantibodies-- --physiology. 2. Autoimmunity--physiology. QW 575 M718]
QR188.3.M67 1991
616.97'8–dc20
DNLM/DLC
for Library of Congress 91-28131
CIP

This book is printed on acid-free paper.

MARCEL DEKKER, INC.
270 Madison Avenue, New York, New York 10016

Current printing (last digit):
10 9 8 7 6 5 4 3 2 1

PRINTED IN THE UNITED STATES OF AMERICA

Series Introduction

The primary function of the immune system is to recognize macromolecules that distinguish self from nonself and preserve the integrity of the body. The response of the immune system is beneficial or detrimental depending on the circumstances. Harmful microorganisms elicit a response designed to destroy or exclude them; transplanted tissues are rejected to the detriment of the host. Only autologous molecules are normally accepted and adopted. Individual integrity is thus preserved.

The ability to separate foreign from self molecules resides in the T lymphocyte, the cell specialized in recognition. Its code is the epitope, the smallest unit of immunologic information. MHC molecules present a fragment of the molecule of 6 to 12 amino acids to the T cells, which make a decision to respond to it as foreign or to ignore it as self.

What forms the basis for this crucial decision? Clearly, it is made on the molecular level. This book deals with the fundamental questions asked by the immune system and the answers supplied by the epitopes. Immunologic health depends upon the answer. When errors occur, when the distinction between self and nonself is not accurately drawn, autoimmune disease may result. Recent advances in our understanding of the molecular basis of self-recognition have highlighted the inherent dangers, but have also revealed fresh opportunitites for avoiding the harmful consequences of autoimmunity. This book is a remarkable collection of essays about the risks and the opportunities that analysis at the molecular basis has brought to the study of autoimmune disease.

Noel R. Rose

Preface

Because immunology was born as a subdiscipline of microbiology it was thought that the major function of the immune system was to defend the host against harmful microbes. From this paradigm two major concepts originated: (1) that the major function of the immune system was to discriminate the self from nonself, and (2) that an eventual antiself reaction was not physiologic. Indeed, for a long time, it was believed that the clones able to recognize the self were deleted or blocked normally and that their activation was an abnormal phenomenon that led to pathologic processes.

Ensuing years have seen the accumulation of findings demonstrating the self-reactive clones are a normal component of the immune repertoire. Furthermore, it has been shown that autoantibodies such as rheumatoid factor occur during conventional antibody responses elicited by a variety of antigens or subsequent to vaccinations. Recognition of idiotypes by both B- and T-cell clones strongly suggests that the immune system is not directed toward exogenous agents alone and that host defense mechanisms against the microbes probably evolved from a more basic and primitive function related to the maintenance of macromolecular homeostasis. Such an evolution in immunologic thinking has been greatly facilitated by the advances in the development of biotechnological tools that permit molecular dissection of the immune system with precision and exactness. This knowledge, however, has for the moment blurred the conventional dividing line between physiologic and pathologic processes of the immune system. This book is a collection of various topics that encompass facets of this "blurred area" where physiologic and autoimmunopathologic processes lose distinction. These processes remain intact during health but go "haywire" for multifactorial reasons, leading to the development of systemic autoimmune disorders.

We would like to express our gratitude to all the authors for their painstaking efforts and their scholarly contributions. Marcel Dekker, Inc. deserves our special thanks for having brought out the volume so elegantly and on time.

Constantin A. Bona
Azad K. Kaushik

Contents

Contributors

M. Abu-Shakra Soroka Medical Center, Beer-Sheva, Israel

David M. Allman University of Pennsylvania School of Medicine, Philadelphia, Pennsylvania

Rosario Billetta University of California at San Diego, San Diego, California

B. Bellon Hôpital Broussais, Paris, France

Constantin A. Bona Mount Sinai School of Medicine, New York, New York

Herbert S. Bresler Biotronic Systems Corporation, Rockville, and The Johns Hopkins School of Hygiene and Public Health, Baltimore, Maryland

C. Lynne Burek The Johns Hopkins School of Hygiene and Public Health, Baltimore, Maryland

Michael P. Cancro University of Pennsylvania School of Medicine, Philadelphia, Pennsylvania

Syamal K. Datta Tufts–New England Medical Center, Boston, Massachusetts

Guillaume Dighiero Pasteur Institut, Paris, France

P. Druet Hôpital Broussais, Paris, France

C. Dubey Hôpital Broussais, Paris, France

Edward Dwyer Hospital for Joint Diseases and Division of Rheumatology, New York University Medical Center, New York, New York

S. B. Ebeling University Hospital Utrecht, Utrecht, The Netherlands

Stacy E. Ferguson University of Pennsylvania School of Medicine, Philadelphia, Pennsylvania

Steven M. Friedman The Hospital for Special Surgery, New York, New York

Uri Galili Medical College of Pennsylvania, Philadelphia, Pennsylvania

Shibnath Ghatak Tufts–New England Medical Center, Boston, Massachusetts

Shannon L. Gleason Dow Chemical Company, Midland, Missouri, and The Johns Hopkins School of Hygiene and Public Health, Baltimore, Maryland

F. H. J. Gmelig-Meyling University Hospital Utrecht, Utrecht, The Netherlands

J.C. Guery Hôpital Broussais, Paris, France

Ellen Heber-Katz The Wistar Institute, Philadelphia, Pennsylvania

F. Hirsch Hôpital Broussais, Paris, France

Kevin J. Horgan The Hospital for Special Surgery, New York, New York

Thereza Imanishi-Kari Tufts–New England Medical Center, Boston, Massachusetts

Kuppuswamy N. Kasturi Mount Sinai School of Medicine, New York, New York

Azad K. Kaushik Ontario Veterinary College, University of Guelph, Guelph, Ontario, Canada and Mount Sinai School of Medicine, New York, New York

Garnett Kelsoe University of Maryland School of Medicine, Baltimore, Maryland

Laura J. Kienker University of Texas Southwestern Medical Center, Dallas, Texas, and University of Pennsylvania School of Medicine, Philadelphia, Pennsylvania

Rudolf C. Kuppers The Johns Hopkins School of Hygiene and Public Health, Baltimore, Maryland

T. Logtenberg University Hospital Utrecht, Utrecht, The Netherlands

Raoul Mayer Mount Sinai School of Medicine, New York, New York

Theresa L. O'Keefe Tufts–New England Medical Center, Boston, Massachusetts

L. Pelletier Hôpital Broussais, Paris, France

David N. Posnett Cornell University Medical College, New York, New York

Sumati Rajagopalan Tufts–New England Medical Center, Boston, Massachusetts

Noel R. Rose The Johns Hopkins School of Hygiene and Public Health, Baltimore, Maryland

A. Saoudi Hôpital Broussais, Paris, France

M. E. M. Schutte University Hospital Utrecht, Utrecht, The Netherlands

Y. Shoenfeld Sheba Medical Center, Tel-Hashomer, Israel

Maurizio Sollazzo University of California at San Diego, San Diego, California

H. Tournade Hôpital Broussais, Paris, France

J. H. van Es University Hospital Utrecht, Utrecht, The Netherlands

Robert Winchester Hospital for Joint Diseases and Division of Rheumatology, New York University Medical Center, New York, New York

Habib Zaghouani Mount Sinai School of Medicine, New York, New York

Maurizio Zanetti University of California at San Diego, San Diego, California

1

A Synopsis of Self-Reactivity

Azad K. Kaushik*
Mount Sinai School of Medicine, New York, New York

I. INTRODUCTION

The phenomenon of natural self-reactivity or autoreactivity, from "horror autotoxicus" to a normal inherent property of a functionally autonomous immune system, has come of an age. "Self-self interactions" between the molecules and cells of the immune system not only underlie the hierarchal acquisition of immune responsiveness during development, e.g., idiotype interactions during emergence of immune repertoire (1), but are also critical to the induction of specific immune responses during adulthood, e.g., major histocompatibility complex (MHC) restriction (2). Yet the immune system normally does not react to self constituents but responds to a diverse number of antigens operationally recognized as "foreign" or detrimental to the host. Such an intricate property of the immune system, contained in the germline and selected by evolutionary forces to host's advantage, is affected by bone marrow–derived B and thymus-derived T lymphocytes that are morphologically similar and originate from common hematopoietic stem cell precursors. Both B and T lymphocytes are functionally connected but use different effector strategies. For example, the immunoglobulin (Ig) molecule, a B-cell antigen receptor and its secreted product, tends to recognize the

**Current affiliation*: Ontario Veterinary College, University of Guelph, Guelph, Ontario, Canada

conformational structure of an antigenic determinant with varying affinities, dissociation constants ranging between 10^{-5} and 10^{-14} M (3). The T-cell antigen receptor (TcR : 4), however, mostly recognizes linear antigenic peptides, degraded and processed by antigen presenting cells (APC), in association with the polymorphic MHC molecules as the restricting element (2). Also, TcR requires certain accessory molecules, i.e., CD2, CD4, LFA-1, and CD8, that enhance their binding ability necessary for T-cell activation (5).

Both T and B lymphocytes use similar basic mechanisms to generate an enormous diversity of receptors capable of recognizing a wide array of antigenic determinants. The potential for generation of such diversity in the T- and B-cell repertoire is contained within the germline gene segments (V, variable; J, junction; D, diversity; and C, constant) that somatically recombine during development to generate receptor molecules unique to each clone. Thus, different specificities exhibited by antibodies arise from heavy- (V_H encoded by VDJC exons) and light- (V_L encoded by VJC exons) chain polypeptides that pair to from the ligand-binding region. Similarly, four polypeptides (α, β, γ, and δ) that form two types of TcR heterodimers (α:β and γ:δ) are encoded by somatically rearranged VDJC (β and δ chains) and VJC (α and γ chains) exons during T-cell development. The magnitude of combinatorial diversity of the TcR is relatively limited, compared to the Ig molecule, because of a small number of TcR V genes. Yet the potential diversity of the TcR ($\alpha:\beta = \sim 10^{15}$; $\gamma:\delta = \sim 10^{18}$) matches that of the Ig molecule ($\sim 10^{11}$). The TcR locus, however, contains more J-region elements than those of the Ig locus. Also, the D region is often translated in all three reading frames in the TcR (β and δ chains) unlike that of the Ig heavy chain. The N-region diversity, noted in the Ig heavy chain only, occurs in both chains of the TcR heterodimers (α:β as well as γ:δ) (4). Importantly, however, a high frequency of somatic mutations have so far been noted to occur in Ig molecules only, thereby further enhancing their already vast ligand-binding specificity (7). In adult mouse, stochastic V_H (8,9) but nonstochastic V_K gene usage (10) has been noted. In addition, genetic evidence has suggested stochastic $V_H + V_K$ pairing (11) in the mitogen-responsive B-cell repertoire. Similar chain pairing in the TcR may also be expected. Therefore, it seems reasonable to assume that the vast potential for diversity of the immune repertoire, contained within the germaine, paradoxically accommodates with the emergence of complementarity or self-reactivities per se.

In this chapter, I shall focus on the occurrence of self-reactivity in the humoral (B-lymphocyte) and cellular (T-lymphocyte) compartments of the immune system and its relevance to tolerance, development of autoimmune disorders, and possible therapeutic implications. The contributions of other molecules, MHC products and cytokines, in the physiology of the immune system and development of autoimmune disorders are discussed elsewhere (12,13) (see Chapter 11).

II. SELF-REACTIVITY AND AUTOIMMUNITY

The phenomenon of immunological self-reactivity refers to self-cognitive and binding properties of cells and/or their secretory products essential to physiological functioning of the immune system and the host's protective ability against an infinite number of foreign antigens. These include the normal occurrence of self-reactive Ig molecules (14–18), called natural autoantibodies (NAAbs), and autoreactive T (19,20) and B lymphocytes in healthy normal individuals (21,22), and nonimmunized normal (23–25) or germ-free animals (26,27). The existence of the latter has sometimes been termed natural autoimmunity or autoreactivity. This marks a conceptual distinction from processes and manifestations of the immune system where presence of autoantibodies or autoreactivity, for historical reasons, was always considered to be of pathologic sequelae. Undoubtedly, the contribution of autoantibodies or autoreactive T cells in the pathogenesis of several autoimmune disorders is well established.

A. Humoral Self-Reactivity

1. Natural Autoantibodies

The first description related to the presence of natural antibodies (NAbs) in the serum of normal individuals can be traced back to the work of Landois (1875), who attempted to understand the mechanisms of shock caused by animal blood transfusion to humans. Subsequently, Landsteiner (1900) discovered the presence of natural hemagglutinins directed against blood group determinants of the ABO system. Based on the demonstration of NAbs against a variety of infectious or noninfectious agents in normal individuals or animals, Boyden (28) defined natural antibodies as a family of molecules present in the body fluids of normal animals which are able to specifically combine with antigens but not with the immunologically acceptable molecules normally present in the body fluids. Nevertheless, NAbs against a number of self antigens (Table 1) have now been described, as the normally circulating Ig, in the blood of normal healthy individuals (15,16,29) or nonimmunized animals (30,31). In general, NAAbs possess specificity against highly conserved structures, e.g., myelin basic protein, nucleic acids, and cytoskeleton proteins. Some NAAbs also bind to synthetic haptens, like 2,4,6-tri-ntriophenyl (TNP), phosphoryl choline (PC), 4-hydroxy,5-iodo,3-nitrophenyl (NIP), α-1-3 dextran, GAT (GLU60,ALA30,TYR10), and α-galactosyl. In fact, NAAbs are of several types: some bind to easily accessible self constituents, like cell surface determinants, extracellular substances, plasma proteins, and hormones (Table 1), whereas others may be directed against autoantigens protected by lack of vascularization (e.g., membrane determinants of spermatozoa) or blood–brain barrier (e.g., murine brain antigen-2). Yet another type of NAAbs are directed against determinants masked by a histochemical barrier. For example,

TABLE 1 Common Autoantigens or Autoconstituents Against Which Natural Autoantibodies Are Demonstrable in Normal Individuals or Nonimmunized Animals

Red blood cells (HB, Hol, I and Spectrin)	Collagen
	Albumin
Thymocytes	Immunoglobulin
Spermatozoa	Thyroglobulin
Chief cells	Transferrin
Parietal cells	Cytokines
Axons	Fetuin
Mitochondria	Cytochrome *c*
Golgi apparatus	Renin
Anterior pituitary	α-Fetoprotein
Smooth muscle	DNA
Corpus luteum	RNA
Islet of Langerhans	Histone
Nervous tissue	Tubulin
MHC (H-2, HLA)	Myosin
Myelin components	Actin

autoantibodies reactive with DNA and cytoskeleton proteins (15–18) (Table 2), bromelain-treated mouse red blood cells (17,32–34) (Table 3), and α-gelactosyl (35) (see Chapter 17).

The NAAbs multispecifically reactive with DNA and cytoskeleton proteins (36) seem to represent germline-encoded affinities against self antigens present in most species normally. These NAAbs comprise a heterogeneous population, exhibiting a variable spectrum of multispecificity (Table 4). Most Ig-V genes (37–43), without any apparent somatic mutations (37,38), encode these NAAbs (Table 4), although a bias for certain V_H (42,44) and V_K (45) gene families has been noted. A V-region or idiotypic connectivity (46) among neonatal murine NAAbs, considered

TABLE 2 Major Characteristics of NAAbs Reactive with DNA and Cytoskeleton Proteins

1. Constitute normal circulating serum Ig (IgM, IgG, IgA) in most species including man, mouse, rabbit, sheep, and fish.
2. Multispecifically recognize structurally dissimilar antigenic determinants (proteins, lipids, and nucleic acids) with low to moderate affinities.
3. Constitute a predominant clonotype in the fetus and newborn and exhibit V-region connectivities.
4. Germline encoded without any apparent somatic mutations.
5. Share a recurrent idiotype, common to several species, with pathologic autoantibodies found in systemic lupus erythematosus.

TABLE 3 Major Characteristics of Murine NAAbs Reactive with BrMRBC

1. Restricted to mouse species, always IgM, and appear late during ontogeny.
2. Monospecifically recognize HB (hidden bromelain) autoantigen exposed on BrMRBC and its soluble analog (SEA-HB) circulating in plasma (TMA ion, also present in phosphatidyl choline, constitutes a subepitope).
3. Secretory cells proplasmacyte type, recently shown to be Ly-1 B cells, are preferentially localized in peritoneal cavity.
4. Germline encoded and genetically restricted ($V_H11:V_K9$) and share a common idiotype (CP).
5. Serum levels elevated in most autoimmune strains (e.g., NZB, BXSB) but essentially predominant in normal CBA/J (2.7% of serum IgM) mice. No direct relationship with autoimmune pathology.

to be important in the development and shaping of the immune repertoire (1), has been demonstrated. These molecules bear an evolutionarily conserved recurrent idiotype (47) that is shared with pathologic autoantibodies found in lupus patients and lupus-prone autoimmune mouse strains (48). An increased serum level of these NAAbs is not always accompanied by the development of autoimmune disorders, however. Their serum levels may also be increased during viral infections (49), chronic diseases (50) (see Chapter 15), cancers (51), monoclonal gammopathies (52), and physical injuries (53). Certain drugs (54) or chemicals (see Chapter 16) may also induce the production of these NAAbs. Thus, these molecules encompass both physiologic and pathologic manifestations of the immune system, and no methods are available to distinguish among those destined for either of the consequences. The significance of these NAAbs has also been considered in immunoregulation (55), housekeeping function (56,57), tolerance (58), and development of immune responses to foreign antigens (16,59).

In contrast to multispecific NAAbs, autoantibodies reactive with bromelain-treated mouse red blood cells (BrMRBC), also germline encoded, have so far been found to occur in mouse species only. These NAAbs occur in most normal and autoimmune mouse strains but are lacking in immunodeficient mice (17,31). Interestingly, however, these NAAbs exhibit an enormous degree of restriction at the level of specificity (relatively monospecific) (60), isotype (IgM only) (57), idiotype (predominantly 'CP' recurrent Id) (61), V gene usage ($V_H11:V_K9$) (62,63), and secretory cells (principally Ly-1 B cells) (64,65) as well as their localization (preferentially peritoneal cavity) (66). These molecules appear late during ontogeny and increase as a function of age (60). Some heterogeneity, however, at the level of idiotype and structure is evident among these NAAbs when strict BrMRBC lytic ability is not taken into account (67,68). The serum levels of anti-BrMRBC NAAbs are enormously increased in NZB mice that suffer from hemolytic anemia, but these do not seem to be directly involved in

TABLE 4 Ig-V Gene Usage Among Murine Natural Autoantibodies

Hybridoma Clone(s)	V_k gene family	V_H gene family	Antibody activity							
			TNP	Actin	Tubulin	Myosin	ssDNA	dsDNA	TMA	BrMRBC
Splenic Origin:										
A2 F9	8	7183		○						
A1 G10	23	Q52	●							
B1 E2	1	J558		○	○		○			
A9 A7	1	Q52	●	●	●	●		○		
A3 D2	4	7183	★	★	○					
A11G8	1	7183	★							
B15D3	N.I	Q52	○							
B13D4	1	Q52	●	○	●	★	★	●		
B1 F5	N.I.	Q52	●	●	○	○				
B8 H5	N.I.	Q52					●	●		
B10B9	1	Q52	●	●	●	★		○		
B6 F2	1	J558	○		●		○	●		
N5 C5	24	J558	●	●		●		●		
N8 F6	19	Q52	●	●		★		●		
N10E9	4	J558	★	●		○				
N8 G2	22	7183	○			★				
Z8 E5	19	J558	●	●	○	●	★	●		
F4 F5	21	J606	●	●		●				
F6 C6	10	36-60								
F9 A7	1	7183	●	●	●	●	○			
F1 B4	22	J558	●	●	★	●				
F11G11	N.I.	Q52	○							
F5-2	21	Q52	●	●	●	●	●	●		
F30-4	N.I.	Q52	★		★	●	●	●		
M15-1	1	J558				●				
M16-13	21	VGAM3.8	○							
M40-1	1	7183	●	●	●	★	●	●		
M34-5	1	36-60	★	○	●	○	●	●		
M25-8	1	7183	●	○	●		●	●		
M25-9	8	7183	●	●	●	●	●	●		
Peritoneal Origin:										
CP8F C4	N.D.	J558				●				
CP8ED2	8	Q52							●	
CP96B1-5	1	J606	★		★		●	●		
CP8CD3	9	V_H11							★	●
CP96B1-7	1	V_H11							★	●
CP95H6	9	V_H11							★	●
CP97C10	10	V_H11							★	●
CP93C11	9	V_H11							★	●
CP9-9A4	19	V_H11							★	●
CP4-99	9	V_H11							★	●
CP5B-3	9	V_H11							★	●

Ni = not identified; ND = not done; Ten V_H (7183,Q52,S107,X24,36-60,VGam3.8,V_H11, J606,3609 and J558) and ten V_K(V_K1, -2, -4, -8, -9, -10, -19, -21, -22, and -24) gene family-specific DNA probes were used. Reactivity pattern: ● = +++; ★ = ++; ○ = +.
Source: Ref. 66.

the pathogenesis of the autoimmune process. Their secondary involvement, as bystander molecules, remains to be excluded, however.

The NAAbs mentioned above are representatives of two different categories of autoantibodies with distinct characteristics and will be discussed for their contributions in immunophysiology and etiopathogenesis of autoimmune diseases.

2. *Self-Reactive B Cells*

The discovery of NAAbs led to an intense search for the B lymphocytes or "natural plasma" cells secreting them. Earlier evidences included the use of plaque-forming cell assays to demonstrate the presence of autoreactive B cells (ABC), e.g., NAAbs against BrMRBC. But the advent of hybridoma technology greatly facilitated the demonstration of ABCs secreting NAAbs in normal healthy individuals (21,22) and nonimmunized (23–25) or germ-free animals (26,27). In addition, NAAbs could be analyzed at immunochemical and molecular level (Table 4). About 10–20% of hybridomas from the spleen or peritoneal cavity of adult normal or autoimmune mice (66) secrete NAAbs reactive with a test panel comprised of common autoantigens, e.g., DNA, actin, tubulin, myosin, albumin, IgG, and BrMRBC (Table 5). It must be mentioned that percent autoreactivity as analyzed by somatic hybridization is expected to increase with an enlargement of the test panel including other autoantigens. Also, the hybridoma technique is unlikely to reveal an actual size of ABC repertoire because of inherent technical difficulties. Nevertheless, this technique unequivocally demonstrates the substantial presence of ABCs normally in the B-cell repertoire. The multispecific NAAbs against DNA and cytoskeleton proteins are predominant in the splenic immune repertoire, while NAAbs reactive with BrMRBC are principally noted in the peritoneal immune repertoire.

Two different approaches have been used to phenotypically single out B cells that secrete autoantibodies. First, a deficient autoantibody production was noted in X-linked immunodeficient (Xid) CBA/N mice that lack a mature subset of B lymphocytes defined by the presence of Lyb-5 surface marker. But the subsequent demonstration of Lyb-5 as a differentiation marker (69) and the presence of an intrinsic B-cell defect in Xid mice (70) confirms that this molecule could not be strictly related to autoantibody-secreting cells. The second approach comprised demonstration of a small subpopulation of normal B cells bearing Ly-1 (human homolog CD5) glycoprotein of 67 kD, initially described as pan T-cell marker, called Ly-1 B cells (65,71). Several observations suggest an important contribution of Ly-1 B cells in the production of autoantibodies: (1) Ly-1 B cells are considerably increased in autoimmune mice like NZB and BXSB, (2) CBA/N Xid mice, deficient in autoantibody secretion, lack functional Ly-1 B subset, (3) an increased frequency of Ly-1 B cells in neonates parallels an increased frequency of activated neonatal ABCs secreting autoantibodies, (4) an increased frequency of Ly-1 B cells in peritoneal cavity parallels predominant anti-BrMRBC

TABLE 5 Profile of Adult Murine Autoreactive B-cell Repertoire as Revealed by Somatic Hybridization

	Mitogen-activated Balb/c		NZB	
Characteristics	Spleen	Peritoneal cavity	Spleen	Peritoneal cavity
% Ig secreting hybridomas	67	60	66	94
% Isotype distribution				
IgM κ	82.5	59.1	64.2	95.1
λ	—	3.0	—	4.9
IgG κ	11.1	1.5 (γ3)	27.4	—
λ	—	—	—	—
IgA κ	—	—	1.1	—
λ	—	—	—	—
Heavy chain^{-} κ	6.3	28.8	6.3	—
λ	—	7.6	1.1	—
% Reactivity with autoantigen panel[a]	11	12	17	16
% Monospecificity	28.6	87.5	81.3	92.3
% Multispecificity	71.4	12.5	18.8	7.7

[a]The autoantigen panel comprised DNA, actin, tubulin, albumin, myosin, rabbit IgG, BrMRBC, TMAion, and TNP hapten (66).

autoantibody secretion (72), and (5) in humans, CD5 B cells, although different from their mouse homolog (Ly-1 B) in several respects, have been related to the production of rheumatoid factors (73). However, certain discrepancies related to Ly-1 B cells and autoantibody production exist: (1) autoimmune-prone MRL 1pr/1pr mice do not exhibit an increased Ly-1 B-cell frequency, (2) anti-BrMRBC specificity is not found in neonates despite the presence of an increased Ly-1 B-cell frequency, (3) not all autoantibody specificities are evident in the peritoneal cavity, rich in Ly-1 B cells (66,72), (4) no increase in the frequency of anti-DNA autoantibody specificity occurs in Ly-1^{+} B cells when compared to Ly-1^{-} B cells (74), and (5) in humans, an increase in the frequency of CD5 B cells has not been observed in patients afflicted with systemic lupus erythematous (SLE) (73). Taken together, these data suggest a relatively important involvement of Ly-1 B cells in autoantibody production, but a further functional or phenotypic heterogeneity might exist in the Ly-1 B subpopulation. In addition, autoantibodies might arise through a number of pathways (Fig. 1), but evidence for certain possibilities might only be partial, and, in some cases, it is not known whether such mechanisms operated in vivo. Molecular approaches, already begun (see

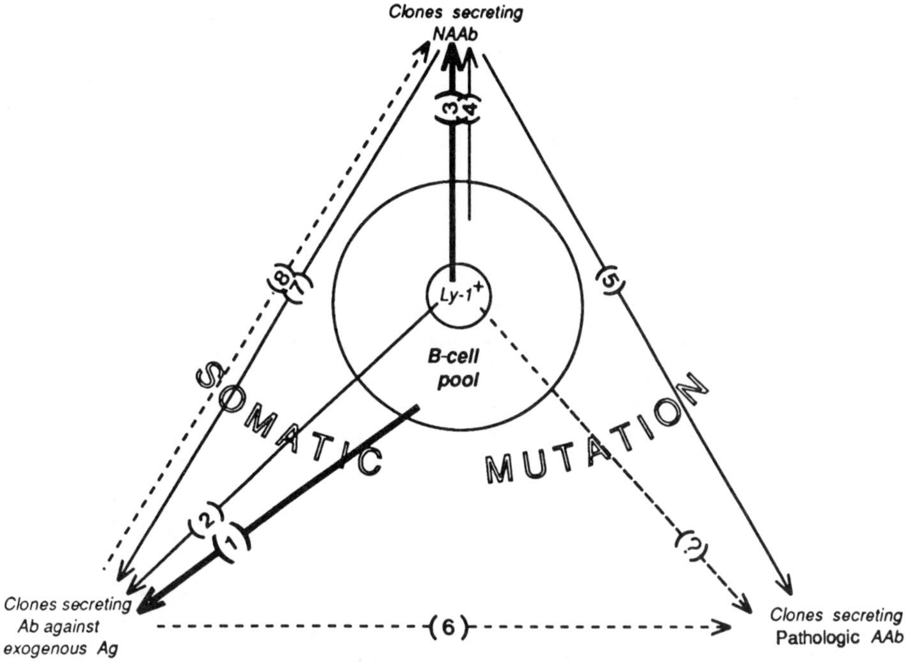

FIGURE 1 Possible pathways through which three types of functionally defined antibodies could arise from the B-lymphocyte pool. These different types of antibodies might overlap in terms of specificity, idiotype, and Ig-V gene usage. References for the arrows are as follows: 1 (65,75); 2 (76); 3 (65,71); 4 (74); 5 (77,78), 6 (79); 7 (59,80); 8 (91).

to help resolve and understand relationships between B-cell subsets and secretion of autoantibodies.

B. T-Cell Autoreactivity

The physiologic existence of NAAbs and the ABCs secreting them generated an interest in the occurrence of self-reactivity among T cells, i.e., whether T cells capable of responding to their own self antigens or MHC molecules, in the absence of a foreign antigen, existed among normal individuals or animals. In fact, the first evidence for occurrence of self-reactivity in T cells came from autologous or syngeneic mixed lymphocyte responses (19). These findings have been confirmed by several laboratories that established autoreactive T-cell lines from healthy individuals or animals. The autoreactive T cells from healthy individuals can be activated in the absence of any identifiable foreign antigen, including absence of any xenogenic serum components (82), by syngeneic and not allogeneic MHC class II stimulators. More recently, V-region connectivities or TcR complementarities have been demonstrated (83). Also, occurrence of autoreactive T cells may not always be accompanied by the development of autoimmune disorders. For example, autoreactive T cells responding to myelin basic protein have been found in the blood of healthy individuals (84).

1. *Reactivity Profile*

Normally, T cells reactive to particular self class II molecules are found in the immature population present in thymus cortex but not in the mature population in the medulla or peripheral lymphocyte pool. Several reports, however, suggest processing and presentation of self antigens by Ia^+ antigen-presenting cells (APC) in vitro. For example, APCs have been shown to present autologous and foreign F protein in vitro (85). Similarly, syngeneic Ig fragments have been shown to be presented in the context of class II molecules in vitro (86). The peripheral nervous system–derived Schwann cells, activated by γ interferon, can present myelin basic protein to T cells in the absence of any exogenous antigen (87). None of these studies, however, showed if these self antigen/Ia complexes could be expressed constitutively in vivo. Recently, murine peritoneal macrophages have been shown to process and potentially present self antigen hemoglobin in vivo (88). Another study suggested specificity of T cells for Ia alone rather than Ia associated with other self antigens (89). These conclusions were based on the observations that glass beads coated with liposomes incorporating affinity purified Ia stimulated autoreactive and alloreactive T-cell hybridomas for IL-2 secretion. In view of the observations that processed peptides may remain associated even with crystalline MHC class I molecules (90), contribution of similar peptides associated with class II molecules, in these studies, to an autoreactive determinant is difficult to rule out. How many self proteins are capable of forming complexes with Ia in vivo needs to be established. At the same time, it could be speculated that self MHC molecules might be processed and presented analogous to other self antigens since it is known that alloreactive cytotoxic T cells can recognize HLA-derived peptides in the context of self MHC molecules (91).

2. *Dynamics of T-Cell Autoreactivity*

It has been suggested that normal autoreactivity is an intrinsic property of T cells originally selected in the thymus and is recalled or revealed following antigen-dependent activation in the periphery (20). Such a physiologically induced state might be transient or relatively stable. Obviously, then, some autoreactive T cells may derive from antigen-stimulated precursors. In fact, the specificity of autoreactive T-cell clones selected from an antigen-primed population, under well-defined conditions, reflects the predominant MHC-restricted specificity of T cells specific for the immunogen (92). Thus, I-E subregion–specific autoreactive T cells are detected at a much higher frequency in populations primed with I-E–restricted antigen than those primed with I-A–restricted antigen (93). Further support comes from the analysis of TcR gene expression in autoreactive T-cell clones selected from cytochrome C–stimulated populations. The diversity of germline TcR V-region genes expressed in the pigeon cytochrome C–specific T-cell repertoire is restricted (94). The $V_\beta 16$ TcR gene predominates in cytochrome C–specific, I-E^k–restricted T cells that have also been selected for I-E^k_α: E^s_β alloreactivity. Autoreactive T cells arose in these cell lines, which also predominantly used $V_\beta 16$ TcR genes. Some evidence also exists that autoreactive specificity is also manifested by some antigen-specific T cells, or that autoreactive T cells might also arise from immature precursors (20). Therefore, it is reasonable to assume tht autoreactive T cells arise physiologically, and their frequent occurrence reinforces the notion of natural self-reactivity as an inherent property of the immune system necessary for its functional autonomy.

III. SELF-REACTIVITY AND TOLERANCE

Most immunologic theories, until now, that attempted to explain the phenomenon of immune responsiveness emphasized the lack of autoreactivity to be the major underlying factor, as reactivity to self was always related to autoimmune disorders. An unequivocal demonstration of self-reactivity, enshrined in the germline, does not support such a long-held view and makes it imperative to delineate mechanisms that allow a host immune system to respond to "foreign" antigens while remaining tolerant to self constituents. An important clue to such mechanisms emerged from the pioneering studies of Owen and colleagues in 1946, with dizygotic twins of cattle, demonstrating that immunologic tolerance is, in fact, an acquired characteristic. Subsequent theories suggested that contact of B or T lymphocytes during development with a self antigen led to either deletion (95) or functional silencing, termed anergy (96), thereby preventing self-reactivity. Alternatively, tolerogenesis might be induced by activation of a distinct population of suppressor cells which would either silence or eliminate mature self-reactive clones (12).

The normal presence of autoreactive B cells and NAAbs, and involvement of some NAAbs in the development of autoimmune disorders, does not apparently support clonal deletion or "anergy" theories. Importantly, however, autoreactive B cells or autoantibodies reactive with certain critical antigens, e.g., blood group antigens, have not been reported so far. Also, mechanisms of clonal deletion or "anergy" of immature B cells operate on high affinity B cells (97), and, thus, low affinity receptors of some NAAb secreting B cells are likely to escape such a control. Certain self-reactive specificities, e.g., anti-BrMRBc autoantibodies, appear late during ontogeny and might be subject to some other similar mechanisms. In addition, somatic hypermutation of Ig genes provides extra diversity that might generate self-reactive B cells of pathologic consequences. For example, an in vitro point mutation in the mouse system myeloma V_H region changed its specificity from antiphosphoryl choline to anti-DNA (79). No direct in vivo evidences are available yet that support these findings. Transgenic mice have provided useful tools to further gain an insight into the mechanisms of tolerogenesis. Two available studies on the fate of autoreactive B cells in transgenic mice provided evidence for both clonal deletion (98) as well as clonal anergy (99). Recent evidences also indicate operation of clonal anergy on mature self-reactive B cells. In transgenic mice, mature peripheral B lymphocytes in lymphoid follicles, like immature B cells, have been found to be rendered tolerant upon encountering self antigens provided receptor occupancy by self antigen exceeded a critical threshold (100). These studies also suggested that clonally silenced self-reactive cells are common in the peripheral B-cell repertoire.

For T cells, thymus plays an important role in the development of tolerogenesis during intrathymic differentiation. The positive selection of T-cell repertoire ensures that mature T cells would recognize an antigen only when it is associated with a self MHC molecule, but this process will also permit differentiation of cells with high affinities for self peptides and self MHC. There is now convincing evidence for clonal deletion of such T cells within the thymus. Studies with monoclonal antibodies directed to TcR restricted by class II MHC, I-E, or bind the products of Mls^a allele of the minor lymphocyte-stimulating locus (Mls) have provided evidence for the existence of cells with such TcR in $I\text{-}E^+$ or Mls^{a+} mice in the immature thymic lymphocyte population but not in the peripheral T-cell population (101–103). Two independent studies, using transgenic mice in which antiself TcR were expressed in the developing T cells, have demonstrated clonal deletion of self-reactive T cells during intrathymic differentiation (104,105). Several in vitro experimental approaches also suggest clonal anergy of autoreactive T cells (12). Whether these mechanisms operate in vivo is not known yet. Transplantation tolerance has also been noted to correlate with high levels of T- and B-lymphocyte activity in the spleen (106), thus sharing some cellular characteristics associated with immune responsiveness. The autoreactive T cells frequently found in normal individuals or animals appear to be an outcome of normal immune processes rather than an escape from the normal mechanisms of tolerogenesis.

Therefore, the presence of autoreactive T or B cells and NAAbs is not in contradiction per se to the mechanisms responsible for the induction of tolerogenesis but reflects their coexistence and, in fact, constitutes the underlying framework of immunophysiologic processes critical to homeostasis, tolerance, and development of immune responses. In other words, the phenomenon of self-reactivity is constitutively interwoven with the immunoregulatory apparatus essential to normal functioning of the immune system.

IV. SELF-REACTIVITY AND AUTOIMMUNE DISORDERS

Autoimmune disorders are of multifactorial origin including genetic and environmental or hormonal factors. Several hypotheses have been put forward that attempt to explain etiopathogenesis of autoimmune disorders. One hypothesis considers disregulation of the immune system (107) as the cause and the target tissue as the victim. Another incriminates molecular mimicry (see Chapter 13) of self antigens by foreign antigenic determinants as the mechanism responsible for breakdown of tolerance. Still another hypothesis considers development of autoimmune disorders as a result of sustained excess antiantigen turnover in the diseased tissue and, thus, does not differ from responses to foreign antigens (108).

A. Natural Autoantibodies and Autoimmune Diseases

The contribution of certain autoantibodies in the development of autoimmune diseases is well established (see Chapter 8). The normal presence of NAAbs adds a new dimension to understanding their contribution in the development of autoimmune disorders. Some of the NAAbs, e.g., NAAbs reactive with BrMRBC, may not be directly involved in the autoimmune process, but their secondary contribution remains to be examined. The NAAbs multispecifically reactive with DNA and cytoskeleton proteins share their specificity pattern and idiotypes with lupus autoantibodies. The possible involvement of these NAAbs in systemic lupus erythematosus, an organ nonspecific autoimmune disorder, is suggested from several findings: (1) multispecific NAAbs have been demonstrated in the tissue lesions of glomerulonephritis in lupus-prone mice (P. Matsiota, personal communication; (109), (2) cross-reactive idiotype related to these NAAbs is shared by lupus NAAbs (48), (3) analysis of serum idiotype profile has been shown to correlate well with the clinical status of several lupus patients (110), and (4) a human monoclonal anti-DNA antibody, bearing 16/6 common idiotype induces SLE-like disease in nonautoimmune prone C3H-SW mice (111). Importantly, however, most pathogenic autoantibodies in SLE exhibit specificity for native DNA. Also, these show isotype switch to IgG, are cationic in nature (112), and exhibit somatic hypermutations in their V regions (78). Similar restricted specificities, isotype switch, and somatic mutations have also been observed for rheumatoid factors involved in the pathogenesis of murine rheumatoid arthritis (77). These observations suggest selection by the autoantigen leading to affinity maturation and, thus, immune responses to target autoantigens are similar to those for exogenous antigens after secondary immunization. It seems that polyclonal B-cell activation, earlier noted for autoantibody secretion (113), precedes the phase during which clonal selection operates leading to the emergence of most isotype switched and somatically mutated pathogenic autoantibodies. The genetic analysis of murine autoantibodies have revealed that organization of both Ig heavy- and light-chain V-region gene complexes of normal and autoimmune prine mice appear similar, based on restriction fragment length polymorphism (RFLP), and systemic autoimmune diseases are not associated with a particular haplotype (42,45,114–116). In fact, both normal and autoimmune mice use similar genes for responses either against self or foreign antigens (42,117) (see Chapter 6). Similar studies in the outbred human populations are difficult to analyze. Nevertheless, some heterogeneity in the human Ig V_H locus has been noted, but its significance is unclear (118). The RFLP pattern of V_K locus in lupus patients has also been found to be normal (119).

B. Self-Reactive T Cells and Autoimmune Disease

The involvement of T cells in the development of autoimmune diseases (see Chapter 9) has been inferred from the following observations: (1) autoreactive T cells are capable of transferring the disease to naive recipients, (2) elimination of T-helper cells can abrogate disease (120), and (3) autoreactive T cells are found in a variety of autoimmune disorders, e.g., myasthenia gravis (121), Graves' disease (122), rheumatoid arthritis (123), etc. But autoreactive T cells have not been demonstrated in all autoimmune diseases, e.g., SLE, where T-cell hyporesponsiveness has been reported (124). The presence of self Ia–specific autoreactive T cells has been shown in the cerebrospinal fluid of patients with multiople sclerosis (125) and in synovial fluid of patients with rheumatoid arthritis (126). In fact, isolation of autoantigen specific T-cell lines from affected individuals does not reveal whether these cells contributed to the primary cause of autoimmune pathology since autoreactive T cells are often recruited in the ongoing specific immune responses. However, injection of self Ia–specific T-cell clones can induce autoimmune skin lesions (127). It seems that normal self Ia–specific autoreactive T cells escape regulatory feedback because of chronic stimulation as a result of aberrant Ia expression noted in several autoimmune diseases (e.g., type 1 diabetes) or concomitant defects in the suppressor T cells. These self Ia–specific T cells, then, might contribute to development of either systemic or organ-specific autoimmune diseases.

Knowledge of organization and genetic variability of TcR gene loci (see Chapter 10) may help determine susceptibility of spontaneous or induced autoimmune diseases. The genetic analysis of hybrids between susceptible (SWR, H_2v) and resistant (B10, H_2b) mice has revealed that one of the determinants of collagen-induced arthritis might be related to the presence of the $V_\beta6$ gene segment in the susceptible mice (120). Similarly, a unique deletion of $C_\beta1$-$D_\beta2$-$J_\beta2$ genetic elements in the β chain of TcR in autoimmune NZB or BXW F_1 mice (128) and a significant skewing for $V_\beta8$ genes of TcR in MRL 1pr/1pr appear to correlate with the development of autoimmune disease (120). Among the four V_α murine haplotypes defined, NZB, SJL, SWR, PL/J, and NOD strains share a common

V_α haplotype (129). In humans, several reports suggest possible associations of RFLPs with various autoimmune diseases, e.g., multiple sclerosis, myasthenia gravis, Graves' disease (120), etc. Most of these studies are of a preliminary nature, and development of improved novel strategies would be necessary to better understand the involvement of autoreactive T cells in autoimmune disorders.

V. THERAPEUTIC IMPLICATIONS

The multispecific NAAbs share a common idiotype, evolutionarily conserved in several species, with lupus autoantibodies. A functional idiotypic connectivity among these murine NAAbs of neonatal origin exists. It would be important to demonstrate whether such a V-region connectivity exists among human multispecific NAAbs. Nevertheless, idiotypic networks have been considered to be important in the immunoregulation of autoimmune responses. Increased levels of anti-idiotypic antibodies have been found among patients afflicted with several systemic or organ-specific autoimmune disorders. Thus, an important strategy would be aimed at bringing the disregulated pathways, whether cause or victim of autoimmune pathogenesis, back to the physiologic threshold of immune processes. Actually, intravenous infusions of IgG prepared from large pools of normal donors have resulted in clinical improvements and/or a decrease in autoantibody titers in several organ-specific autoimmune diseases. It is known that these therapeutic Ig contain anti-idiotypic antibodies against a variety of autoantibodies, e.g., anti-DNA, antithyroglobulin, anti-intrinsic factor, and anti-factor VIII autoantibodies (130). These reagents seem to provide control mechanisms of autoimmune responsiveness either through immunoregulatory circuits or by preventing binding of autoantibodies to their respective autoantigens, and perhaps both. Importantly, however, the size of the Ig pool would determine the probability of expression of desired anti-idiotypic activities. Pools of genetically defined, engineered, and conformationally shaped proteins, analogous to normal Ig, might provide better refined approaches towards treatment of autoimmune diseases in the future. Such passive administration of anti-idiotypic antibodies may be necessary at regular intervals to continuously revitalize the normal immunoregulatory circuits.

Whether V-region connectivities observed in some multispecific NAAbs extend to T-cell clones is not yet known. The possibility of using attenuated autoimmune T-cell clones as immunogens to prevent or revert autoimmune diseases has been suggested (131). T cells expressing $\alpha\beta$ TcR for antigen can elicit anti-idiotypic antibodies that might regulate T-cell function. Thus, strategies aimed at exploiting the normal immunoregulatory properties of autoreactive T cells could be developed to prevent autoimmune diseases. Certain homogeneity in the receptors of T cells generated in several experimentally induced autoimmune disorders has been observed. Two studies used synthetic TcR V-region peptides to induce specific regulatory immunity that resulted in successful prevention of experimental allergic encephalomyelitis (132,133). Similar studies could be extended to other autoimmune diseases like rheumatoid arthritis. Molecular characterization of the TcR of self Ia-reactive T cells should provide important insights into their immunoregulatory properties and whether these could be exploited for prevention of systemic or organ specific autoimmune diseases. Importantly, however, immunotherapy with peptides will have to take into account the extensive MHC polymorphism in the outbred human population as well as possible effects upon the beneficial protective ability of the host.

ACKNOWLEDGMENTS

I thank Dr. Brenda Hall and Dr. Yukiko Saitoh for their valuable help in the preparation of this manuscript, and Ms. Anita Spingarn for her skillful secretarial assistance.

REFERENCES

1. Kearney, J. F., and M. Vakil. 1986. Idiotype directed interactions during ontogeny play a major role in the establishment of the adult B cell repertoire. *Immunol. Rev.*, *94*: 39–49.
2. Zinkernagel, R. M., and P. C. Doherty. 1979. MHC restricted cytotoxic T cells: Studies on the biological role of polymorphic major transplantation antigens during T cell restricted specificity, function and responsiveness. *Adv. Immunol.*, *27*: 52.
3. Steward, M. W., and J. Steensgaard. 1983. *Antibody Affinity: Thermodynamic Aspects and Biological Significance*. CRC, Bocca Raton, FL.
4. Davis, M. M., and P. J. Bjorkman. 1988. T cell antigen receptor genes and T cell recognition. *Nature, 334*: 395–402.
5. Springer, T. A., M. L. Dustin, T. K. Kishimoto, and S. D. Marlin. 1987. The lymphocyte function associated LFA-1, CD2 and LFA-3 molecules. Cell adhesion receptors of the immune system. *Ann. Rev. Immunol.*, *5*: 223–252.
6. Tonegawa, S. 1983. Somatic generation of antibody diversity. *Nature, 302*: 575–581.
7. Siekevitz, M., C. Kocks, K. Rajewsky, and R. Dildrop. 1987. Analysis of somatic mutation and class switching in naive and memory B cells generating adoptive primary and secondary responses. *Cell, 48*: 757.
8. Dildrop, R., U. Krawinkel, E. Winter, and K. Rajewsky. 1985. V_H gene expression in murine lipopolysaccharide blasts distributes over the nine known V_H gene groups and may be random. *Eur. J. Immunol.*, *15*: 1154.
9. Schulze, D. H., and G. H. Kelsoe. 1987. Genotypic analysis of B cell colonies by *in situ* hybridization. Stoichiometric expression of three V_H families in adult C57 BL6 and Balb/c mice. *J. Exp. Med.*, *166*: 163.
10. Kaushik, A., D. H. Schulze, C. Bona, and G. Kelsoe. 1989. Murine V_K gene expression does not follow the V_H paradigm. *J. Exp. Med.*, *169*: 1859–1864.

11. Kaushik, A., D. H. Schulze, F. A. Bonilla, C. Bona, and G. Kelsoe. 1990. Stochastic $V_H{}^+V_K$ pairing occurs among polyclonally activated cell clones. *Proc. Natl. Acad. Sci. USA, 87*: 4932–4936.
12. Nossal, G. J. V. 1989. Immunologic tolerance: Collaboration between antigen and lymphokines. *Science, 245*: 147–152.
13. Feldmann, M. 1989. Molecular mechanisms involved in human autoimmune diseases: Relevance of chronic antigen presentation, class II expression and cytokine production. *Immunology* (Suppl.), *2*: 66–71.
14. Bussard, A. E. 1966. Antibody formation in non-immune peritoneal cells after incubation in gum containing antigen. *Science, 153*: 887–888.
15. Avrameas, S., B. Guilbert, and G. Dighiero. 1981. Natural antibodies against tubulin, actin, myoglobulin, thyroglobulin, fetuin, albumin and transferrin are present in normal human sera and monoclonal immunoglobulins from multiple myeloma and Waldenstrom's macroglobulinaemia may express similar antibody specificities. *Ann. Immunol. (Inst. Pasteur), 132c*: 231.
16. Dighiero, G., P. Lymberi, B. Guilbert, T. Ternynck, and S. Avrameas. 1986. Natural autoantibodies constitute a substantial part of normal circulating immunoglobulins. *Ann. N.Y. Acad. Sci., 475*: 135–145.
17. Dighiero, G., A. Kaushik, P. Poncet, and X. R. Ge. 1987. Origin and significance of autoantibodies. *Concepts Immunopathol., 4*: 42–76.
18. Tomer, Y., and Y. Shoenfeld. 1988. The significance of natural autoantibodies. *Immunol. Invest., 17*: 389–424.
19. Weksler, M. E., C. E. Moody, and R. W. Kozak. 1981. The autologous mixed lymphocyte reaction. *Adv. Immunol., 31*: 271.
20. Zauderer, M. 1989. Origin and significance of autoreactive T cells. *Adv. Immunol., 45*: 417–437.
21. Shoenfeld, Y., S. C. Hsu-Lin, J. E. Gabriels, L. E. Silberstein, B. C. Furie, B. D. Stollar, and R. W. Schwartz. 1982. Production of autoantibodies by human-human hybridomas. *J. Clin. Invest., 70*: 205–208.
22. Cairns, E., J. Block, and D. A. Bell. 1984. Anti-DNA autoantibody producing hydridomas of normal human lymphoid cell origin. *J. Clin. Invest., 74*: 880.
23. Pages, J. M., and A. E. Bussard. 1978. Establishment and characterization of permanent murine hybridoma secreting monoclonal autoantibodies. *Cell. Immunol., 41*: 188.
24. Dighiero, G., P. Lymberi, J. C. Mazie, S. Rouvy, G. S. Butler-Brown, R. G. Whalen, and S. Avrameas. 1983. Murine hybridomas secreting natural monoclonal antibodies reacting with self antigens. *J. Immunol., 131*: 2267.
25. Probhakar, B. S., J. Saegusa, T. Onodera, and A. L. Notkins. 1984. Lymphocytes capable of making monoclonal autoantibodies that react with multiple organs are a common feature of the normal B cell repertoire. *J. Immunol., 133*: 2815.
26. Underwood, J. R., J. S. Pedersen, P. J. Chalmers, and G. H. Toh. 1985. Hybrids from normal germfree nude and neonatal mice produce monoclonal autoantibodies to eight different intracellular structures. *Clin. Exp. Immunol., 60*: 417.
27. Box, N. A., and C. G. Meenuwsen. 1989. B cell repertoire in adult antigen free and conventional neonatal mice I. Preferential utilization of the C_H-proximal V_H gene family 7183. *Eur. J. Immunol., 19*: 1811–1815.

28. Boyden, S. V. 1966. Natural antibodies and the immune response. *Adv. Immunol.*, *5*: 1.
29. Hooper, B., S. Whittingham, and J. D. Mathews. 1972. Autoimmunity in a rural community. *Clin. Exp. Immunol.*, *12*: 79.
30. Karsenti, E., B. Guilbert, M. Bornens, and S. Avrameas. 1977. Antibodies to tubulin in normal non-immunized animals. *Proc. Natl. Acad. Sci. USA*, *74*: 3997.
31. Kaushik, A., P. Poncet, and A. Bussard. 1986. Autoantibodies against bromelainized mouse erythrocyte: Strain distribution of idiotype expression and relative peritoneal cell activity. *Cell. Immunol.* *102*: 323–334.
32. Cunningham, A. J. 1974. Large number of cells in normal mice produce antibody components of isologous erythrocytes. *Nature* (London), *252*: 749.
33. Pages, J. M., and A. E. Bussard. 1976. Precommitment of normal mouse peritoneal cells by erythrocyte antigens in relation to autoantibody production. *Nature* (London), *257*: 316.
34. Huetz, F., and P. Poncet. 1989. Immunocompetence of peritoneal B cells. *Res. Immunol.*, *140*: 75–87.
35. Galili, U., E. A. Rachmilewitz, A. Peleg, and I. Flechner. 1984. A unique natural human IgG antibody with α-galactosyl specificity. *J. Exp. Med.*, *160*: 1519.
36. Ternynck, T., and S. Avrameas. 1986. Murine natural monoclonal autoantibodies: A study of their polyspecificities and their affinities. *Immunol. Rev.*, *94*: 99–112.
37. Baccala, R., Quang, V., B. Guilbert, T. Ternynck, and S. Avrameas. 1989. Two murine natural polyreactive autoantibodies are encoded by non-mutated germline genes. *Proc. Natl. Acad. Sci. USA*, *86*:4624–4628.
38. Holmberg, D., A. Andersson, L. Carlsson, and S. Forsgren. 1989. Establishment and functional implications of B cell connectivity. *Immunol. Review*, *110*: 89–103.
39. Bellon, B., A. Lory-Manheimer, M. Monestier, T. Moran, A. Dimitriu-Bona, F. Alt, and C. Bona. 1987. High frequency of autoantibodies bearing cross-reactive idiotope among hydridomas using V_H7183 genes prepared from normal and autoimmune strains. *J. Clin. Invest.*, *79*: 1044–1053.
40. Painter, C., M. Monestier, B. Bonin, and C. Bona. 1986. Functional and molecular studies of V genes expressed in autoantibodies. *Immunol. Rev.*, *94*: 75–98.
41. Monestier, M., A. Lory-Manheimer, B. Bellon, C. Painter, H. Dang, N. Talal, M. Zanetti, R. Schwartz, D. Pisetsky, R. Kuppers, N. Rose, J. Brochier, L. Klareskog, R. Holmdahl, B. Erlanger, F. Alt, and C. Bona. 1986. Shared idiotopes and restricted V_H genes characterize murine autoantibodies of various specificities. *J. Clin. Invest.*, *78*: 753–759.
42. Bona, C. A. 1988. V genes encoding autoantibodies molecular and phenotypic characteristics. *Ann. Rev. Immunol.*, *6*: 237–358.
43. Dighiero, G., A. Lim, M.-P. Lembezat, A. Kaushik, L. Andrade, and A. Freitas. 1988. Comparative study of V_H gene family usage by newhorn Xid and non-Xid mice, newborn and adult NZB mice, and by splenic and peritoneal cavity B cell compartments. *Eur. J. Immunol.*, *18*: 1979–1983.
44. Logtenberg, T., F. M. Young, J. H. VanEs, H. J. Gemalig-Meyling, and F. W. Alt. 1989. Autoantibodies encoded by the most J_H-proximal human immunoglobulin heavy variable region gene. *J. Exp. Med.*, *170*: 1347–1355.

45. Kasturi, K., M. Monestier, R. Mayer, and C. Bona. 1988. Biased usage of certain V_K gene families by autoantibodies and their polymorphism in autoimmune mice. *Molec. Immunol.*, *25*: 213.
46. Holmberg, D., S. Forsgren, F. Ivars, and A. Coutinho. 1984. Reactions among IgM antibodies derived from normal mice. *Eur. J. Immunol.*, *14*: 435.
47. Morgan, A., D. A. Isenberg, Y. Naparstek, J. Rauch, D. Duggan, R. Khiroija, N. A. Staines, and A. Schattner. 1985. Shared idiotypes are expressed on mouse and human anti-DNA autoantibodies. *Immunology, 56*: 393.
48. Madio, M. P., Schattner, A., Schattner, M., and R. S. Schwartz. 1986. Lupus serum and normal human serum contain anti-DNA antibodies with the same idiotypic marker. *J. Immunol.*, *137*: 2535.
49. Aaronson, S. A., and J. R. Stephenson. 1974. Wide spread natural occurrence of high titers of neutralizing antibodies to a specific class of endogenous mouse type C virus. *Proc. Natl. Acad. Sci. USA, 71*: 1957.
50. Galvao-Castro, B. S. A., J. A. Ferreira, K. F. Marzochi, M. C. Marzochi, S. G. Coutinho, and M. H. Lambert. 1984. Polyclonal activation circulating immune complexes and autoimmunity in human American visceral leishmaniasis. *Clin. Exp. Immunol.*, *56*: 58.
51. Nowinski, R. C., and S. L. Kochler. 1974. Antibody to leukaemia virus: Widespread occurrence in inbred mice. *Science, 185*: 869.
52. Dighiero, G., B. Guilbert, and S. Avrameas. 1982. High incidence of monoclonal Ig exhibiting antibody activity against actin and tubulin and sharing antibody specificities with natural antibodies. *J. Immunol.*, *128*: 2788.
53. Schattner, A. 1987. The origin of autoantibodies. *Immun. Lett.*, *14*: 143.
54. Ochi, T., E. A. Goldings, P. E. Lipski, and N. Ziff. 1983. Immunomodulatory effect of procainamide in man. *J. Clin. Invest.*, *71*: 36.
55. Holmberg, D., and A. Coutinho. 1985. Natural antibodies and autoimmunity. *Immunol. Today, 6*: 356.
56. Grabar, P. 1975. Autoantibodies and immunological theories: An analytical review. *Clin. Immunol. Immunopathol.*, *4*: 453.
57. Kaushik, A., T. Matthes, and G. Dighiero. 1988. Do natural autoantibodies play an important role in the elimination of senescent or damaged red blood cells? *Blood Cells, 14*: 161–170.
58. Cohen, I. R., and A. Cooke. 1986. Natural autoantibodies might prevent autoimmune disease. *Immunol. Today, 7*: 363.
59. Naparstek, Y., J. Andre-Schwartz, T. Manser, L. J. Wysocki, L. Bretiman, B. Stollar, M. Gefter, and R. S. Schwartz. 1986. A single germline V_H gene segment of normal A/J mice encodes autoantibodies characteristics of systemic lupus erythematosus. *J. Exp. Med.*, *16*: 614.
60. Poncet, P., M. P. Kocher, J. Pages, J. C. Taton, and A. E. Bussard. 1985. Monoclonal autoantibodies against red blood cells. A family of structurally related molecules. *Molec. Immunol.*, *22*: 541.
61. Bussard, A. E., M. A. Vinit, and J. M. Pages. 1976. Immunochemical characterization of the autoantibodies produced by mouse peritoneal cells in culture. *Immunochemistry, 14*: 1.

62. Reininger, L., P. Ollier, P. Poncet, A. Kaushik, and J. C. Jaton. 1987. Novel V genes encode virtually identical variable regions of six murine monoclonal anti-bromelain treated red blood cell autoantibodies. *J. Immunol., 138*: 316.
63. Reininger, L., A. Kaushik, S. Izui, and J. C. Taton. 1988. A member of a new V_H gene family encodes anti-bromelainized mouse red blood cell autoantibodies. *Eur. J. Immunol., 18*: 1521.
64. Bussard, A. E., and J. Pages. 1976. The peritoneal cell phenomenon: Its general significance in cellular immunology. *Ann. Immunol., 127C*: 583.
65. Hayakawa, K., R. R. Hardy, D. R. Parks, and L. A. Herzenberg. 1983. The Ly-1 B cell subpopulation in normal, immunodefective and autoimmune mice. *J. Exp. Med., 157*: 202.
66. Kaushik, A., A. Lim, P. Poncet, X. R. Ge, and G. Dighiero. 1988. Comparative analysis of natural antibody specificities among hybridomas originating from spleen and peritoneal cavity of adult NZB and Balb/c mice. *Scand. J. Immunol., 27*: 461–471.
67. Pennell, C. A., L. W. Arnold, G. Haughton, and S. H. Clarke. 1988. Restricted Ig variables gene expression among Ly-1^+ normal B cell lymphomas. *J. Immunol., 141*: 2788.
68. Conger, J. D., H. J. Sage, and R. B. Corley. 1988. Diversity in the available repertoire of murine antibodies reactive with bromalain treated isologous erythrocytes. *J. Immunol., 143*: 4044–4052.
69. Smith, M. R., L. J. Yaffe, D. L. Kastner, and A. D. Steinberg. 1986. Evidence that Lyb 5 is a differentiation antigen in normal and Xid mice. *J. Immunol., 136*: 1194.
70. Ohriner, W. D., and J. J. Cebra. 1985. Antigens apparently non-immunogenic for xid/Y mice cause the development of specific splenic plasmablasts and of fusion partners for SP2 cells giving hybridomas that secrete antibodies. *Eur. J. Immunol., 15*: 906.
71. Herzenberg, L. A., A. M. Stall, P. A. Lalor, C. Sidman, W. A. Moore, D. R. Parks, and L. A. Herzenberg. 1986. The Ly-1 B cell lineage. *Immunol. Rev., 93*: 81.
72. Dighiero, G., P. Poncet, T. Matthes, and A. Kaushik. 1987. Is autoantibody production related to particular B cell subsets and variable region genes? *Pathol. Immunopathol. Res., 6*: 371–389.
73. Calvert, J. E., M. F. Duggan, S. W. G. Smith, A. L. Givan, and P. Bird. 1988. The $CD5^+$ B cell: A B cell lineage with a central role in autoimmune diseases? *Autoimmunity, 1*: 223–240.
74. Conger, J. D., B. L. Pike, and G. J. V. Nossal. 1987. Clonal analysis of the anti-DNA repertoire of murine B lymphocytes. *Proc. Natl. Acad. Sci., 84*: 2931.
75. Rajewsky, K., I. Forster, and A. Cumano. 1987. Evolutionary and somatic selection of the antibody repertoire in the mouse. *Science, 238*: 1088–1094.
76. Forster, I., and K. Rajewsky. 1987. Expansion and functional activity of Ly-$1B^+$ cells upon transfer of peritoneal cells into allotype congenic newborn mice. *Eur. J. Immunol., 17*: 521.
77. Shlomchik, M. J., A. Marshak-Rothstein, C. B. Wolfowicz, T. L. Rothstein, and M. G. Weigert. 1987. The role of clonal selection and somatic mutation in autoimmunity. *Nature* (London), *328*: 805.
78. Schlomchik, M., M. Masulli, H. Shan, M. Z. Radic, D. Pisetsky, A. Marshak-

Rothstein, and M. Weigart. 1990. Anti-DNA antibodies from autoimmune mice arise by clonal expansion and somatic mutation. *J. Exp. Med., 171*: 265–297.
79. Giusti, A. M., N. C. Chien, D. J. Zack, S. V. Shin, and M. D. Schraff. 1987. Somatic diversification of S107 from an anti-phosphocholine to an anti-DNA autoantibody is due to a single base change in its heavy chain variable region. *Proc. Natl. Acad. Sci. USA, 84*: 2926.
80. Manser, T., J. W. Lawrence, M. N. Margolies, and M. L. Gefter. 1987. Evolution of antibody variable region struture during the immune response. *Immunol. Rev., 96*: 41.
81. Bos, N. A., C. G. Meenuwsen, P. V. Winggaarden, and R. Bermer. 1989. B cell repertoire in adult antigen free and conventional neonatal Balb/c mice II. Analysis of antigen binding capacities in relation to V_H gene usage. *Eur. J. Immunol., 19*: 1817–1822.
82. Yamashita, V., and E. M. Shevach. 1980. The syngeneic mixed leukocyte reaction: The genetic requirements for the recognition of self resemble the requirements for the recognition of antigen in association with self. *J. Immunol., 124*: 1773.
83. Sim, G. K., and A. A. Augustin. 1983. Internal images of major histocompatibility antigens on T cell receptors and their role in the generation of the T-helper cell repertoire. *Ann. N.Y. Acad. Sci., 418*: 272.
84. Tournier-Lasserve, E., G. A. Hashim, and M. A. Bach. 1988. Human T cell response to myelin basic protein in multiple sclerosis patients and healthy subjects. *J. Neurosci. Res., 19*: 149–156.
85. Winchester, G., G. H. Sunshine, N. Nardi, and N. A. Mitchison. 1984. Antigen presenting cells do not discriminate between self and non-self. *Immunogenetics, 19*: 487–491.
86. Bogen, B., B. Malissen, and W. Haas. 1986. Idiotype specific T cell clones that recognize syngeneic Ig fragments in the context of class II molecules. *Eur. J. Immunol., 16*: 1373–1378.
87. Wekerle, H., M. Schwab, C. Linington, and R. Meyermann. 1986. Antigen presentation in the peripheral nervous system: Schwann cells present endogenous myelin autoantigens to lymphocytes. *Eur. J. Immunol., 16*: 1551–1557.
88. Lorenz, R. B., and P. M. Allen. 1988. Direct evidence for functional self protein/Ia molecule complex *in vivo. Proc. Natl. Acad. Sci. USA, 85*: 5220–5223.
89. Coeshott, C. M., R. W. Chesnut, R. T. Kubo, S. F. Grammer, D. M. Tenis, and M. M. Grey. 1986. Ia specific mixed lymphocyte reactive T cell hybridomas: Analysis of their specificity by using purified class II MHC molecules in a synthetic membrane system. *J. Immunol., 136*: 2832.
90. Bjorkman, P. J., M. A. Saper, B. Samraoui, W. S. Bennett, J. L. Strominger, and D. C. Wiley. 1987. The foreign antigen binding site and T cell recognition regions of class I histocompatibility antigens. *Nature* (London), *329*: 512.
91. Parkham, P., C. Clayberger, S. L. Zorn, D. S. Ludwig, and A. M. Krensky. 1987. Inhibition of alloreactive cytotoxic T lymphocytes by peptides from the α-2 domain of HLA-A2. *Nature* (London), *325*: 625.
92. Faherty, D. A., D. R. Johnson, and M. Zauderer. 1985. Origin and specificity of autoreactive T cells in antigen induced populations. *J. Exp. Med., 161*: 1293.

93. Sproviero, J. F., M. J. Imperiale, and M. Zauderer. 1981. Clonal analysis of F_1 hybrid helper T cells. Ia sub-region encoded hybrid determinants restrict the activity of keyhole limpet hemocyanin-specific helper T cells. *J. Exp. Med., 154*: 1255.
94. Fink, P., L. Matis, D. McElligot, M. Bookman, and S. Hedrick. 1986. Correlations between T cell specificty and the structure of the antigen receptor. *Nature* (London), *321*: 219.
95. Burnet, F. M. 1959. *The Clonal Selection Theory of Acquired Immunity*. Cambridge University Press, Cambridge, Eng.
96. Nossal, G. J. V. 1983. Cellular mechanisms of immunologic tolerance. *Ann. Rev. Immunol., 1*: 33–62.
97. Riley, R. L., and N. R. Klinman. 1986. The affinity threshold for antigenic triggering differs for tolerance susceptible unimature precursors vs mature primary B cells. *J. Immunol., 136*: 3147–3154.
98. Nemazee, D. A., and K. Burki. 1989. Clonal deletion of B lymphocytes in a transgenic mouse bearing anti-MHC class-I antibody genes. *Nature* (London), *337*: 562–566.
99. Goodnow, C. C., J. Crosbie, S. Adelstein, T. B. Lavoie, S. J. Smith-Gill, R. A. Brink, M. Prichard-Briscoe, J. S. Wotherspoon, R. H. Loblay, K. Raphael, R. J. Trent, and A. Basten. 1988. Altered immunoglobulin expression and functional silencing of self-reactive B lymphocytes in transgenic mice. *Nature* (London), *336*: 73–76.
100. Goodnow, C. C., J. Crosbie, M. Jorgensen, R. A. Brink, and A. Basten. 1989. Induction of self-tolerance in mature peripheral B lymphocytes. *Nature* (London), *342*: 385–391.
101. Kappler, J. W., N. Roehm, and P. Marrack. 1987. T cell tolerance by clonal elimination in the thymus. *Cell, 49*: 273–280.
102. Kappler, J. W., V. Staerz, J. White, and P. Marrack. 1988. Self tolerance eliminates T cells specific for the Mls modified products of the major histocompatibility complex. *Nature* (London), *332*: 34–40.
103. McDonald, M. R., R. Sneider, R. K. Lees, R. C. Howe, A. Acha-Orbea, M. Fetenstein, R. M. Zinkernagel, and H. Hengartner. 1988. T cell receptor V_β use predicts reactivity and tolerance to Mls^a encoded antigens. *Nature* (London), *332*: 40–45.
104. Kisielow, P., H. Bluthmann, V. D. Staerz, M. Steinmetz, and H. von Boehmer. 1988. Tolerance in T cell receptor transgenic mice involves deletion of non-mature $CD4^+$ 8^+ thymocytes. *Nature* (London), *333*: 742–746.
105. Sha, W. C., C. A. Nelson, R. D. Newberry, D. M. Kranz, J. H. Russell, and D. Loh. 1988. Positive and negative selection of an antigen receptor on T cells in transfenic mice. *Nature* (London), *336*: 73–76.
106. Bandeira, A., A. Coutinho, C. Carnaud, F. Jacquemart, and L. Forni. 1989. Transplantation tolerance correlates with high levels of T and B lymphocyte activity. *Proc. Natl. Acad. Sci. USA, 86*: 272–276.
107. Kantor, F. S. 1988. Autoimmunities: Diseases of dysregulation. *Hosp. Practice* (July 15): 75–84.
108. Wilkin, T. 1989. Autoimmunity: Attack or defense? *Autoimmunity, 3*: 57–73.
109. Pankewycz, O. G., P. Migliorini, and M. Madio. 1987. Polyreactive autoantibodies are nephritogenic in murine lupus nephritis. *J. Immunol., 139*: 3287.

110. Isenberg, D. A., Y. Shoenfeld, M. P. Madio, J. Rauch, M. Reichlin, B. D. Stollar, and R. S. Schwartz. 1984. Anti-DNA antibody idiotypes in systemic lupus erythematosus. *Lancet, ii*: 417–422.

111. Mendlovic, S., B. Stefan, Y. Shoenfeld, M. Ben-bassat, A. Meshorer, R. Bakimer, and E. Mozes. 1988. Induction of a systemic lupus erythematosus like disease in mice by a common human anti-DNA idiotype. *Proc. Natl. Acad. Sci. USA, 85*: 2260–2264.

112. Gavalchin, J., R. A. Seder, and S. K. Datta. 1987. The NZB x SWR model of lupus nephritis I. cross-reactive idiotypes of monoclonal anti-DNA antibodies in relation to antigenic specificity, charge and allotype. Identification of interconnected idiotype families inherited from the normal SWR and autoimmune NZB parents. *J. Immunol., 138*: 128–137.

113. Dziarski, R. 1982. Preferential induction of autoantibody secretion in polyclonal activation by peptidoglycan and lipopolysaccharide I. *In vitro* studies. *J. Immunol., 128*: 1018–1025.

114. Kofler, R., R. M. Perlmutter, D. J. Noonan, F. J. Dixon, and A. N. Theofilopoulos. 1985. Ig heavy chain variable region gene complex of lupus mice exhibits normal restriction fragment length polymorphism. *J. Exp. Med., 162*: 346.

115. Kofler, R., R. Strohal, R. S. Balderas, M. E. Johnson, D. J. Noonan, M. A. Duchosal, F. J. Dixon, and A. N. Theofilopoulos. 1988. Immunoglobulin K-light chain variable region complex organization and Ig genes encoding anti-DNA autoantibodies in lupus mice. *J. Clin. Invest., 82*: 852–860.

116. Bona, C., K. N. Kasturi, R. Mayer, and V. Fidanza. 1988. V genes usage by autoantibodies and their polymorphism in autoimmune mice. *Autoimmunity, 2*: 29–53.

117. Kofler, R., D. J. Noonan, D. E. Levy, M. C. Wilson, N. P. H. Moller, F. J. Dixon, and A. N. Theofilopoulos. 1985. Genetic elements used for a murine lupus anti-DNA autoantibody are closely related to those for antibodies to exogenous antigens. *J. Exp. Med., 161*: 805.

118. Dijk, K. W. V., H. W. Schroeder, R. M. Perlmutter, and E. C. B. Milner. 1989. Heterogeneity in the human Ig V_H locus. *J. Immunol. 142*: 2547–2554.

119. Zouali, M., M. P. Madio, R. T. Canoso, and B. D. Stollar. 1989. Restriction fragment analysis of the V_K locus in human lupus. *Eur. J. Immunol. 19*: 1757–1760.

120. Kumar, V., D. H. Kono, J. L. Urban, and L. Hood. 1989. The T cell receptor repertoire and autoimmune diseases. *Ann. Rev. Immunol., 7*: 657–682.

121. Hohfeld, R., K. V. Toyka, K. Heinenger, H. Gross-Wilde, and I. Kalies. 1984. Autoimmune human T lymphocytes specific for acetylcholine receptor. *Nature* (London), *310*: 244–246.

122. Londei, M., G. F. Bottazzo, and M. Feldmann. 1985. Human T cell clones from autoimmune thyroid glands: specific recognition of autologous thyroid cells. *Science, 228*: 85–89.

123. Londei, M., C. Savill, A. Verhoef, F. Brennan, V. Duance, R. N. Maini, and M. Feldmann. Persistence of collagen type II specific T cell clones in the synovial membrane of a patient with rheumatoid arthritis. *Proc. Natl. Acad. Sci. USA, 86*: 636–640.

124. Rosenthal, C. J., and E. C. Franklin. Depression of cellular mediated immunity

in systemic lupus erythematosus: Relation to disease activity. *Arthritis Rheum.*, *18*: 207–217.

125. Brinbaum, G., L. Kotilinek, M. Schwartz, and M. Sternad. 1984. Spinal fluid lymphocytes responsive to autologous and allogeneic cells in multiple sclerosis and control individuals. *J. Clin. Invest.*, *74*: 1307.
126. Schlesier, M., C. Ramb-Lindhaver, M. Gartner, and H. H. Peter. 1984. Analysis of T cell cultures and clones from a patient with classic rheumatoid arthritis—Evidence for the existence of autoreactive T cell clones in blood and synovial fluid. *Rheumatol. Int.*, *4* (Suppl.), 1.
127. Shiohara, T., N. Moriya, T. Mochizuki, and M. Nagashima. 1987. Lichenoid tissue reaction (LTR) induced by local transfer of Ia reactive T cell clones. II. LTR by epidermal invasion of cytotoxic lymphokine producing autoreactive T cells. *J. Invest. Dermatol.*, *89*: 8.
128. Kotzin, B. L., V. L. Barr, and E. Palmer. 1985. A large deletion within the T cell receptor B chain gene complex in New Zealand white mice. *Science, 229*: 167–171.
129. Singer, P. A., R. J. McVilly, R. S. Balderas, F. J. Dixon, and A. N. Theofilopoulos. 1988. T cell receptor α-chain variable region haplotypes of normal and autoimmune laboratory mouse strains. *Proc. Natl. Acad. Sci.*, *85*: 7729–7733.
130. Rossi, F., G. Dietrich, and M. D. Kazatchkine. 1989. Anti-idiotypes against autoantibodies in normal immunoglobulins: Evidence for network regulation of human autoimmune responses. *Immunol. Rev.*, *110*: 315.
131. Ben-nun, A., H. Wekerle, and I. R. Cohen. 1981. Vaccination against autoimmune encephalomyelitis with T lymphocyte live cells reactive against myelin basic protein. *Nature, 292*: 60–61.
132. Vandenbark, A., G. Hashim, and H. Offner. Immunization with a synthetic T cell receptor V-region peptide protects against experimental autoimmune encephalomyelitis. *Nature* (London), *341*: 541-544.
133. Howell, M. D., S. T. Winters, T. Olee, H. C. Powell, D. J. Carlo, and S. W. Brostoff. 1989. Vaccination against experimental allergic encephalomyelitis with T cell receptor peptides. *Science, 246*: 668–670.

2

B-Cell Repertoire Development

Michael P. Cancro, Laura J. Kienker,* Stacy E. Ferguson, and David M. Allman
University of Pennsylvania School of Medicine, Philadelphia, Pennsylvania

I. INTRODUCTION: REPERTOIRE DEVELOPMENT DEFINED

Repertoire development is the process through which the receptor-bearing (Ig or TcR) lymphocyte pool is generated and maintained. Current concepts of repertoire development are based on the notion of clonal selection (1,2), which dictates that immune specificity is afforded through the clonal distribution of variable-region pairs (IgV_LV_H among B cells and TcR V_α V_β or V_γ V_δ among T cells). Accordingly, the assessment of repertoire development involves defining the mechanisms that shape the *distribution* of V-region pairs within the lymphocyte pool. These mechanisms include heritable ontogenetic events, clonal turnover, and ligand-mediated events, all of which may dictate or alter the relative representation of specificities within this distribution. Each of these areas may be examined individually but must ultimately be considered in concert, since their combined effects determine the exact distribution of specificities at a given point.

**Current affiliation*: University of Texas Southwestern Medical Center, Dallas, Texas

II. THE GENERATION OF RECEPTOR-EXPRESSING B CELLS—OVERVIEW

While a detailed treatment of genetic and cellular events in the differentiation of functional B cells is beyond the scope of this chapter, some general principles should be reviewed.

During early development, the differentiation of mammalian B cells occurs in three sites: fetal liver, spleen, and bone marrow. Subsequently, the bone marrow serves as the primary site of B-cell generation (see Refs. 3–5 for review).

The generation of surface Ig^+ B lymphocytes from hematopoietic stem cells requires the rearrangement of heavy- and light-chain gene segments to form functional genes. The first rearrangement joins D and J_H segments to form a DJ_H complex. This generally occurs on both chromosomes and is followed by either DJ_H replacement, where an upstream D segment joins to a downstream J_H segment, or by V_H rearrangement, to form a complete V_HDJ_H gene. Once a productive rearrangement is achieved, the Ig heavy chain is translated. The translation of a complete heavy chain is associated with the arrest of further V_H to DJ_H rearrangements, and with the initiation of light-chain gene rearrangement, where a V_L gene segment is rearranged to a J_L segment. Once light chains are translated, membrane-bound immunoglobulin is expressed on the cell surface (reviewed in detail in Refs. 6–8).

Receptor diversity within the primary B-cell pool is thus generated through: (1) the availability of multiple gene segments allowing many permutations *within* heavy (V_HDJ_H) and light (V_LJ_L) chains; (2) combinatorial association of heavy and light chains; and (3) "junctional" variability created by imprecise V_H-D, D-J_H, and V_L-J_L junctions. Based upon these strategies and estimates of the total number of available gene segments, the genome affords a *potential* repertoire of greater than 10^8 V_L-V_H pairs.

Understanding repertoire development requires analyses of the expression and relative representation of these potential specificities as a function of time.

III. PROBLEMS OF REPERTOIRE ASSESSMENT

Several aspects of repertoire development pose particularly challenging problems of experimental design and interpretation. Four issues of particular concern must thus be addressed initially: (1) the extent of repertoire diversity, both during ontogeny and at steady state, since this defines the heterogeneity of the distribution being examined; (2) the degree to which population and distribution assessments can be extrapolated to reflect the behavior of clones during B-cell differentiation; (3) the dynamics of the receptor-bearing B-cell pool; and (4) the plasticity of the receptor-bearing B-cell pool.

A. The Extent of B-Cell Repertoire Diversity

B cells rapidly expand in number during late development and achieve a steady state some time after parturition. A first-order consideration in examining repertoire development is establishing the diversity, in terms of clonally distributed V_LV_H pairs, within the steady-state population.

Early estimates of the adult murine B-cell repertoire were made from the frequency and clonotypic diversity of cells responsive to several antigens, as assessed through limiting dilution methods (9,10, and reviewed in Ref. 11). Isoelectric focusing, fine specificity analysis, and anti-idiotypic reagents were applied to distinguish V_LV_H species. Studies of the adult murine repertoires responsive to nitrophenacetyl (NP), beta-galactosidase, phosphorylcholine (PC), influenza hemagglutinin (HA), and 2, 4-dinitrophenyl (DNP) yielded estimates in the range of 2×10^7 total specificities in the adult B-cell pool (12–16). These estimates have proven generally accurate, if not somewhat low, and highlight the central question in assessing development of the B-cell repertoire: From the inception of B-cell production to the achievement of a steady state encompassing greater than 10^7 clonally distributed specificities, what is the behavior of the repertoire in terms of relative representation of particular specificities (clonal composition) and total array of specificities (diversity)?

B. Limitations of Population Assessments

The B-cell pool is a dynamic *population* of cells derived from multiple stem cell clones. While the differentiation scheme outlined in Section II described the generation of a single receptor-bearing cell, most examinations of repertoire development focus on analyses of B-cell populations, rather than following individual clones through the process of differentiation. This results in potential interpretive pitfalls, which should be briefly considered.

First, although largely synchronous (in terms of the production of B-lineage cells) in early development, the stem cell compartment achieves asynchrony quickly. Thus, the B-cell *population's* behavior may fail to reveal the order of events within a stem cell clone, except during the early, synchronous stages. Second, extrapolation from population data to the level of developing clones is constrained by a lack of knowledge in several critical areas. For example, the precise length of time between initial V_H to DJ_H rearrangement and the generation of a mature B cell, the number of divisions (equal or unequal) required, and the number of receptor-bearing progeny produced by a single progenitor (pro-pre-B cell) are unknown. Finally, the relationship of different B-cell subsets, as defined by surface markers, functional criteria, or antigen priming status, are also presently unknown (17).

C. The Dynamics of the B-Cell Pool

Although the precise numbers remain debated, B-cell clones show a turnover rate of between 1 week and 2 months, based on a variety of experimental approaches (18–23). It remains unclear whether subsets of B cells with different half-life properties exist, as well as to what extent discrepancies in these estimates reflect differences in experimental design. Regardless of these discrepancies, the B-cell pool's turnover rate is relatively rapid and thus must be carefully considered in the examination of developmental properties of the population.

This relatively rapid turnover rate implies that the clonal composition (the distribution of V_LV_H pairs within the pool) may change with time. Therefore, when the kinetics of repertoire development are examined, changes in diversity or composition with time must be viewed in the context of a constantly renewed pool of cells.

D. The Potential for Induced Effects—Plasticity of the B-Cell Repertoire

The plasticity of the B-cell repertoire reflects its potential sensitivity to ligand-driven events. Through a variety of mechanisms, particular members of the potential repertoire may be precluded from representation, while others may be expanded in their representation enormously. Further, these events are an ongoing process, mediated by the current array of available ligands (self, exogenous antigen, etc.). Thus, the relative contributions of ligand-driven events, which are superimposed upon the array of clonally distributed specificities afforded by genotype, must be addressed. The issue of ligand-induced perturbations of the developing repertoire will not be discussed in detail here. However, such events interdigitate with ligand-independent ontogenetic processes in shaping the repertoire and should be carefully considered, especially with respect to the generation or control of autoreactivity.

IV. THE B-CELL REPERTOIRE DURING ONTOGENY AND EARLY LIFE

A. Early Repertoire Development

1. *Heritable Emergence of Specificities*

Clonal specifities emerge in a heritable, nonrandom fashion during fetal and neonatal development. Early studies with sheep, opossum, and inbred mice showed that the ability to respond to certain antigens arises at particular times during development (24–28). Adoptive-transfer systems, in which B cells were intentionally supplied with competent accessory and helper cells, established this sequential acquisition of immune responsiveness as a property intrinsic to available responsive B cells. Whether particular *clonotypes* (cells bearing receptors comprised of particular $V_L V_H$ pairs) emerge at certain points was rigorously tested in several model antigen systems, primarily through limiting dilution analyses of B cells from inbred mice (29–36). These experiments all showed that clonotypes emerged in an ordered fashion. Further, the patterns of emergence were reproducible among genetically identical individuals, indicating a heritable basis for these developmental patterns.

Finally, entire funtional repertoires responsive to particular antigens were studied either by using animal models which have limited repertoire diversity, such as frogs (44,45) or bursectomized chickens, or by establishing systems for extensive fine-specificity analysis, such as the murine response to influenza hemagglutinin (37–39). These studies confirmed and extended previous observations of heritable patterns of clonal emergence by demonstrating that the *distribution* of clonotypes within a response was restricted and reproducible among genetically identical individuals of the same age.

2. *Heritable Patterns of Turnover*

Age-related changes were observed quite readily among predominant clonotypes responsive to many antigens, suggesting that the distribution or clonal composition of the repertoire undergoes turnover during early development. However, dilution rather than clonal turnover remained an explanation for these observations, since only a single responsive clonotype was assessed, and the number of responsive B cells was increasing during the developmental period studied. More recently, both the absolute number and diversity of HA-specific B-cell precursors were shown to remain relatively constant between 1 and 2 weeks of age (40,41), but the clonal composition differed. These observations confirmed and extended the earlier observations and showed that a rapid and regular turnover in the distribution of clonotypes indeed occurs during early development. In addition, because the distribution of clonotypes at each age was reproducible among genetically identical individuals, it was clear that not only the emergence of specificities, but also their turnover patterns, were under heritable control.

Together, these observations indicate a heritable developmental scheme through which the repertoire emerges. (The work summarized above is reviewed in greater detail in Refs. 42–44.)

3. *Multiple Genes and Repertoire Ontogeny*

Since heritable ontogenetic mechanisms operate during the initial development of the B-cell repertoire, the nature and number of genes involved are of interest. Studies have now shown that the clonal emergence and turnover patterns are mediated by multiple, unlinked loci (45–47). These studies demonstrated that distinct patterns of clonotypic emergence could be distinguished among inbred strains. Further, repertoire development in their F_1 progeny, although consistent among F_1s, was distinct from either parental strain's developmental pattern.

Among the genes controlling repertoire ontogeny, one of these is linked to or within the heavy-chain structural gene complex on murine chromosome 12. The remaining loci remain unmapped, but might be light-chain structural genes or loci that dictate the manner in which V_L and V_H genes are expressed (48).

These observations raise an important point for studies of outbred populations. Although it could clearly be seen that multiple unlinked genes control repertoire ontogeny by examining F_1 individuals from *inbred* mice, such patterns may be difficult to perceive in outbred populations, since the likelihood of generating genetically identical members of filial generations (comparable to F_1s derived from two inbreds) is slight. Thus, although broad rules may apply to outbred populations, such as the utilization of particular V gene families at certain developmental points (see below), it seems improbable that particular antigenic specificities will be characteristic of certain developmental stages in the neonatal B-cell pool of outbred populations.

B. V_H Gene Expression During Early Development

Since the patterns of clonal emergence are heritable, and at least some of the genes responsible segregate with heavy-chain structural genes, it was clear that assessments of variable region gene use within the developing repertoire might provide insight regarding the mechanisms underlying these phenomena.

These studies first required a detailed knowledge of the murine V_H gene pool and its organization and subsequent analyses of the relative representation of these genes within the emerging B-cell repertoire.

1. J_H-Proximal V_H Genes

The majority of murine heavy-chain variable-region gene segments have been defined and grouped into families according to nucleotide sequence homology. V_H gene segments with greater than 80% homology are considered family members. At least 13 families have now been described, and these vary in "complexity" (relative number of family members based on genomic Southern blot) from 1 to perhaps 1000 members. Further, the relative chromosomal map order of these V_H gene families has been established with some certainty (49–52). In BALB/c and C57BL mice, members of the V_H7183 and V_HQ52 families are those most proximal to D, J_H, and C_H. Many studies have examined whether the representation of these families is stochastic (i.e., only a function of family complexity) or instead appears skewed toward the use of particular families at particular developmental stages.

Numerous findings indicate that a preferential utilization of the V_H7183 and V_HQ52 families occurs during early B-cell development (53–63). For example, Abelson virus transformed pre–B-cell lines, and fetal pre-B cells preferentially rearrange V_H gene segments belonging to these families (57–62).

In other experiments, hybridomas from neonatal liver utilized J_H *distal* V_H gene segments at a higher frequency than hybridomas derived from fetal liver, suggesting that more distal V_H gene segments are utilized as development progresses. Since the chromosomal order of V_H families seems correlated with the time during development when each is expressed, the program of heavy-chain V_H gene segment rearrangement has been presumed to follow the order of V_H genes.

Similar heavy-chain variable-region chromosomal maps, as well as analyses of V_H family representation, are now also available in human model systems. The results suggest that J_H proximal V_H genes also predominate during early human development (63–66). Of particular interest is the observation that the J_H-proximal V_H family in the human is the homolog of the murine V_H7183 family, suggesting that this family's chromosomal position, in order to foster its over-representation in the early B-cell pool, may have been selectively preserved.

2. *Stochastic Distribution of V_H Genes in Adult B-Cells*

In contrast to the skewed distribution of V_H representation seen during early development, a stochastic distribution of V_H gene representation is generally observed when adult splenic B cells have been examined (67,68). While some deviation from a purely stochastic distribution has been noted in some strains of mice, these are not so striking as to suggest preferential expression mechanisms. Instead these distinctions are thought to reflect either ligand-driven expansion events, tolerogenic events, or differences in IgH-V haplotypes (e.g., the number of usable members in each family may vary between haplotypes).

The basis for this apparent "randomization" may be that in the mature individual, rearrangement of gene segments is itself a random process. Alternatively, this could reflect the continued preferential rearrangement strategies within stem cell clones, but asynchrony in the production of receptor-bearing B cells from the stem cell pool. Finally, it might reflect ligand-driven events that expand clonotypes representative of all V_H families.

3. *Preferential V_H Gene Usage in the Stem Cell Compartment*

Although the most J_H-proximal *Igh-V* genes participate in early rearrangements, how long such preferential events persist and whether they are evident within the antigen-responsive B-cell pool remain unclear. Recent studies suggest that preferential representation of J-proximal V_H genes may be evident within the B-cell pool for some time and may actually continue throughout life. When hydridomas representative of predominant HA specificites at 1 versus 2 weeks of age were compared, a marked preferential V_H gene representation was observed at both ages: V_H7183 appeared preferentially among hybridomas representative of 1 week of age, whereas V_HX24, V_H36-60, and V_HS107 were preferentially expressed at 2 weeks of age (62). Interestingly, the temporal order of family prevalence observed closely matches the murine V_H gene family order. These findings linked the heritable, age-related turnover of clonotypes (see Sec. IV.A.) with changes in V_H family predominance, and showed that nonrandom *shifts* in V_H gene representation occur within the neonatal antigen-responsive B-cell pool.

Studies that examined V_H message levels normalized to full-length μ transcripts have now shown that a disproportinate segment of the marrow pre–B-cell pool appears to be transcribing J_H-proximal V_H families (69).

Neither the marked shift in V_H predominance between 1 and 2 weeks of age nor the skewed representation of J_H-proximal V_H families in adult pre-B cells are consistent with completely random processes being operative even during later stages of development. The possible basis for these observations is discussed below.

4. V_L Gene Utilization Within the Developing B-Cell Pool

While not as well characterized as the V_H gene pool, the relative gene order within the V_κ cluster in mice is resolved to a degree where similar questions may be asked about V_κ expression during ontogeny. In such studies, the evidence suggests that the J_κ-proximal V_κ genes are not preferentially used during early development (70–72). Nonetheless, several laboratories have reported that certain V_κ families deviate from stochastic representation based on family size. Whether these reflect distinctions in the rearrangement and expression strategies at the kappa locus or are instead a reflection of ligand-driven expansion remains unclear.

V. LIGAND-DRIVEN EVENTS MAY SHAPE THE REPERTOIRE

The foregoing has addressed our knowledge of mechanisms at work in generating the primary, presumably unperturbed repertoire. As indicated earlier, however, these events simply provide a moving window of availability upon which ligand-driven events may operate to selectively expand or delete particular specificities. Although beyond the scope of this chapter, ligand-driven events must thus be considered an integral part of the development of the B-cell repertoire. Further, such events may have profound effects upon the repertoire over lengthy periods. For example, negative events may be mediated by ligand challenge. Early studies established that the interaction of B cells with ligand may under certain circumstances lead to irreversible anergy or death of a B-cell clone. The precise role of this process in the avoidance of self-reactivity is debated, although it is clear that this process may occur in vivo and may be mediated by endogenously synthesized molecules. In contrast, ligand may also act to expand and preserve the representation of particular specificities within the repertoire.

VI. OVERVIEW—CURRENT THOUGHTS AND REMAINING PROBLEMS

Nonrandom representation of V_H families within the primary, antigen-responsive B-cell pool can best be accommodated by models involving either the temporally controlled expression of V_H gene segments or intrinsic clonal expansion and deletion events based on V_H gene utilization that change with age. Intrinsic, receptor-driven clonal expansion and deletion events, mediated by anti-idiotypic interactions or self-reactivity, remain an alternative explanation for shifts in nonrandom representation of V_H families. However, these would necessarily involve a cascade of V_H-specific interactions triggered by the initial preferential expression of V_H7183.

It is tempting to speculate about the underlying reasons for patterned expression of immunoglobulin variable-region genes. Patterns may merely reflect an evolutionarily neutral rearrangement mechanism in which V_H genes are utilized based on their relative proximity to J_H.

Alternatively, either the mechanism per se or the gene order of V_H families may have been selectively favored, inasmuch as it gurantees the steady-state representation of most V_H families (even small ones) at all times in the adult, whereas completely random rearrangement mechanisms would not absolutely ensure this. Specifically, random gene rearrangement could allow several asynchronous B-cell progenitors to simultaneously rearrange the same V_H gene segment, limiting overall diversity—especially the likelihood of continous representation of very small families—in the available B-cell repertoire. In contrast, patterned, successive rearrangements, coupled with an asynchronous progenitor pool, would always yield a stochastic distribution of specificities containing representatives of most, if not all, families. Thus, only during early development, when there is a synchronous commitment to the B-cell lineage, would skewing towards certain V_H families be evident within the antigen-responsive B-cell pool. Significantly, during this period maternal antibodies are present that likely provide protection.

Finally, the patterned rearrangement mechanism coupled with a selected *Igh-V* locus organization might ensure that particular specificities are reproducibly expressed at particular times. The early B-cell repertoire has been reported to contain a disproportionate number of autoreactive and autoanti-idiotypic specificities, and such antibodies may be necessary for the development of the B-cell repertoire (73–74). The precise resolution of these mechanisms should yield insight regarding the relationship of normal developmental processes to autoreactivity and self/nonself discrimination in the B-cell compartment.

REFERENCES

1. Burnet, F. M. 1959. *The Clonal Selection Theory of Acquired Immunity*. Vanderbilt University Press, Nashville.
2. Jerne, N. K. 1954. The natural selection theory of antibody formation. *Proc. Natl. Acad. Sci. USA, 41*: 849–853.
3. Gowans, J. L., and E. J. Knight. 1964. The route of recirculation of lymphocytes in rat, *Proc. Royal Soc. Series B, 159*: 257.
4. Quesenberry, P., and L. Levitt. 1979. Hematopoietic stem cells *N. Engl. J. Med., 301*: 819–868.
5. Osmond, D. G. 1986. Population dynamics of bone marrow B-lymphocytes *Immunological Rev., 93*: 103–124.
6. Tonegawa, S. 1983. Somatic generation of antibody diversity. *Science, 302*: 575–581.
7. Blackwell, T. K., and F. W. Alt. 1988. Immunoglobulin genes. In *Molecular Immunology* (B. D. Hames and D. M. Glover, eds.). IRL Press, Washington, D.C.
8. Lewis, S., and M. Gellert. 1989. The mechanism of antigen receptor gene assembly. *Cell, 59*: 585–588.
9. Klinman, N. R. 1969. Antibody with homogeneous antigen binding produced by splenic foci in organ culture. *Immunochemistry, 6*: 757–759.
10. Lefkovits, I., and H. Waldmann. 1979. *Limiting Dilution Analysis of Cells in the Immune System*. Cambridge University Press, Cambridge.
11. Sigal, N. H., and N. R. Klinman. 1976. The B-cell clonotype repertoire. *Adv. Immunol., 26*: 255–324.
12. Nossal, G. J. V., J. W. Stocker, B. Pike, and J. W. Goding. 1977. Hapten-specific B-lymphocytes: Enrichment, cloning, receptor analysis, and tolerance induction. *Cold Spring Harbor Symp. Quant. Biol., 41*: 237–248.
13. Kreth, H. W., and A. R. Williamson. 1973. The extent of diversity of anti-hapten antibodies in inbred mice: Anti-NIP (4-hydroxy-5-iodo-3-nitrophenacetyl) antibodies in CBA/H mice. *Eur. J. Immunol., 3*: 141–147.
14. Kohler, G. 1976. Frequency of precursor cells against the enzyme B-galactosidase: An estimate of the BALB/c strain antibody repertoire. *Eur. J. Immunol., 6*: 340–347.
15. Cancro, M. P., W. Gerhard, and N. R. Klinman. 1978. The diversity of the influenza-specific primary B-cell repertoire in BALB/c mice. *J. Exp. Med., 147*: 776–787.
16. Owen, J. A., N. H. Sigal, and N. R. Klinman. 1982. Heterogeneity of the BALB/c IgM anti-phosphorylcholine antibody response. *Nature* (Lond.), *295*: 347–348.
17. Cancro, M. P., and S. E. Ferguson. 1989. Probing the cellular basis for immunologic memory: Approaching functional distinctions between primed and unprimed B-cell populations. *Seminars in Immunol., 1*: 79–86.
18. Sprent, J., and A. Basten. 1973. Circulating T and B lymphocytes of the mouse. II. Lifespan. *Cell. Immunol., 7*: 40–59.
19. Sprent, J., and J. F. A. P. Miller. 1972. Thoracic duct lymphocytes from nude mice: Migratory properties and life-span. *Eur. J. Immunol., 2*: 384–387.
20. Freitas, A. A., and A. Coutinho. 1981. Very rapid decay of mature B lymphocytes in the spleen. *J. Exp. Med., 154*: 994–999.
21. Freitas, A. A., B. Rocha, and A. A. Coutinho. 1986. Two major classes of mitogen-reactive B lymphocytes defined by life span. *J. Immunol., 136*: 466–469.

22. Freitas, A. A., B. Rocha, L. Forni, and A. Coutinho. 1982. Population dynamics of B lymphocytes and their precursors: Demonstration of high turnover in the central and peripheral lymphoid organs. *J. Immunol.*, *128*: 54–60.
23. Freitas, A. A., B. Rocha, and A. A. Coutinho. 1986. Life span of B lymphocytes: The experimental basis for conflicting results. *J. Immunol.*, *136*: 470–476.
24. Silverstein, A. M., J. W. Uhr, K. L. Kraner, and R. J. Lukes. 1963. Fetal response to antigenic stimulus. II. Antibody production by the fetal lamb. *J. Exp. Med.*, *117*: 799–812.
25. Yung, L. L. L., T. C. Wyn-Evans, and E. Diener. 1973. Ontogeny of the murine immune system: Development of antigen recognition and immune responsiveness. *Eur. J. Immunol.*, *3*: 224–228.
26. Rowlands, D. T., D. Blakeslee, and E. Angala. 1974. Acquired immunity in opossum (*Didelphis virginiana*) embryos. *J. Immunol.*, *112*: 2148–2153.
27. Sherwin, W. K., and D. T. Rowlands. 1974. Development of humoral immunity in lethally irradiated mice reconstituted with fetal liver. *J. Immunol.*, *113*: 1353–1360.
28. Sherwin, W. K., and D. T. Rowlands. 1975. Determinants of the hierarchy of humoral immune responsiveness during ontogeny. *J. Immunol.*, *115*: 1549–1554.
29. Press, J. L., and N. R. Klinman. 1973. Enumeration and analysis of antibody-forming cell precursors in the neonatal mouse. *J. Immunol.*, *111*: 829–835.
30. Press, J. L., and N. R. Klinman. 1974. Frequency of hapten-specific B cells in neonatal and adult murine spleens. *Eur. J. Immunol.*, *4*: 155–159.
31. Klinman, N. R., and J. L. Press. 1975. The characterization of the B-cell repertoire specific for the 2,4-dinitrophenyl and 2,4,6-trinitrophenyl determinants in neonatal BALB/c mice. *J. Exp. Med.*, *141*: 1133–1146.
32. Gearhart, P., N. Sigal, and N. Klinman. 1975. Heterogeneity of the BALB/c antiphosphorylcholine antibody response at the precursor cell level. *J. Exp. Med.*, *141*: 56–71.
33. Sigal, N. H., P. J. Gearhart, J. L. Press, and N. R. Klinman. 1976. Late acquisition of a germline antibody specificity. *Nature* (Lond.), *259*: 51–52.
34. Sigal, N. H., A. R. Pickard, E. S. Metcalf, P. J. Gearhart, and N. R. Klinman. 1977. Expression of phosphorylcholine-specific B cells during murine development. *J. Exp. Med.*, *146*: 933–948.
35. Sigal, N. H. 1977. The frequency of p-azophenyl- arsonate and dimethylaminoapthalene-sulfonyl-specific B cells in neonatal and adult BALB/c mice. *J. Immunol.*, *119*: 1129–1133.
36. Bona, C., J. J. Mond, K. E. Stein, S. House, R. Lieberman, and W. E. Paul. 1979. Immune response to levan. III. The capacity to produce anti-inulin antibodies and cross-reactive idiotypes appears late in ontogeny. *J. Immunol.*, *123*: 1484–1490.
37. DuPasquier, L., and M. R. Wabl. 1978. Antibody diversity in amphibians: Inheritance of isoelectric focusing antibody patterns in isogenic frogs. *Eur. J. Immunol.*, *8*: 428–433.
38. Huang, H. V., and W. J. Dreyer. 1978. Bursectomy *in ovo* blocks the generation of immunoglobulin diversity. *J. Immunol.*, *121*: 1738–1747.
39. Cancro, M. P., D. E. Wylie, W. Gerhard, and N. R. Klinman. 1979. Patterned acquisition of the antibody repertoire: diversity of the hemagglutinin-specific B-cell repertoire in neonatal BALB/c mice. *Proc. Natl. Acad. Sci. USA*, *76*: 6577–6581.

40. Thompson, M. A., and M. P. Cancro. 1982. Dynamics of B cell repertoire formation: Normal patterns of clonal turnover are altered by ligand interaction. *J. Immunol.*, *129*: 2372–2376.
41. Thompson, M. A., S. Raychaudhuri, and M. P. Cancro. 1983. Restricted adult clonal profiles induced by neonatal immunization: Influence of suppressor T cells. *J. Exp. Med.*, *158*: 112–125.
42. Cancro, M. P., M. A. Thompson, S. Raychaudhuri, and D. Hilbert. 1984. Ontogeny of the HA-responsive repertoire: Interaction of heritable and inducible mechanisms in the establishment of phenotype. In *Idiotypy in Biology and Medicine* (H. Kohler, P. A. Casenave, and J. Urbain, eds.). Academic Press, New York, pp. 143–175.
43. Cancro, M. P., M. A. Thompson, and D. M. Hilbert. 1983. Developmental aspects of B-cell repertoire phenotype. *Surv. Immunol. Res.*, *2*: 62.
44. Klinman, N. R., and P. J. Linton. 1988. The clonotype repertoire of B-cell subpopulations. *Adv. Immunol.*, *42*: 1–93.
45. Cancro, M. P. 1982. Multiple loci mediate B cell repertoire ontogeny: Analysis of the hemagglutinin-specific repertoires in neonatal C.B20 and (C.B20 × B10.D2)F_1 mice. *J. Immunol.*, *128*: 1307–1310.
46. Cancro, M. P., and N. R. Klinman. 1981. B cell repertoire ontogeny: Heritable but dissiimlar development of parental and F_1 repertoires. *J. Immunol.*, *126*: 1160–1164.
47. Wu, G. E., and C. J. Paige. 1988. V_H gene family utilization is regulated by a locus outside of the V_H region. *J. Exp. Med.*, *167*: 1499–1504.
48. Schatz, D. G., M. A. Oettinger, and D. Baltimore. 1989. The V(D)J recombination activating gene, RAG-1. *Cell*, *59*: 1035–1048.
49. Brodeur, P. H., and R. Riblet. 1984. The immunoglobulin heavy chain variable region (Igh-V) locus in the mouse. I. One hundred Igh-V genes comprise seven families of homologous genes. *Eur. J. Immunol.*, *14*: 922–930.
50. Blankenstein, T., and U. Krawinkel. 1987. Immunoglobulin V_H region genes of the mouse are organized in overlapping clusters. *Eur. J. Immunol.*, *17*: 1351–1357.
51. Brodeur, P. H., G. E. Osman, J. J. Mackle, and T. M. Lalor. 1988. The organization of the mouse Igh-V locus. Dispersion, interspersion, and the evolution of V_H gene family clusters. *J. Exp. Med.*, *168*: 2261–2278.
52. Pennell, C. A., K. M. Sheehan, P. H. Brodeur, and S. H. Clarke. 1989. Organization and expression of V_H gene families preferentially expressed by Ly1 (CD5) B-cells. *Eur. J. Immunol.*, *19*: 2115–2121.
53. Yancopoulos, G. D., S. V. Desiderio, M. Paskind, J. F. Kearney, D. Baltimore, and F. W. Alt. 1984. Preferential utilization of the most J_H-proximal V_H gene segments in pre-B cell lines. *Nature* (Lond.), *311*: 727–733.
54. Alt, F. W., G. D. Yancopoulos, T. K. Blackwell, C. Wood, E. Thomas, M. Boss, R. Coffman, N. Rosenberg, S. Tonegawa, and D. Baltimore. 1984. Ordered rearrangement of immunoglobulin heavy chain variable region segments. *EMBO J.*, *3*: 1209–1219.
55. Perlmutter, R. M., J. F. Kearney, S. P. Chang, and L. E. Hood. 1985. Developmentally controlled expression of immunoglobulin V_H genes. *Science*, *227*: 1597–1601.
56. Yancopoulos, G. D., and F. W. Alt. 1986. Regulation of the assembly and expression of variable-region genes. *Ann. Rev. Immunol.*, *4*: 339–368.

57. Alt, F. W., T. K. Blackwell, R. A. DePinho, M. G. Reth, and G. D. Yancopoulos. 1986. Regulation of genome rearrangement events during lymphocyte differentiation. *Immunol. Rev., 89*: 5–30.
58. Malynn, B. A., J. E. Berman, G. D. Yancopoulos, C. A. Bona, and F. W. Alt. 1987. Expression of the immunoglobulin heavy-chain variable gene repertoire. *Curr. Top. Microbiol. Immunol., 135*: 75–94.
59. Yancopoulos, G. D., B. A. Malynn, and F. W. Alt. 1988. Developmentally regulated and strain-specific expression of murine V_H gene families. *J. Exp. Med., 168*: 417–435.
60. Jeong, H. D., J. L. Komisar, E. Kraig, and J. M. Teale. 1988. Strain-development expression of V_H gene families. *J. Immunol., 140*: 2436–2441.
61. Jeong, H. D., and J. M. Teale. 1988. Comparison of the fetal and adult functional B cell repertoires by analysis of V_H gene family expression. *J. Exp. Med., 168*: 589–603.
62. Kienker, L. J., J. M. Korostoff, and M. P. Cancro. 1988. Patterns of IgH-V region expression among neonatal hemagglutinin responsive B cells. Evidence for non-random V_H gene representation during later stages of development. *J. Immunol., 141*: 3634–3641.
63. Lai, E. R. K. Wilson, and L. E. Hood. 1989. Physical maps of the mouse and human immunoglobulin like loci. *Adv. Immunol., 46*: 1–59.
64. Krawinkel, U. T. Christoph, and T. Blankenstein. Organization of the IgV_H locus in mice and humans. *Immunol. Today, 10*: 339–343.
65. Capra, D. J., and Tucker, P. H. 1989. Human immunoglobulin heavy chain genes. *J. Biol. Chem., 264*: 12,745–12,748.
66. Schoeder, H. W., Jr., J. L. Hillison, and R. M. Perlmutter. 1987. Early restriction of the human antibody repertoire. *Science, 238*: 791–793.
67. Shulze, D. H., and Kelsoe, G. 1987. Genotypic analysis of B-cell colonies by *in situ* hybridization. Stoichiometric expression of three V_H families in adult C57BL/6 and BALB/c mice. *J. Exp. Med., 166*: 163–172.
68. Jeong, H. D., and J. M. Teale. 1988. Strain dependent expression of V_H gene families. *J. Immunol., 140*: 2436–2441.
69. Malynn, B. A., G. D. Yancopoulos, J. E. Barth, C. A. Bona, and F. W. Alt. 1990. Biased expression of JH proximal VH genes occurs in the newly generated repertoire of neonatal and adult mice. *J. Exp. Med., 170*: 843.
70. Lawler, A. M. J. F. Kearny, M. Keuhl, and P. J. Gearhart. 1989. Early rearrangements of genes encoding the murine immunoglobulin kappa chains, unlike genes encoding heavy chains, use variable gene segments dispersed throughout the locus. *Proc. Natl. Acad. Sci. USA, 86*: 6744–6748.
71. Teale, J. M., and E. G. Morris. 1989. Comparison of V-kappa gene family expression in adult and fetal B-cells. *J. Immunol., 143*: 2768–2772.
72. Kaushik, A. D. Schulze, C. Bona, and G. Kelsoe. 1989. Murine V-kappa gene expression does not follow the V_H paradigm. *J. Exp. Med., 169*: 1859–1864.
73. Holmberg, D. 1987. High connectivity, natural antibodies preferentially use 7183 and QUPC 52 V_H families. *Eur. J. Immunol., 17*: 399–403.
74. Vakil, M., H. Sauter, C. Paige, and J. F. Kearney. 1986. *In vivo* suppression of perinatal multispecific B cells results in a distortion of the adult B cell repertoire. *Eur. J. Immunol., 16*: 1159–1165.

3

Autoreactive B-Cell Repertoire

Guillaume Dighiero
Pasteur Institute, Paris, France

I. INTRODUCTION

In 1900, experimental work by Ehrlich and Morgenroth showed that isoantibodies (to blood group antigens of homologous erythrocytes) readily developed in animals, although all attempts at immunization with the animals' own erythrocytes failed (1). These pioneering observations led Ehrlich to propose the notion of "horror autotoxicus" (2). During this period (1900–1901) Landsteiner, while trying to define blood group determinants, discovered the constant presence of natural antibodies which were always directed against absent blood group determinants and never against their own erythrocytes (3). In 1949, Burnet (4), strongly influenced by Owen's studies (5) of dizygotic twins, postulated that autoreactive lymphocytes were purged during embryonic life to provide self tolerance. According to this concept, autoantibodies are always harmful and correspond to the expression of mutant forbidden clones able to circumvent the process of immunologic regulation. However, during the last several years, considerable data have accumulated, raising doubts concerning the clonal deletion theory as a general explanation for tolerance since (1) autoimmune diseases can be induced by injecting organ extracts (6); (2) numerous autoantibodies have been demonstrated under normal conditions (7); (3) the presence of normal autoreactive B cells can also be demonstrated

(8); and (4) autoantibodies have been induced from normal B lymphocytes upon mitogenic stimulation (9).

Although in recent years considerable progress has been achieved in the understanding of the autoreactive B-cell repertoire, critical issues await elucidation: (1) What are the rules regulating expression of this repertoire early in ontogeny and during fetal life, and are there special subpopulations of B cells involved in the production of such antibodies? (2) What is the relationship between natural autoantibodies (NAAbs) and pathologic autoantibodies, and between NAAbs and induced antibodies? and (3) Why does this autoreactive B-cell repertoire frequently achieve malignant transformation?

In this chapter, we shall discuss currently available data on the subject, which could help to elucidate these problems. Our review will focus mainly on the discussion of two well-documented models of natural autoimmunity in the study in which we have been involved. These two models include polyreactive autoantibodies and autoantibodies directed against blood erythrocytes. After presentation of these two models, we shall discuss the following issues:

1. The relationship between natural and induced antibodies and between natural and pathologic antibodies.
2. B-cell subpopulations involved in the production of autoantibodies.
3. Malignant transformation of this autoreactive B-cell repertoire.

II. POLYREACTIVE AUTOANTIBODIES

While preparing specific sera against tubulin, Karsenti et al. (10) observed the presence of naturally occurring autoantibodies in the sera of normal unimmunized animals. Subsequently, in collaboration with Guilbert and Avrameas (11), we immobilized nine different antigens (tubulin, actin, thyroglobulin, myoglobin, fetuin, albumin, transferrin, collagen, and cytochrome *c*) on ACA beads. Sera from normal donors were successfully run through the nine immunoadsorbents, from which in all cases we eluted lgs (IgG 70%, IgM and IgA 15% each) with antibody specificity directed against immobilized antigen. Lutz and Wipf (12), nearly at the same time, were able to demonstrate the constant presence of NAAbs against spectrin. These results agree with those of other grops reporting the presence, in normal serum, of NAAbs directed against brain antigens (13), thymus cells (14), lymphocytes (15), IgG (15), carbohydrate (16), collagen, gelatin, normal erythrocytes, thyroid components, and gastric parietal cells (15,17).

The presence of NAAbs under normal conditions implies, of necessity, the presence of autoreactive B lymphocytes. In order to demonstrate the presence of these B-cell precursors, we employed hybridoma technology to fuse unimmunized BALB/c splenocytes with nonsecreting myelomas. The Ig-secreting hybrids were tested for antibody activity against a panel of antigens mainly constituted by cytoskeleton proteins, DNA, and TNP (18,19). Results indicated the presence, with high frequency, of hybridomas with NAAB specificity. Subsequently, Monier et al. (20) reported similar results with BALB/c mice, and Prabhakar et al. (21) reported hybridomas derived from B lymphocytes of SJL/J or BALB/cJ mice which showed multiple organ reactivity. Idiotypic studies showed that these NAAbs displayed a high degree of connectivity (22–31). In humans, Shoenfeld et al. (32,33) reported, for the first time, this type of autoantibody from B lymphocytes of lupic patients. Soon after, Notkins' group reported the presence of multiple-organ–reactive human monoclonal autoantibodies derived from normal B lymphocytes (34,35). These results have been confirmed and exhausted by several groups using either hybridoma technology, EBV immortalization, or both (36–39).

One interesting and puzzling characteristic of these polyreactive natural autoantibodies is their broad reactivity. The simultaneous binding of these antibodies to several different cytoskeleton proteins, DNA, and different haptens, or to multiple organs, has been clearly demonstrated (11,17,18,21,33–35,37,40–47). This widespread reactivity raises the question of which epitope(s) are recognized by these antibodies. Since no obvious homologies exist between such dissimilar molecules as proteins, nucleic acids, and polysaccharides which can all be recognized by the same NAABs, no definitive explanation for these cross-reactivities is presently available. The possibility that the antibody site simultaneously accommodates several different antigens has been advanced on the basis of results derived from crystallographic studies (48). It has also been speculated that charge distribution within the antibody site could account for immunological cross-reactions with diverse and unrelated substances sharing similarities in charge distribution (49). Finally, the possibility that antibodies and antigens could cooperate to establish a better interaction through conformational changes has also been hypothesized (49).

During the last several years, considerable work has been performed to better define the genetic origins of polyreactive NAAbs. Expression of V_H gene families in adult mice appears to follow the same general principles governing response to foreign antigens (50–52). In that sense, the frequency of expression of different V_H gene families is in agreement with the reported complexity of the system and follows a stochastic process (52,53). However, in the fetus and neonate, there is overexpression of 3′ V_H families (7183 and Q52) (53–55). The same overexpression of these D-proximal families has been initially claimed in the case of murine autoantibodies, but has not been further confirmed (52).

Results are less clear concerning V_K gene family expression in mice. Overexpression of V_K1, V_K4, V_K8, V_K10, and V_K19 has been reported in autoantibodies derived from autoimmune disease–prone mouse strains and from normal strains (56).

As genetic restriction is a common finding among induced antibodies that bind to some haptens, it was important to define whether genetic restriction could exist among autoantibodies of a given specificity. Despite results indicating some restriction at the level of V_H and V_K usage, for autoantibodies with anti-Fc IgG and DNA activity (57), no clear correlation has yet been demonstrated (58). In a recent study performed on 71 hybridomas derived from our laboratory with autoantibody activity against DNA and cytoskeleton proteins, no preferential V_H gene usage was apparent, and only a slight predominance of V_K1, V_K4, V_K8, V_K10, and V_K19 was found for V_K family genes (59,60).

Heavy- and light-chain sequences from several NAAbs derived from normal and lupus mice are presently available. Baccala et al. (49) recently reported the nucleic acid sequence of the first two polyreactive NAAbs derived from BALB/c mice and found that both polyreactive NAAbs were encoded by unmutated germline genes. Interestingly, they found that the two unmutated germline genes employed by these NAAbs had been reported previously to be used for antibodies against exogenous antigens, indicating that autoantibodies and induced antibodies could derive from the same genetic repertoire. Studies of murine rheumatoid factors (RF) and anti-DNA antibodies did not succeed in showing differences between autoantibodies obtained from normal and autoimmune mouse strains (61–64). Schlomchik et al. (65,66) reported that IgG RF and anti-DNA hybridomas derived from different MRL Ipr/Ipr mice were clonally unrelated. However, for a given mouse, they originated from a single or very few B-cell clones, which diversified by somatic mutation, and the distribution of which suggested positive selection by antigen.

Taken together, these results indicate that there is no convincing evidence favoring the idea that autoantibodies use abnormal germline genes or particular somatic mechanisms to generate their diversity. On the contrary, they appear to follow the same general rules that govern the expression of antibodies directed against exogenous antigens.

III. AUTOANTIBODIES DIRECTED AGAINST BLOOD ERYTHROCYTES

In both normal and autoimmune strains of mice, a number of spontaneously occurring autoantibodies against different erythrocyte antigens, i.e., Hb, X, HOL, and I, have been described (67,68). Anti-X autoantibodies have been described in the NZB mouse and appear to be related to the characteristic autoimmune hemolytic anemia observed in this strain (67–69). Anti-Hb autoantibodies observed in all studied mouse strains except CBA/N do not seem to be associated with any pathological syndrome (70,71).

A normal unimmunized mouse possesses B cells secreting antibodies against its own erythrocytes, previously treated with the proteolytic anzyme bromelain; this can be demonstrated by a direct plaque-forming cell assay and seric hemolytic titer (71,72). The antigen unmasked by bromelain represents a normal hidden autoantigen called HB autoantigen, though its precise structure remains undefined (73,74).

The B lymphocytes secreting these autoantibodies appear late during ontogeny and are principally localized in the peritoneal cavity (75–78). Mouse hydridomas secreting IgM autoantibodies against bromelain-treated mouse red blood cells (BrMRBC) have been established both from the peritoneal cavity and from splenic B cells in different mouse strains (79). These NAAbs share a recurrent idiotype called CP, which appears to be shared by all monoclonal IgM obtained until now, whatever the mouse strain concerned. This recurrent idiotype is present in the sera of nearly all mouse strains and is undetectable in the CBA/N mouse (80).

In humans, naturally occurring antibodies to red cell membrane constituents, such as band 3 (81,82), spectrin (12), and a rare glycosphingolipid (83) (Galα (1→3) Gal) were isolated from human sera and polyspecific IgG preparations. Anti-Gal antibodies have been postulated by Galili (83) to be implicated in the removal of senescent red blood cells, in which a cryptic B epitope like the Galα 1→3 gal epitope is exposed as the cells age, and which could subsequently bind the anti-Gal antibody. In addition, autoantibodies directed against I antigen are currently found in low titers in normal human serum (84).

As opposed to polyrective NAAbs, which do not appear to preferentially employ a particular V_H and V_K family, anti-BrMRBC antibodies appear to use a highly restricted set of V_H and V_K genes. The complete nucleotide sequences of seven anti-BrMRBC antibodies derived from NZB, CBA/J, and BALB/c mice revealed that all seven antibodies employed the same V_H, D, JH, V_K, and JH gene segments. The V_H regions were derived from a new V_H family (V_H11) which has only two members. The D segment appeared to be derived from the germline D gene SP2 family, and J_H was derived from J_H1 germline gene segments. V_K9 and J_K2 family genes appeared to be used to derive the K light chain. Interestingly, the seven heavy- and light-chain sequences reported appeared to be almost identical (85).

In humans, the amino acid sequence of several anti-I cold agglutinins revealed restricted usage of V_KIII and V_H4 family genes (86, 87), which we shall discuss later.

Taken together, these results indicate that:

1. NAAbs and autoreactive B cells constitute a substantial part of the available and expressed B-cell repertoire.
2. These NAAbs express recurrent idiotypes and frequently appear early during ontogeny. These initial results suggested a germinal origin, now extensively confirmed by structural studies.
3. The binding activities of these NAAbs are directed against highly conserved molecules including cytoskeleton proteins, nucleic acids, myelin basic protein, cytochrome c, transferrin.

4. Since NAAbs are directed against self molecules, they fulfill the definition of autoantibodies; however, they are not autospecific, since they typically bind to epitopes localized in phylogenetically conserved regions of antigens.
5. As the autoreactive B-cell repertoire constitutes a substantial part of the normal B-cell repertoire, the clonal deletion theory can no longer be accepted as the only general explanation for self tolerance. However, to our knowledge, autoantibodies directed against very critical antigens defining polymorphism (e.g., the A antigen in the case of a subject belonging to the A group or against polymorphic antigens of the major histocompatibility system) have not been described until now. Therefore, clonal deletion mechanisms cannot at the present time be completely excluded in such cases.

A. Relationship Between NAAbs and Induced Antibodies and Between NAAbs and Pathological Autoantibodies

In 1983 (18), while reporting our results with murine hybridomas displaying NAAB activity and derived from BALB/c mice, we concluded as follows:

> If correct, this hypothesis would imply that these B cells carry a polyspecific receptor capable of fixing several different antigens. During active immunization, the binding of a given antigen to this receptor would then induce the corresponding B cell by a series of divisions and mutations, which, under the selective pressure of the antigen, would lead to the production of highly specific antibodies for a given epitope of these antigens. In that case, these B cells and their receptors would then be encoded by the germ-line, and the natural polyspecific antibodies would constitute the synthesized products secreted by these cells.

This provocative hypothesis assumed that NAAbs were the product of the germline repertoire and that they constituted a template upon which Ag-driven selection and somatic mutation could operate to derive highly specific immune antibodies.

This germline origin was substantiated during the following years, since: (1) polyreactive NAAbs appear to predominate early during ontogeny (19) even in germ-free animals (88); (2) NAAbs express recurrent idiotypes (22–31) and appear to be highly interconnected (26); and (3) structural studies have demonstrated their germinal origin (49,58,62–64) and showed that these autoantibodies are encoded by structural genetic elements similar to those employed by nonautoimmune autoantibodies (52).

The template hypothesis is still awaiting experimental verification. Only indirect evidence has been obtained so far. Naparstek et al. (89) have studied a set of antibodies that use the $V_H Id^{CR}$ gene, employed for the antiarsonate system. They have found that germline-encoded antibodies of this system to not bind arsonate, but display a polyreactive pattern of binding by reacting with DNA and cytoskeleton proteins. Upon immunization with arsonate, the $V_H Ig^{CR}$ gene undergoes somatic mutations, allowing it to become a high affinity antiarsonate antibody. This process is accompanied by loss of NAAb activity. Guilbert et al. (90) studied hybridomas derived from mice previously immunized with several different antigens and reported that, besides hybrids binding to specific immunizing antigen, they also obtained hybrids binding to specific antigen as well as to self antigen, suggesting that the latter could be an intermediate stage between the preimmune and specifically immune repertoire. In our laboratory, Matthes et al. (91) have recently compared the epitopes recognized on tubulin by natural polyspecific autoantibodies and by induced antibodies. They found that whereas NAAbs recognized the same or closely overlapping epitopes in the central part of both α and β subunits of tubulin, induced antibodies recognized very different epitopes located either in amino-terminal or carboxyl-terminal parts of the tubulin subunits. Whether these results indicate a different genetic origin for NAAbs and induced antibodies or the occurrence of extensive somatic mutations in induced antibodies is an unsolved issue.

An alternative hypothesis to the template theory is that these NAAbs constitute a polylogenetically strongly conserved system which might make up the first defense barrier. In that sense, these widely reacting antibodies which probably are of low affinity could allow some degree of protection. In primitive animals with no possibility of further diversification of the immune system, they could constitute the unique defense system. This primitive system could have been conserved during evolution, since it allows some protection; meanwhile, the immune system developed more specific antibodies. Whatever the case, verification of these hypotheses requires careful experimentation at the single-cell level, which has not yet been carried out.

Two alternative views have been advanced to explain autoantibody production in autoimmune diseases (92). The first proposes that they are the consequence of polyclonal stimulation of normal autoreactive B cells, resulting in increased levels of autoantibodies (93). The second view assumes that pathological autoantibodies are a consequence of an antigen-driven selection process of autoreactive B cells which, under the selective pressure of the antigen, undergo somatic mutations (65,66).

The polyclonal activation model is supported by the fact that (1) spontaneous polyclonal stimulation is constantly observed during systemic autoimmune diseases (94–96); (2) polyclonal B-cell stimulation, upon mitogenic stimulation, induces production of autoantibodies against DNA, against the Fc of IgG, and against erythrocytes (92,96–100); (3) chronic polyclonal stimulation can induce autoimmune disease in genetically nonprone mice (9,96–100); and (4) autoantibodies derived by hybridoma technology from lupic mice and lupus patients are frequently encoded by germline genes (52).

Antigen-driven autoantibody production is supported by the following: (1) The results of Shlomchik et al. on murine hybridomas with anti-DNA (66) and RF activity (65) derived from MRL/Ipr,Ipr lupic mice. The nucleotide sequence of IgG and IgA monoclonal antibodies showed evidence of numerous somatic mutations clearly predominating in the CDR regions, indicating a positive selection by antigen. (2) Except in the case of cold agglutinin disease, most paraproteins with autoantibody activity described until now have not been associated with autoimmune manifestations (17,41,42). (3) The concentration of autoantibodies appears to be disproportionally increased when compared to other antibodies (92,96).

Indeed, both explanations are complementary (101). It can be speculated that in the case of systemic autoimmune disease, there is initially polyclonal B-cell stimulation followed by an antigen-driven somatic mutation selection process, resulting in the production of IgG autoantibodies which probably constitute pathologic autoantibodies. In the case of organ-specific autoimmune diseases, polyclonal B-cell activation is probably not relevant.

B. B-Cell Subpopulations Involved in the Production of Autoantibodies

Mouse Ly-1 B cells (102) and their human counterpart $CD5^+$ B cells (103) have been postulated to correspond to distinct B-cell subsets particularly involved in the production of autoantibodies. The Ly-1 marker, initially reported to identify a T-helper subset (104), was subsequently shown to be a pan-T-cell marker present on a small subpopulation of murine B cells (105). This subpopulation accounts for 1–2 and 5–10% of splenocytes in BALB/c and NZB mice, respectively (106). They largely predominate in the peritoneal B-cell population (20–40% in BALB/c and 40–80% in NZB) (107).

Phenotypically, Ly-1 B cells are characterized by high IgM, low IgD surface membrane Ig expressed along with most well-known B-cell markers (102). During ontogeny, Ly-1 B cells predominate in the fetus and neonate. Studies, mainly performed in Herzenberg's laboratory, indicated that:

1. $Ly\text{-}1^+$ B cells can survive longer in culture than $Ly\text{-}1^-$ B cells (102).
2. Ly-1 B cells cannot be reconstituted in lethally irradiated mice with adult bone marrow cells. These experiments suggest a different origin for $Ly\text{-}1^+$ B cells (108,109).
3. Ly-1 B cells may be involved mainly in production of autoantibodies (102,110).

Several findings are in agreement with the latter assumption: (1) There is increased frequency of $Ly\text{-}1^+$ B cells in NZB (106) and motheaten autoimmune prone strains (111); (2) a lack of Ly-1 B cells parallels a lack of autoantibody secretion in CBA/N Xid mice (102,106); (3) increased frequency of Ly-1 B cells in newborn mice is in agreement with the increased frequency of NAAB precursors, as observed by somatic hybridization (19,112); and (4) an increased frequency of Ly-1 B cells in the peritoneal cavity (107) parallels an increased frequency of anti-BrMRBC activity in this particular compartment (77).

However, some discrepancies concerning Ly-1 B cells and autoantibody production exist: (1) the lupus-prone mouse strain MRL Ipr/Ipr does not exhibit a high frequency of Ly-1 B cells (94,96,101,113); (2) Xid mice, which are known not to express the Ly-1 marker on B cells, display a frequency of NAAb precursors similar to that observed in non-Xid mice (114); (3) the frequency of NAAb precursors in the peritoneal cavity enriched in Ly-1 B cells was found not to be higher than that observed with the splenic repertoire in which Ly-1 B cells constitute a minor population (115); (4) Conger et al. (116) have shown that neither CBA/J cells nor NZB Ly-1^+ B spleen cells exhibited a high frequency of anti-ssDNA forming clones compared to CBA spleen cells or NZB Ly-1^- B spleen cells, respectively; and (5) a study based on detection of the mRNA transcript of the Ly-1 gene by Northern blotting among hybridomas with NAAb specificity derived from several mouse stains indicated that NAAb arise from both Ly-1^+ and Ly-1^- B-lymphocyte subsets (60).

The human counterpart of the Ly-1^+ B cell is the $CD5^+$ B cell. Ly-1 and CD5 molecules have similar primary structures, and, in both species, this molecule is also expressed on all T cells (117). $CD5^+$ B cells account for at least 15% of normal B cells (103) and, like Ly-1 B cells, they predominate in the fetus and neonate (118,119). As is the case for Ly-1 B cells, they have been claimed to be mainly involved in autoantibody secretion (120) since: (1) after purification by cytofluorometry, $CD5^+$ B cells infected with EBV under limiting dilution conditions accounted for the vast majority of lymphocytes committed to the production of NAAb (120–122), and (2) three different groups, including our laboratory, recently unequivocally demonstrated that $CD5^+$ B-CLL lymphocytes are frequently involved in the production of these polyreactive NAAbs (123–125).

Although these results indicate that $CD5^+$ B cells are involved in production of NAAbs, the frequency of precursors of polyreactive NAAbs in normal healthy subjects is similar to that found in subjects suffering from autoimmune diseases, such as Hashimoto's disease and systemic lupus erythematosus (120). In these patients, the frequency of B-cell precursors of high affinity IgG autoantibodies directed, respectively, against thyroid antigens and ssDNA is considerably higher than normals, and the latter antibodies appear to be produced by $CD5^-$ B cells (120).

In summary, although there is some evidence that murine Ly-1^+ B cells and its human counterpart $CD5^+$ B cells may constitute a separate lineage, evidence presently available is not conclusive, and the possibility that CD5 constitutes an activation marker cannot be completely ruled out. The involvement of $CD5^+$ B cells in the production of NAAbs has been demonstrated, but there is some evidence indicating that $CD5^-$ B cells may also be involved. Whether $CD5^+$ B cells play an important role in autoimmune disease remains an unsolved issue.

C. Malignant Transformation of the Autoreactive B-Cell Repertoire

During recent years, considerable evidence has accumulated indicating that autoreactive B cells frequently undergo malignant transformation. This evidence arose from the study of monoclonal immunoglobulins (MIgs) and from studies of chronic lymphocytic leukemia (CLL) B lymphocytes.

1. Antibody Activity of MIgs

MIgs correspond to normal products whose counterpart can be found in the heterogenous normal Ig compartment. The antibody-like activity of MIgs has been described against a large number of antigens, e.g., bacterial antigens, plasma proteins, tissue antigens, and nonbilogical haptens (126). However, an unexpected, very high frequency of activity has been reported against: (1) the Fc fraction of IgG (rheumatoid factor (RF) (127); (2) I blood group antigen (cold agglutinins (CA)) (84,126); and (3) cytoskeleton proteins and DNA (polyreactive autoantibodies) (42).

a. MIgs with RF Activity. Since the first report by Kritzman et al. (128) of a monoclonal IgMK paraprotein with anti-IgG activity, a considerable number of similar cases have been reported, and the frequency of this specificity has been estimated at more than 10% of total IgM paraproteins (127). Most monoclonal components with reported RF activity were found to form a cryoprecipitate (126). Almost all cases corresponds to IgMK MIgs, but rare cases of human monoclonal IgG and IgA with RF activity and cryoprecipitable have been described (129,130).

Pioneer work from Kunkel's laboratory demonstrated the presence of cross-reactive idiotypic (CRI) specificities among these MIgs (131). Sixty percent of these MIgs displaying RF activity were found to share a major CRI called Wa; 20% belonged to a less common CRI designated Po, and a few expressed a more rare CRI, named Bla (132).

In recent years, several studies, mainly emanating from the group of Dennis Carson, have defined the genetic origin of MIg in serologic and structural terms (133–140).

These studies were mainly focused on MIgs sharing the Wa CRI. It was found that:

1. Amost all Wa + RF share the 17109 CRI related to light chains and the G6 idiotype related to heavy chains.
2. They constantly express the minor subgroup V_KIIIb light chain.
3. The V_K light chain is derived from a single germinal gene (Hum Kv 325),

since most Wa + paraproteins display an identical or nearly identical light chain sequence, as shown by 13 complete light-chain sequences.

4. There is strong sequence homology among μ chains expressing the Wa idiotype. Most of them use the V_H1 family (80%), and a minority use V_H2 and V_H3 families

Although information derived from Po + RF MIg is less extensive, they appear to constantly use a V_K germinal gene (Hum Kv 328) and to use a conserved VH3 sequence.

b. MIgs with CA Activity. CA paraproteins are almost always IgMK paraproteins, which usually react with a set of antigenic determinants directed against the Ii system, or compound antigens including Ii (AI, HI, etc). Their activity is increased by cold, but thermal amplitude is variable (84).

As for RF cryoglobulins, CRI associated with light and heavy chains have been described. By studying the N-terminal sequence of isolated K chains of 9 CA, Capra et al. (86) first reported that a majority of them belonged to the V_KIII subgroup. Subsequently, it could be established that the majority of CA employ the V_H4 family (87). The amino acid sequence of light chains revealed striking similarities. Interestingly, some CA used the same Hum Kv 325 germinal gene employed by Wa + RF paraproteins, indicating that antigenic specificity against IgG or anti-I was supplied by heavy chains (87).

c. MIgs with Polyreactive Activity. Prompted by our results with normal human serum in the early 1980s, we screened 612 MIgs for the presence of antibody activity directed against cytoskeleton protein and DNA. Our results indicated that about 6% of all MIgs and 10% of IgM paraproteins bound to these antigens, and that most of them displayed a polyreactive pattern of binding comparable to that found in normal serum, indicating that MIgs frequently correspond to expansion of a clone normally producing a NAAb (42). Delaggi et al. (141) also reported the presence of IgM paraproteins binding to intermediate filaments, and Shoenfeld et al. (142) found that more than 10% of MIgs shared the 16-6 CRI derived from a monoclonal Ig with anti-DNA activity.

The presence of shared CRI among these polyreactive MIgs favors their germinal origin (31,142). Although the structure of these paraproteins is unknown, studies of monoclonal NAAbs derived from normal and autoimmune mice and humans suggest that they have a germinal origin. The use of multiple V_H and V_L genes has been reported for monoclonal NAAbs.

D. Antibody Activity of the CLL B Lymphocyte

CLL is a malignancy arising from clonal expansion of morphologically small mature B lymphocytes expressing the CD5 antigen (143). This latter characteristic, as well as the high frequency with which hypogammaglobulinemias and immune-associated phenomena are observed, distinguish B-CLL from other B-cell malignancies (144). Recent evidence arising from studies with phorbol ester stimulation indicate that the $CD5^+$ B cell proliferating in CLL is frequently involved in NAAb production (123–124).

In our laboratory, we recently fused lymphocytes from 27 B-CLL patients with the nonsecreting X-63 murine myeloma. Our results indicate that about half of the CLL patients secrete NAAbs with RF activity, while about 20% of them display polyreactive NAAb activity (125).

In a recent study, Kipps et al. (145,146) found that a high proportion of B-CLL cells expressing K at the membrane reacted with a murine anti-idiotypic antibody raised against a monoclonal IgM RF, expressing the Wa idiotype. Analysis of kappa light-chain variable-region genes expressed by leukemic cells sharing idiotype Wa enabled these authors to demonstrate that they used the germinal unmutated Hum Kv 325 germinal gene (145). Similar restriction was found when V_H genes were analyzed (146).

In summary, these results reveal that there is an high frequency of B malignancies displaying antibody activity against RF, CA, cytoskeleton proteins and DNA. Malignant transformation appears to occur frequently among B cells which exhibit an autoreactive activity and express germline genes. Since autoreactive B cells constitute a substantial part of the normal B-cell repertoire and are frequently in an "activated" state, this could explain why these clones are often obtained by hybridoma technology. This "activated" state could also render the clones highly susceptible to malignant transformation.

IV. CONCLUDING REMARKS

There has been considerable progress in our understanding of the autoreactive B-cell repertoire during the last decade. There is considerable evidence indicating that autoreactive B cells constitute a substantial part of the B-cell repertoire. These autoreactive B cells create the so-called "NAAbs" characterized by broad and puzzling reactivity, mainly directed against highly conserved public epitopes. They fulfill the definition of an autoantibody since they are self-reactive, although they are not self-specific. As yet, NAAbs directed against determinants of polymorphism have not been reported.

These NAAbs are encoded by the germline repertoire, as attested by their early appearance during ontogeny, their expression of cross-reactive idiotypes, and their sequences.

The relationship between NAAbs and induced antibodies need to be further elucidated. No important differences in the use of V genes have been reported. It has been postulated that germline-encoded NAAbs constitute a template for induced antibodies, which may be derived from NAAbs by an antigen-driven somatic mutation process. Alternatively, NAAbs may represent a phylogenetically conserved system, which, through low-affinity, broadly reacting antibodies could serve as a first barrier of defense while the immune system is engaged in producing antibodies of higher specificity. There is no definite evidence favoring one or the other hypothesis, and careful experiments at the single cell levels are needed to answer this question.

The relationship between NAAbs and pathologic autoantibodies is also presently unclear. Whether pathologic autoantibodies are the consequence of polyclonal stimulation, resulting in increased levels of germline-encoded NAAb, or whether they are derived via an antigen-driven somatic mutation process operating in NAAb precursors is not well established. Probably both mechanisms are involved, at least in systemic autoimmune diseases.

Ly-1 $CD5^+$ B cells have been postulated to constitute a particular B-cell subset mainly implicated in the production of NAAbs. However, it is unclear whether CD5 is a marker defining a particular subset of B cells or whether it constitutes an activation marker. The involvement of $CD5^+$ B cells in autoantibody production is now well substantiated, but there is evidence indicating that $CD5^-$ B cells could also secrete autoantibodies.

Studies on the antibody function of paraproteins and some B-cell malignancies, such as CLL, indicate that the autoreactive B-cell repertoire frequently undergoes malignant transformation. About 25% of IgM paraprotein and at least 10% of IgG and IgA paraproteins display rheumatoid factor, cold agglutinin, or polyreactive activity. Similar results have been observed when $CD5^+$ CLL B lymphocytes are induced to secrete Ig. The activation of this autoreactive B-cell repertoire through continuous challenge by self antigens could create suitable conditions for the occurrence of mutations and chromosomal translocations.

REFERENCES

1. Ehrlich, P., and Morgenroth, J. 1957. On haemolyzins: Third communication, in *The Collected Papers of Paul Ehrlich*, Vol. 2. Pergamon, London, pp. 205, 224, 246, 278.
2. Ehrlich, P., and Morgenroth, J. 1957. On haemolysins: Fifth communication, in *The Collected Papers of Paul Ehrlich*, Vol. 2. Pergamon, London, p. 253.
3. Landsteiner, K. 1900. *The Specificity of Serological Reactions*, Vol. 27. Harvard University Press, Cambridge, Mass., p. 357.
4. Burnet, M. F. 1959. *The Clonal Selection Theory of Acquired Immunity*. Cambridge University Press, London, New-York.
5. Owen, R. D. 1945. Immunogenetic consequences of vascular anastomoses between bovine cattle twins, *Science, 102*: 400.
6. Rose, N. R., and Witebsky, E. 1956. Studies on organ specificity: V changes in the thyroid glands of rabbits following acute immunization with rabbit tyroid extracts. *J. Immunol., 76*: 417.
7. Hooper, B., Whittingham, S., and Mathews, J. D. 1972. Autoimmunity in a rural community. *Clin. Exp. Immunol., 12*: 79.

8. MacKay, I. R. 1983. Natural autoantibodies to the forbidden clones to the rear? *Immunol. Today, 4*: 340.
9. Izui, S., Lambert, P. H., and Founie, G. L. 1977. Features of systemic lupus erythematosus in mice infected with bacterial lipopolysaccharides. *J. Exp. Med., 145*: 1115.
10. Karsenti, E., Guilbert, B., Bornens, M., and Avrameas, S. 1977. Antibodies to tubulin in normal nonimmunized animals. *Proc. Nat. Acad. Sci. USA, 74*: 3997.
11. Guilbert, B., Dighiero, G., and Avrameas, S. 1982. Naturally occurring antibodies against nine common antigens in normal humans. I. Detection, isolation and characterization. *J. Immunol., 128*: 2799.
12. Lutz, H. U., and Wipf, G. 1982. Naturally occurring auto-antibodies to skeletal proteins from human red blood cells. *J. Immunol., 128*: 1695.
13. Martin, S. E., and Martin, W. J. 1975. Interspecies brain antigen detected by naturally occurring mouse anti-brain auto-antibody. *Proc. Natl. Acad. Sci. USA, 72*: 1036.
14. Martin, W. J., and Martin, S. E. 1975. Thymus reactive IgM auto-antibodies in normal mouse sera. *Nature, 254*: 716.
15. Walford, R. L. 1969. *The Immunologic Theory of Aging*. Munksgaard, Copenhagen.
16. Sela, B. A., Wang, J. L., and Edelman, G. M. 1975. Antibodies reactive with cell surface carbohydrates. *Proc. Natl. Acad. Sci. USA, 72*: 1127.
17. Dighiero, G., Lymberi, P., Guilbert, B., Ternynck, T., and Avrameas, S. 1986. Natural auto-antibodies constitute a substantial part of normal circulating immunoglobulins. *Ann. N.Y. Acad. Sci., 475*: 135.
18. Dighiero, G., Lymberi, P., Mazié, J. C., Rouyre, S., Butler-Browne, G. S., Whalen, R. G., and Avrameas, S. 1983. Murine hybridomas secreting natural monoclonal antibodies reacting with self antigens. *J. Immunol., 131*: 2267.
19. Dighiero, G., Lymberi, P., Holmberg, D., Lundquist, I., Coutinho, A., and Avrameas, S. 1985. High frequency of natural autoantibodies in normal newborn mice. *J. Immunol., 134*: 765.
20. Monier, J. C., Brochier, J., Moreira, A., Sault, C., and Roux, B. 1984. Generation of hybridoma antibodies to double-stranded DNA from non-autoimmune BALB/c strain: studies on anti-idiotype. *Immun. Lett., 8*: 61.
21. Prabhakar, B. S., Saegusa, J., Onodera, T., and Notkins, A. L. 1984. Lymphocytes capable of making monoclonal autoantibodies that react with multiple organs are a common feature of the normal B cell repertoire. *J. Immunol., 133*: 2815.
22. Rauch, J., Murphy, E., Roths, J. B., Stollar, B. D., and Schwartz, R. S. 1982. A high frequency idiotypic marker of anti-DNA autoantibodies in MR-Ipr/Ipr mice. *J. Immunol., 129*: 236.
23. Tron, F., Le Guern, C. L., Cazenave, P. A., and Bach, J. F. 1982. Intrastrain recurrent idiotypes among anti-DNA antibodies of (NZB/NZW)F1 hybrid mice. *Eur. J. Immunol., 12*: 761.
24. Marion, T. N., Lawton, A. R., Kearney, J. F., and Briles, D. E. 1982. Anti-DNA autoantibodies in (NZB × NZW)F1 mice are clonally heterogenous, but a majority share a common idiotype. *J. Immunol., 128*: 668.
25. Isenberg, D. A., Shoenfeld, Y., Madaio, M. R., Rauch, J., Reichlin, M., and Stollar, B. D. 1983. Z-DNA specific antibodies in human systemic lupus erythematosus. *J. Clin. Invest., 71*: 314.

26. Holmberg, D., Forsgren, S., Ivars, F., and Coutinho, A. 1984. Reactions among IgM antibodies derived from normal, neonatal mice. *Eur. J. Immunol., 14*: 435.
27. Lymberi, P., Dighiero, G., Ternynck, T., and Avrameas, S. 1985. A high incidence of cross-reactive idiotypes among murine natural autoantibodies. *Eur. J. Immunol., 15*: 702.
28. Morgan, A., Isenberg, D. A., Naparstek, Y., Rauch, J., Duggan, D., Khiroga, R., Staines, N. A., and Schattner, A. 1985. Shared idiotypes are expressed on mouse and human anti-DNA autoantibodies. *Immunology, 56*: 393.
29. Kearney, J. F., and Vakil, M. 1986. Idiotype directed interactions during ontogeny play a major role in the establishment of the adult B cell repertoire. *Immunol. Rev. 94*: 39.
30. Monestier, M., Manheimer-Lory, A., Bellon, B., Painter, C., Dang, H., Talal, N., Zanetti, M., Schwartz, R., Pisetsky, D., Kuppers, R., Rose, N., Brochier, J. Klareskog, L., Holmdahl, R., Erlanger, B., Alt, F., and Bona, C. Shared idiotopes and restricted immunoglobulin variable region heavy chain genes characterize murine autoantibodies of various specificities. *J. Clin. Invest., 78*: 753.
31. Matthes, T., and Dighiero, G. 1988. Detection of private and recurrent idiotopes on natural antitubulin antibodies by monoclonal anti-idiotopic antibodies. *J. Immunol., 140*: 148.
32. Shoenfeld, Y., Hsu-lin, S. C., Gabriels, J. E., Silberstein, L. E., Furie, B. C., Stollar, B. D., and Schwartz, R. S. 1982. Production of autoantibodies by human-human hybridomas. *J. Clin. Invest., 70*: 205.
33. Shoenfeld, Y., Rauch, J., Massicotte, H., Datta, S. K., André-Schwartz, J., Stollar, B. D., and Schwartz, R. S. 1983. Polyspecificity of monoclonal lupus autoantibodies produced by human-human hybridomas. *N. Engl. J. Med., 308*: 414.
34. Satoh, J., Prabhakar, B. S., Haspel, M. V., Ginsberg-Fellner, F., and Notkins, A. L. 1983. Human monoclonal autoantibodies that react with multiple endocrine organs. *N. Engl. J. Med., 309*: 217.
35. Haspel, M. V., Onodera, T., Prabhakar, B. S., McClintock, K. E., Ray, U. R., Yagihashi, S., and Notkins, A. L. 1983. Multiple organ-reactive monoclonal autoantibodies. *Nature, 304*: 74.
36. Cairns, E., Block, J., and Bell, D. A. 1984. Anti-DNA autoantibody producing hydridomas of normal human lymphoid cell origin. *J. Immunol., 74*: 880.
37. Rubin, R. L., Balderas, R. S., Tan, E. M., Dixon, F. J., and Theofilopoulos, A. N. 1984. Multiple autoantigen binding capabilities of mouse monoclonal antibodies selected for rheumatoid factor activity. *J. Exp. Med., 159*: 1429.
38. Rauch, J., Massicotte, H., and Tannenbaum, H. 1985. Hybridoma anti-DNA autoantibodies from patients with rheumatoid arthritis and systemic lupus erythematosus demonstrate similar nucleic acid binding characteristics. *J. Immunol., 136*: 180.
39. Haskard, D. O., Gul, V., Morgan, A., Kataaha, P., Staines, N. A., and Archer, J. R. 1985. Human monoclonal autoantibodies from patients with rheumatoid arthritis against cellular constituents. *Clin. Exp. Immunol., 61*: 496.
40. Lafer, E. M., Rauch, J., Andrzewski, C., Mudd, D., Furie, B., Furie, B., Schwartz, R. S., and Stollar, B. D. 1981. Polyspecific monoclonal lupus autoantibodies reactive with both plynucleotides and phospholipids. *J. Exp. Med., 153*: 897.
41. Dighiero, G., Guilbert, B., and Avrameas, S. 1982. Naturally occurring antibodies

against nine common antigens in human sera: II. High incidence of monoclonal Ig exhibiting antibody activity against actin and tubulin and sharing antibody specificities with natural antibodies. *J. Immunol.*, *128*: 2788.

42. Dighiero, G., Guilbert, B., Fermant, J. P., Lymberi, P., Danon, F., and Avrameas, S. 1983. Thirty-six human monoclonal immunoglobulins (MIg) with antibody activity against cytoskeleton proteins, thyroglobulin and native DNA. Immunological studies and clinical correlations. *Blood, 62*: 264.
43. André-Schwartz, J., Datta, S. K., Shoenfeld, Y., Isenberg, D. A., Stollar, B. D., and Schwartz, R. S. 1984. Binding of cytoskeletal proteins by monoclonal anti-DNA lupus autoantibodies. *Clin. Immunol. Immunopathol.*, *31*: 261.
44. Faaber, P., Capel, P. J. A., Rijke, G. P. M., Vierwindent, G., Van Der Putte, L. B. A., Koene, R. A. P. 1984. Cross reactivity of nti-DNA antibodies with proteoglycans. *Clin. Exp. Immunol.*, *55*: 502.
45. Rauch, J., Tannenbaum, H., Stollar, B. D., and Schwartz, R. S. 1984. Monoclonal anticardiolipin antibodies bind to DNA. *Eur. J. Immunol.*, *14*: 529.
46. Jacob, L., Tron, F., Bach, J. F., and Louvard, D. A. 1984. A monoclonal anti-DNA antibody also binds to cell surface proteins. *Proc. Natl. Acad. Sci. USA, 81*: 3843.
47. Poncet, P., Matthes, T., Billecocq. A., and Dighiero, G. 1988. Immunochemical studies of polyspecific natural autoantibodies: charge lipid reactivity. Fab'2 fragments activity and complement fixation. *Mol. Immunol.*, *25*: 981.
48. Amit, A. G., Mariuzza, R. A., Phillips, S. E., and Poljak, R. J. 1986. Three dimensional structure of an antigen-antibody complex at 28A resolution. *Science, 233*: 747.
49. Baccala, R., Vo Quang, T., Gilbert, M., Ternynck, T., and Avrameas, S. 1989. Two murine polyreactive antibodies are encoded by nonmutated germ-line genes. *Proc. Natl. Acad. Sci. USA, 8*: 4624.
50. Brodeur, P., and Riblet, R. 1984. The immunoglobulin heavy chain variable region (Igh-V) locus in the mouse. I. One hundred Igh-V genes comprise seven families of homologus genes. *Eur. J. Immunol.*, *14*: 922.
51. Painter, C., Monestier, M., Brown, B., and Bona, C. A. 1986. Functional and molecular studies of V genes expressed in autoantibodies. *Immunological Reviews, 94*: 75.
52. Kofler, R., Dixon, F. J., and Theofilopoulos, A. N. 1987. The genetic origin of autoantibodies. *Immunol. Today, 8*: 374.
53. Dighiero, G., Lim, A., Lembezat, M. P., Kaushik, A., Andrade, L., and Freitas, A. 1989. Comparative study of VH gene family usage by newborn Xid and non Xid mice, newborn NZB and adult NZB mice and by splenic and peritoneal cavity B cell compartments. *Eur. J. Immunol.*, *18*: 1979.
54. Yancopoulos, G. D., Desiderio, S. V., Paskind, M., Kearney, J. F., Baltimore, D., and Alt, F. 1984. Preferential utilization of the most JH-proximal VH gene segments in pre-B-cell lines. *Nature, 311*: 727.
55. Holmberg, D. 1987. High connectivity natural antibodies preferentially use 7183 and QPC52 VH families. *Eur. J. Immunol.*, *17*: 399.
56. Bona, C. 1988. V genes encoding autoantibodies, molecular and phenotypic characteristic. *Ann. Rev. Immunol.*, *6*: 327.

57. Shlomchik, M. J., Nemazee, D. A., and Sato, V. L. 1986. Variable region sequence of murine IgM anti-IgG1 monoclonal autoantibodies (rheumatoid factors): A structural explanation for the high frequency of IgM anti-IgG B cells. *J. Exp. Med., 164*: 407.
58. Kofler, R., Noonars, D. I., Levy, D. E., Wilson, M. C., Moller, N. P. H., Dixon, F. J., and Theofilopoulos, A. N. 1985. Genetic elements utilized for a murine lupus anti-DNA autoantibody are closely related to those for antibodies to exogenous antigens. *J. Exp. Med., 161*: 805.
59. Kasturi, K., Monestier, M., Meyer, R., Bona, C. A. 1988. Biased usage of certain VK gene families by autoantibodies and their polymorphism in autoimmune mice. *Molec. Immunol., 25*: 213.
60. Kaushik, A., Meyer, R., Fidanza, V., Lim, A., Bona, C., and Dighiero, G. 1990. Ly1 and V gene expression among hybridomas secreting natural autoantibody. *J. Autoimmunity*, in press.
61. Dersimonian, H., Schwartz, R. S., Barret, K. J., and B. D. Relationship of human variable region heavy chain germline genes to genes encoding anti-DNA autoantibodies. *J. Immunol., 139*: 2490.
62. Trepicchio, W., Jr., Maruya, A., and Barrett, K. J. 1987. The heavy chain genes of a lupus anti-DNA autoantibody are encoded in the germ line of a nonautoimmune strain of mouse and conserved in strains of mice polymorphic for this gene locus. *J. Immunol., 139*: 3139.
63. Aguado, M. T., Balderas, R. S., Rubin, R. L., Duchosal, M. A., Kofler, R. Birshtein, B. K., Secher, D. S., Dixon, F. J., and Theofilopoulos, A. N. Specificity and molecular characteristics of monoclonal IgM rheumatoid factors from arthritic and non-arthritic mice. *J. Immunol., 139*: 1080.
64. Sanz, I., Casali, P., Thomas, J. W., Notkins, A. L., and Capra, J. O. 1989. Nucleotide sequences of eight human natural autoantibody VH regions reveal apparent restricted use of VH families. *J. Immunol., 142*: 4054.
65. Schlomchik, M. J., Marshall-Rothstein, A., Wolfowicz, C. B., Rothstein, T. L., and Weigert, M. G. 1987. The role of clonal selection and somatic mutation in autoimmunity. *Nature, 328*: 805.
66. Schlomchik, M. J., Aucoin, A. H., Pisetsky, D. S., and Weigert, M. G. 1987. Structure and function of anti-DNA autoantibodies derived from a single autoimmune mouse. *Proc. Natl. Acad. Sci. USA, 84*: 9150.
67. Linder, E. J., and Edginton, T. S. 1972. Antigenic specificity of anti-erythrocyte autoantibody responses by NZB mice. Identification and partial characterization of two erythrocyte surface antigens. *J. Immun., 108*: 1615.
68. De Heer, D. H., and Edgington, T. S. 1976. Cellular events associated with the immunogenesis of anti-erythrocyte autoantibody responses of NZB mice. *Transplant Rev., 31*: 116.
69. De Heer, D. H., Pages, J. M., and Busssard, A. E. 1980. Specificity of anti-erythrocyte autoantibodies secreted by a NZB-derived hybridoma and NZB peritoneal cells. *Cell Immunol., 49*: 135.
70. Pages, J. M., and Bussard, A. E. 1975. Precommitment of normal mouse peritoneal cells by erythrocyte antigens in relation to autoantibody production. *Nature, 257*: 316.
71. Lord, E., and Dutton, R. W. 1975. The properties of plaque forming cells from

autoimmune and normal strains of mice with specificity for autologous erythrocyte antigens. *J. Immun.*, *115*: 1199.

72. Gisler, R. H., Pages, J. M., and Bussard, A. E. 1975. Spontaneous development of plaque forming cells against sheep erythrocytes by mouse peritoneal cells in culture. *Ann. Immunol. Paris*, *126C*: 231.
73. Cox, K. O., Baddams, J., and Evans, A. 1977. Studies of the antigenicity and immunogenicity of bromelain pretreated red blood cells. *Aust. J. Exp. Biol. Med. Sci.*, *55*: 27.
74. Linder, E. J., and Edgington, T. S. 1973. Immunobiology of the autoantibody response. I. Circulating analogues of erythocyte autoantigens and heterogeneity of the autoimmune response of NZB mice. *Clin. Exp. Immunol.*, *13*: 279.
75. Bussard, A. E. 1966. Antibody formation in non-immune peritoneal cells after incubation in gum containing antigen. *Sciences*, *153*: 887.
76. Cox, K. O., Evans, D., Brooks, D., and Cunliffe, D. A. 1979. In vitro investigation of autoantibody secreting peritoneal cells and their regulation. *Immunology*, *38*: 355.
77. Bussard, A. E., Vinit, M. A., and Pages, J. M. 1976. Immunochemical characterization of the autoantibodies produced by mouse peritoneal cells in culture. *Immunochemistry*, *14*: 1.
78. Pages, J. M., and Bussard, A. E. Precommitment of normal mouse peritoneal cells to erythocyte antigens in relation to autoantibody production. *Nature*, *257*: 316.
79. Pages, J. M., and Bussard, A. E. 1978. Establishment and characterization of permanent murine hybridoma secreting monoclonal autoantibodies. *Cell Immunol.*, *41*: 188.
80. Poncet, P., Kocher, H. P., Pages, J., Jaton, J. C., and Bussard, A. E. 1985. Monoclonal autoantibodies against mouse red blood cells. A family of structurally restricted molecules. *Mol. Immunol.*, *22*: 541.
81. Kay, M. M. B. 1984. Localization of senescent cell antigen on band 3. *Proc. Natl. Acad. Sci. USA*, *81*: 5753.
82. Lutz, H. U., Bussolino, F., and Flepp, R. 1987. Naturally occurring anti-band 3 antibodies and complement together mediate phagocytosis of oxidatively stressed human erythrocytes. *Proc. Natl. Acad. Sci. USA*, *84*: 7368–7372.
83. Galili, U., Rachmilewitz, E. A., and Peleg, A. 1984. A unique natural human IgG antibody with anti-galactosyl specificity. *J. Exp. Med.*, *160*: 1519.
84. Pruzanski, W., and Shumak, K. H. 1977. Biologic activity of cold reacting autoantibodies. *N. Engl. J. Med.*, *297*: 538.
85. Reininger, L., Ollier, P., and Poncet, P. 1987. Novel V genes encode virtually variable regions of six murine monoclonal anti-bromelin-treated red blood cell autoantibodies. *J. Immunol.*, *138*: 316.
86. Capra, J. D., Williams, R. C., Feizi, T., and Kunkel, H. G. 1972. Light chain sequences of human IgM cold agglutinin. *Proc. Natl. Acad. Sci. USA*, *69*: 40.
87. Silverman, G. J., Goni, F., Fernandez, J., Che, P. J., Frangione, B., and Carson, D. A. 1988. Distinct patterns of heavy chain variable region subgroup use by human monoclonal autoantibodies of different specificity. *J. Exp. Med.*, *168*: 2361.
88. Bos, N. A., Meenwsen, C. G., Hoojikaas, H., Benner, R., Wostman, B. S., and

Pleasants, J. R. 1987. Early development of Ig secreting cells in young of germ Balb/mice fed a chemically defined ultrafiltered diet. *Cell Immunol.*, *105*: 235.

89. Napastek, Y., André-Schwartz, J., Manser, T., Wysocki, L. J., Breitman, L., Stollar, B. D., Gefter, M., and Schwartz, R. S. 1986. A single germline VH gene segment of normal A/J mice encodes autoantibodies characteristic of systemic lupus erythematosus. *J. Exp. Med.*, *164*: 614.
90. Guilbert, B., Mahana, W., Gilbert, M., Mazié, J. C., and Avrameas, S. 1985. Presence of natural autoantibodies in hyperimmunized mice. *Immunology*, *56*: 401.
91. Matthes, T., Wolff, A., Soubiran, P., Gros, F., and Dighiero, G. 1988. Antitubulin antibodies. II. Natural autoantibodies and induced antibodies recognize different epitopes on the tubulin molecule. *J. Immunol.*, *141*: 3135.
92. Dziarski, R. 1988. Autoimmunity: polyclonal activation or antigen induction? *Immunology Today*, *9*: 340.
93. Klinman, D., and Steinberg, A. D. 1987. Systemic autoimmune disease arises from polyclonal B-cell activation. *J. Exp. Med.*, *165*: 1755.
94. Theofilopoulos, A. N., and Dixon, F. J. 1985. Murine models of systemic lupus erythematosus. *Adv. Immunol.*, *37*: 269.
95. Schwartz, R. S., and Stollar, B. D. 1985. Origins of anti-DNA autoantibodies. *J. Clin. Invest.*, *75*: 321.
96. Schwartz, R. S., and Datta, S. K. 1989. Autoimmunity and autoimmune diseases. In *Fundamental Immunology*, 2nd ed.
97. Cunningham, A. J. 1974. Large numbers of cells in normal mice produce antibody components of isologus erythrocytes. *Nature*, *252*: 749.
98. Izui, S., Zaldivar, N. M., Scher, I., and Lambert, P. H. 1977. Mechanism for induction of anti-DNA antibodies by bacterial lipopolysaccharides in mice. I. Anti-DNA induction by LPS without significant release of DNA in circulating blood. *J. Immunol.*, *119*: 2151.
99. Playfair, J. H. 1982. Immunity to malaria. *Br. Med. Bull.*, *38*: 153.
100. Kazyumba, G., Berney, M., and Brighouse, G. 1986. Expression of the B cell repertoire and autoantibodies in human african trypanosomiasis. *Clin. Exp. Immunol.*, *65*: 10.
101. Dighiero, G, Kaushik, A., Poncet, P., and Ge, X. R. 1987. Origin and significance of autoantibodies. *Concepts in Immunopathology*, *4*: 42.
102. Herzenberg, L. A., Stall, A. M., Lalor, P. A., Sidman, C., Mosse, W. A., Parly, D. R., and Herzenberg, L. A. 1986. The Ly1-B cell lineage. *Immunol. Rev.*, *93*: 81.
103. Hardy, R., and Hayakawa, K. 1986. Development and physiology of Ly-1 B and its human homolog, Leu-1B. *Immunol. Rev.*, *93*: 53.
104. Cantor, H., and Boyse, E. A. 1975. Functional subclasses of T lymphocytes bearing different Ly antigens. I. The generation of functionally distinct T-cell subclasses in a differentiation process independent of antigen. *J. Exp. Med.*, *141*: 1376.
105. Manohar, V., Brown, E., Leiserson, W. M., and Chused, T. M. 1982. Expression of Ly-1 by a subset of B lymphocytes. *J. Immun.*, *129*: 532.
106. Hayakawa, K., Hardy, R. R., and Parks, D. R. 1983. The Ly-1 B cell subpopulation in normal immunodefective and autoimmune mice. *J. Exp. Med.*, *157*: 202.
107. Hayakawa, K., Hardy, R. R., and Herzenberg, L. A. 1986. Peritoneal Ly-1 B cells:

genetic control, autoantibody production, increased lambda light chain expression. *Eur. J. Immunol.*, *16*: 450.

108. Hayakawa, K., Hardy, R. R., Herzenberg, L. A., and Herzenberg, L. A. 1985. Progenitors for Ly-1 B cells are distinct from progenitors for other B cells. *J. Exp. Med.*, *161*: 1554.
109. Hayakawa, K., Hardy, R. R., Stall, A. M., Herzenberg, L. A., and Herzenberg, L. A. 1986. Immunoglobulin bearing B cells reconstitute and maintain the murine Ly-1 B cell lineage. *Eur. J. Immunol.*, *16*: 1313.
110. Hayakawa, K., Hardy, R. R., Honda, M., Herzenberg, L. A., Steinberg, A. D., and Herzenberg, L. A. 1984. Ly-1 B cells: Functionally distinct lymphocytes that secrete IgM autoantibodies. *Proc. Natl. Acad. Sci. USA*, *81*: 2494.
111. Sidman, C. L., Shultz, L. D., Hardy, R. R., Hayakawa, K., and Herzenberg, L. A. 1986. Production of immunoglobulin isotypes by Ly-1^+ B cells in viable motheaten and normal mice. *Science*, *232*: 1423.
112. Dighiero, G., Lim, A., Poncet, P., Kaushik, A., Ge, X. R., and Mazié, J. C. 1987. Age-related natural antibody specificities among hybridoma clones originating from NZB spleen. *Immunology*, *62*: 341.
113. Dighiero, G., Poncet, P., Matthes, T., and Kaushik, A. 1987. Is autoantibody production related to particular B cell subsets and variable region genes? *Pathol. Immunopathol. Res.*, *6*: 371.
114. Dighiero, G., Poncet, P., Rouyre, S., and Mazié, J. C. 1986. New-born Xid mice carry the genetic information for the production of natural autoantibodies. *J. Immunol.*, *136*: 4000.
115. Kaushik, A., Lim, A., Poncet, P., Ge, X. R., and Dighiero, G. 1988. Comparative analysis of natural antibody specificities among hybridomas originating from spleen and peritoneal cavity of adult NZB and BALB/c mice. *Scand. J. Immunol.*, *27*: 461.
116. Conger, J. D., Pike, B. L., and Nossal, G. J. V. 1987. Clonal analysis of the anti-DNA repertoire of murine B lymphocytes. *Proc. Natl. Acad. Sci. USA*, *84*: 2931.
117. Huang, H. J., Jones, N. H., and Strominger, J. L. 1987. Molecular cloning of Ly-1, a membrane glycoprotein of mouse T lymphocytes and a subset of B cells: Molecular homology to its human counterpart Leu-1/T1 (CD5). *Proc. Natl. Acad. Sci. USA*, *84*: 204.
118. Bofil, M., Janossy, G., Janossa, M., Burford, G. D., Seymour, G. J., Wernet, P., and Kelemen, E. 1985. Human B cell development H. Subpopulations in the human fetus. *J. Immunol.*, *134*: 1531.
119. Antin, J. H., Emerson, S. P., Martin, P., Gaddol, N., and Ault, K. A. 1986. Leu 1 (CD5) B cells, a major lymphoid subpopulation in human fetal spleen: phenotypic and functional studies. *Immunology*, *136*: 505.
120. Casali, P., and Notkins, A. L. 1989. Probing the human B-cell repertoire with EBV: Polyreactive and $CD5^+$ B lymphocytes. *Ann. Rev. Immunol.*, *7*: 513.
121. Hardy, R. R., and Hayakawa, K., Shimizu, M., Yamasaki, K., and Kishimoto, T. 1987. Rheumatoid factor secretion from human Leu-1^+ B cells. *Science*, *236*: 81.
122. Casali, P., Burastero, S. E., Nakamura, M., Inghirami, G., and Notkins, A. L. 1987. Human lymphocytes making rheumatoid factors and antibodies to single stranded DNA belong to the Leu-1^+ B cell subset. *Science*, *236*: 77.

123. Bröker, B. M., Klajman, A., Youinou, P., Jouquan, J., Worman, C. P., Murphy, J., Mackenzie, L., Quartey-Papafio, R., Blaschek, M., Collins, P., Lal, S., and Lydyard, P. M. 1988. Chronic lymphocytic leukemic (CLL) cells secrete multispecific autoantibodies. *J. Autoimmunity, 1*: 469.
124. Sthoeger, Z. M., Wakai, M., Tse, D. B., Vinciguerra, V. P., Allen, S. L., Budman, D. R., Lichtman, S. M., Schulman, P., Weiselberg, L. R., and Chiorazzi, N. 1989. Production of autoantibodies by CD5-expressing B lymphocytes from patients with chronic lymphocytic leukemia. *J. Exp. Med., 169*: 255.
125. Borche, L., Lim, A. Binet, J. L., and Dighiero, G. Evidence that chronic lymphocytic leukemia B lymphocytes are frequently committed to productions of natural autoantibodies. (submitted).
126. Seligmann, M., and Brouet, J. C. 1973. Antibody activity of human myeloma globulins. *Semin. Hematol., 10*: 163.
127. Crowley, J. J., Goldfien, R. D., Schrohenlober, R. E., Spiegelberg, H. L., Silverman, G. J., Mageed, R. A., Jefferis, R., Koopman, W. J., Carson, D. A., and Fong, S. 1988. Incidence of three cross-reactive idiotypes on human rheumatoid factor paraproteins. *J. Immunol., 140*: 3411.
128. Kritzman, J., Kunkel, H. G., McCarthy, J., and Mellors, R. C. 1961. Studies of a Waldenström-type macroglobulin with rheumatoid factor properties. *J. Lab. Clin. Med., 57*: 905.
129. Abraham, G. N., Clark, R. A., and Vaughan, J. M. 1972. Characterization of an IgA rheumatoid factor binding properties and reactivity with the subclasses of human G globulin. *Immunochemistry, 9*: 301.
130. Klein, M., Danon, F. Brouet, J. C., Signoret, Y., and Seligmann, M. 1972. Etude immunochimique de 130 cryoglobulines humaines. *Rev. Eur. Etude Clin. Biol., 17*: 948.
131. Agnello, V., Joslin, F. G., and Kunkel, H. G. 1972. Cross idiotypic specificity among monoclonal IgM anti-gammaglobulins. *Scand. J. Immunol., 1*: 283.
132. Kunkel, H. G., Agnello, V., Joslin, F. G., Winchester, R. J., and Capra, J. D. 1973. Cross idiotypic specificity among monoclonal IgM proteins with anti-gammaglobulin activity. *J. Exp. Med., 137*: 331.
133. Capra, J. D., and Kehoe, D. G. 1974. Structure of antibodies with shared idiotyp: the complete sequence of the heavy chain variable regions of two anti-gammaglobulins. *Proc. Natl. Acad. Sci. USA, 71*: 4032.
134. Goni, F, Chen, P. P., Pons-Estel, B., Carson, D. A., and Frangione, B. 1985. Sequence similarities and cross-idiotypic specificity of L chains among human monoclonal IgM-K with anti-gammaglobulin activity. *J. Immunol., 135*: 4073.
135. Newkirk, M. M., Mageed, R. A., Jefferis, R., Chen, P. P., and Capra, J. D. 1987. Complete amino acid sequences of variable regions of two human IgM rheumatoid factors. BOR and KAS of the Wa idiotypic family reveal restricted use of heavy and light chain variable and joining region gene segments. *J. Exp. Med., 166*: 550.
136. Chen, P. P., Robbins, D. L., Jirik, F. R., Kipps, T. J., and Carson, D. A. 1987. Isolation and characterization of a light chain variable region gene for human rheumatoid factors. *J. Exp. Med., 166*: 1900.
137. Chen, P. P., Albrandt, K., Kipps, T. J., Radoux, V., Liu, F. T., and Carson, D.A.

1987. Isolation and characterization of human V_KIII germline genes: implications for the molecular basis of human V_KIII light chain diversity. *J. Immunol.*, *139*: 1727.

138. Agnello, V., Goni, F., Barnes, J. L., de la Vega, M. T., and Frangione, B. 1987. Human rheumatoid factor crossidiotypes. II. Primary structure-dependent cross reactive idiotype. PSL2-CRI, present on Wa monoclonal rheumatoid factor is present on Bla and other IgMk monoclonal autoantibodies. *J. Exp. Med.*, *165*: 263.
139. Silverman, G. J., Goldstein, R. D., Chen, P. P., Mageed, R. A., Jefferis, R., Goni, F., Frangione, B., Fong, S., and Carson, D. A. 1988. Idiotypic and subgroup analysis of human monoclonal rheumatoid factors: implications for structural and genetic basis of autoantibodies in humans. *J. Clin. Invest.*, *82*: 469.
140. Chen, P. P., Fong, S., Goni, F., Silverman, G. J., Fox, R. I., Liu, M. F., Frangione, B., and Carson, D. A. 1988. Cross-reacting idiotypes on cryoprecipitating rheumatoid factor. *Springer Semin. Immunopathol.*, *10*: 35.
141. Dellagi, K., Brouet, J. C., and Danon, F. 1979. Cross idiotypic antigens among monoclonal immunoglobulin M from patients with Waldenström's macroglobulinemia and polyneuropathy. *J. Clin. Invest.*, *64*: 1530.
142. Shoenfeld, Y., Amital Teplizki, H., Mendlovic, S., Blank, M., Mozes, E., and Isenberg, D. A. 1989. The role of the human anti-DNA idiotype 16/6 in autoimmunity. *Clin. Immunol., Immunopathol.*, *51*: 313.
143. Boumsell, L., Bernard, A., and Lepage, V. 1978. Some chronic lymphocytic leukemia cells bearing surface immunoglobulins share determinants with T cells. *Eur. J. Immunol.*, *8*: 900.
144. Dighiero, G. 1988. An attempt to explain disordered immunity and hypogammaglobulinemia in CLL. *Nouv. Rev. Franç.* Hématol., 30: 283.
145. Kipps, T. J., Tomhave, E., Chen, P. P., and Carson, D. A. 1988. Autoantibody associated K light chain variable region gene expressed in chronic lymphocytic leukeia with little orno somatic mutation, implications for etiology and immunotherapy. *J. Exp. Med.*, *167*: 840.
146. Kipps, T. J., Tomhave, E., Pratt, L. F., Duffy, S., Chen, P. P., and Carson, D. A. 1989. Developmentally restricted immunoglobulin heavy chain variable region gene expressed at high frequency in chronic lymphocytic leukemia. *Proc. Natl. Acad. Sci. USA*, *86*: 5913.

4

The Contribution of The Ly-1 B-cell Subset to Self-Reactivity

Raoul Mayer and Habib Zaghouani
Mount Sinai School of Medicine, New York, New York

I. CD5 B CELLS—HYSTORICAL PERSPECTIVE

A. The Discovery of CD5 on B-Cell Malignancies

CD5 is a pan-T lymphocyte differentiation antigen with a molecular weight of 67 kD. In 1978 the presence of Leu-1 (human CD5 cytodifferentiation antigen) was first reported on B cells in a human leukemia study (1). This expression was confined to Ig^+ cells from B-CLL patients and small lymphocytic lymphoma (SLL) patients (2–6). Ig^+ cells from acute leukemias, Burkitt's lymphomas, and other B-cell proliferative disorders were all negative. In the same year Lanier and his collaborators (7) reported a high incidence of murine B-cell lymphomas in a new strain of mouse called B10-H-2^a H-4^b (2^a4^b), which were induced by hyperimmunization with sheep red blood cells (SRBC). Several malignant B-lymphoma lines were obtained (CH lines) from these mice (8–9). At about the same time, Slavin and Strober (10) also reported a case of murine B-cell leukemia (BCL1) which developed spontaneously in an old BALB/c mouse and was characterized by prominent splenomegaly and a very high lymphocyte count ($>200{,}000/\mu l$). BCL1 has been subsequently used as a model of human BCLL based on phenotypic and morphologic markers. All these mouse B-cell malignancies are characterized by variable expression of Ly-1 (mouse CD5 cytodifferentiation antigen), marked splenomegaly, lymph node enlargement, transplantability using as few as two cells, and no involvement of the thymus or bone marrow.

B. Characterization of Ly-1 B Cells in Normal Animals

In the case of mouse and human B-cell malignancies expressing CD5 on their surface, their large numbers in the spleen and other lymphoid organs made them easily detectable by staining. Since the CD5 B cells are extremely rare in normal animals and human subjects, their detection proved to be difficult. With improved immunofluorescence techniques, particularly the development of FACS, the Ly-1 B population in mice was better characterized. The Ly-1–expressing B cells were detected in the spleen and peripheral blood at a very low frequency (1–2%) in most adult mouse strains tested (11). A paradoxical enrichment (10–40%) was found among peritoneal B cells (12). A large fraction of these B cells were found to produce autoAbs specific for autologous erythrocytes (13–14). Ly-1 B cells are, however, undetectable in the bone marrow, lymph nodes, and Peyer's patches (11–12). In a recent report, sorted thymic B cells, which constitute a small percentage of total thymic lymphocytes, were shown to be of the phenotype Ly-1^+, Ia+,B220 low, and MAC-1^+ (15). Therefore, it appears that most thymic B cells have the Ly-1^+ phenotype. When young mice (1 week old) were studied, a higher proportion (>30%) of Ly-1 B cells was found among splenic and peritoneal IgM^+ cells (11–12). This high proportion of IgM^+ Ly-1 B cells is, however, maintained throughout adulthood only in the peritoneum (12). When grown in culture, Ly-1 B-cell lines multiply rapidly and show genomic amplification and increased transcription of the *c-myc* gene (16–17). While most B cells die after a short time when cultured in vitro, Ly-1 B cells demonstrate prolonged survival and spontaneous IgM secretion (16).

C. Ly-1 B Cells as a Separate Lineage

Bone marrow reconstitution experiments showed a dichotomy in the differentiation of Ly-1^+ and Ly-1^- B cells probably originating at the stem cell level. Liver cells from fetal mice (the liver is the site of hematopoiesis in some stages of fetal development) reconstituted both sets, while bone marrow cells originating from adult animals were able to reconstitute only the Ly-1^- B cell population (18). As a corollary to these results, it was shown that IgM^+ B cells from adult peritoneum or Ig^+ B cells from newborn mice were able to reconstitute almost exclusively the Ly-1^+ population (12). In view of these very significant reconstitution experiments, most researchers today regard the Ly-1 B cells as a distinct subset of B cells which appears early in ontogeny, migrates to the periphery, and is maintained independently of the bone marrow. These characteristics as well as the ability to spontaneously secrete Ig when cultured in vitro clearly distinguish the Ly-1^{+} B-cell subset from the conventional, Ly-1^{-} B-cell subset.

D. Studies in Autoimmune Inbred Mouse Strains

The Ly-1 B-cell subset was studied in a variety of inbred mouse strains, particularly several immunodefective strains. One of the common features shared by these mice is spontaneous autoantibody production. At one end of the spectrum, SJL, xid, and CBA/N mice show a lower level of expression (12,19,20). The proportion of Ly-1 B cells is distinctly higher in NZB mice (11,21). Interestingly, an oligoclonal proliferation of the Ly-1 B subset was observed in NZB mice (22–24). This spontaneous proliferation is extreme in the peritoneum and later involves the spleen and lymph nodes. The observed splenomegaly was shown to be due mostly to Ly-1 B cells (22–24). Phenotypical analysis on NZB peritoneal B cells revealed hyperdiploidy, which is believed to represent a premalignant stage (22–24). This may very well be due to a selective expansion of the Ly-1 B cells as a functionally distinct subset. A large fraction of the IgM Ig spontaneously secreted by NZB mice are autoantibodies with specificities restricted to Fc gamma, ssDNA, and thymocytes (25). It therefore appears that Ly-1 B cells in NZB mice are responsible for the spontaneous autoantibody production of the IgM isotype. The viable motheaten me^{v} autoimmune strain carries a mutation mapping to chromosome 6 (26–27). These mice die at a young age, and display severe immunodeficiency and autoimmunity (27). Even though the overall number of B cells is decreased, nearly all of them are Ly-1^{+} (28). The high level of spontaneous autoantibody production observed in me^{v} mice must also be due to the Ly-1 B cells since this subset is predominant in me^{v} mice. Painter et al. (29) analyzed the self-reactivity of a panel of hybridomas obtained from me^{v} mice. Interestingly, more than 60% of these hybridomas produce autoAbs specific for autoantigens. These findings therefore suggest that a high proportion of me^{v} Ly-1 B cells immortalized by the fusion event produce autoantibodies, but as a corollary not all Ly-1 B cells product autoAbs. The distribution of V gene utilization in this panel of hybridomas was, however, random. Sidman et al. (30) showed that in this strain the increased Ig secretion is promoted by a B-cell–derived maturation factor uniquely elevated in me^{v} mice. Interestingly enough, when normal strains were examined, a close correlation between the Ly-1 B expression and autoantibody secretion was observed. Following in vivo LPS stimulation, a large fraction of Ly-1^{+} sorted B cells were shown to be specific for bromelain-treated mouse red blood cells (BrMRBC) (19). These cells are consistently enriched in the peritoneal cavity of normal adult mice (31⅔32). The same correlation between Ly-1 expression and bromelain-treated mouse erythrocyte (BrMRBC) specificity was observed among the CH mouse lymphoma lines; almost all CH murine B-lymphoma lines show erythrocyte specificities and Ly-1 expression

(33–25). Further, detailed analysis identified the phosphotydilcholine determinant on RBC membranes as the epitope recognized by antibodies produced by CH mouse lymphomas which bound BrMRBC (35).

E. Molecular Cloning of Ly-1 and Leu-1

Recently the genes for the Ly-1 and the Leu-1 cytodifferentiation antigens have been cloned (36–37). Both proteins are 471 amino acids long with 63% overall amino acid homology. Interestingly, there is a gradient of increasing homology. The first amino-terminal subregion has 43% identity, the second 58%, and the carboxy-terminal subregion 90%. Two of the three potential glycosylation sites at the amino terminal and the two at the carboxy terminal are conserved. The sequence is consistent with an extracellular amino-terminal region of 347 amino acids, followed by a hydrophobic transmembrane segment of 31 amino acids and a carboxy-terminal intracellular segment of 93 amino acids. The N-terminal region is relatively rich in cysteine and is separated into two homologous domains by a hinge-like region rich in proline and threonine residues. The 23 cysteine residues are present in very similar locations in the two sequences. This molecular information represents a strong argument that murine Ly-1 and human CD5 B-cell subsets are functionally related.

F. Possible Physiologic Role of CD5 and the CD5 B-Cell Subset

The physiologic function of the vast majority of lymphocyte cytodifferentiation antigens is presently unknown. There are a few examples of CD molecules for which a role in cell-cell interaction (LFA-1, ICAM, CD4, and CD8), intracellular signal transduction (CD3), or ligand binding (CD21,CD23) has been demonstrated. Unfortunately, despite the extensive characterization of the CD5 B-cell subset in both mice and humans, its physiologic role is poorly understood. In the murine system, Griffith et al. (38) recently demonstrated the constitutive phosphorylation of CD5 and implicated protein kinase C in this process. While phorbol esters have an enhancing effect on CD5 expression, concanavalin A (ConA) has an opposite action. Furthermore, CD5 was found to be induced upon in vitro activation of both B and T lymphocytes and has been associated with the upregulation of T-cell activation when used in conjunction with other T-cell stimuli (39–40). In addition, sorted Ly-1$^+$ B cells demonstrated a higher stimulation index of both proliferative and immunoglobulin secretory responses after IL-5 treatment as compared to Ly-1$^-$ B cells (41). IL-4, on the other hand, was found to downregulate the surface expression of CD5 on normal and leukemic B cells (42–43). Finally, Ansar-Ahmed et al. (44) have shown that estrogen increases the net number of CD5$^+$ B cells and augments the autoAb production by sorted CD5$^+$ B cells obtained from autoimmune mice. This finding might explain the effect of sex hormones on the manifestation of autoimmune phenomena.

In conclusion, present data suggest that the expression of CD5 in both T and B lymphocytes is associated with lymphocyte activation. Obviously, this concept applies only to $CD5^+$ B cells and has no bearing on conventional $CD5^-$ B cells. Various soluble mediators (IL-5, IL-4, estrogen) affect the expression of the CD5 antigen and/or cell activation. Since all available data are based on in vitro experiments, the in vivo role of CD5 in lymphocyte activation remains to be determined, possibly by transgenic mouse experiments.

II. THE EXPRESSION OF Ly-1 GENE AND POLYPEPTIDE IN HIGHLY PURIFIED B CELLS AND HYBRIDOMAS PRODUCING AUTOANTIBODIES OBTAINED FROM NORMAL AND AUTOIMMUNE-PRONE MURINE STRAINS

A. Historical Perspective and Significance of Present Studies

Ly-1 B cells constitute a small (1–3%) but distinct subset of B cells in normal mice. This B-cell subset is enlarged in NZB (30–40%) mice and predominant in me^V (>90%) ice (11,28), two autoimmune-prone mouse strains. Preliminary studies have suggested that Ly-1 B cells play an important role in experimental murine autoimmunity. The production of RF and certain autoAbs, such as DNA, RF, Br-MRBC, and thymocyte specific (19), is attributed mostly to this B-cell subset. The hybridoma technology allows the random immortalization of autoimmune B cells from normal and autoimmune animals as well as human subjects. In view of the weak expression of the Ly-1 antigen on the membrane of B cells, it was difficult to directly correlate the Ly-1 phenotype with the production of specific types of autoAbs. All prior work implicating the Ly-1 B-cell subset in autoAb production was done exclusively by surface staining being based on the indirect association, seen in a limited number of murine strains, between an increased proportion of Ly-1 B cells and a high frequency of autoAb production. Using more sensitive molecular techniques in a previous study we were able to identify Ly-1 transcripts in autoAb-producing hybridomas obtained from MRL/1pr mice and therefore make a Ly-1 phenotypic assignment based on the detection of gene expression (45–46). The Ly-1 phenotypic assignment of the hybridomas was initially done by Northern blot analysis. A representative panel of Ly-1^+ hybridomas was further studied by immunofluorescence and Western analysis. The questions addressed in the present study were:

1. Whether the hybridoma Ly-1 transcripts detected with the Ly-1 cDNA probe in Northern analysis are indeed derived from the same gene as the corresponding Ly-1 transcripts identified in thymocytes.
2. Whether there is a relationship between the detection of hybridoma Ly-1 gene transcripts and the detection of polypeptides reacting with monoclonal anti–Ly-1 antibodies in immunofluorescence and Western analysis.

3. Whether there is a relationship between the hybridoma Ly-1 phenotype as determined by Northern analysis, the strain of origin (normal vs. autoimmune-prone strain), and the specificities of the autoAbs produced by these hybridomas.

B. Expression of the Ly-1 Gene in Thymocytes, Motheaten Enriched B Cells, and Hybridomas

The expression of the Ly-1 gene in total, nuclear, and cytoplasmic RNA extracted from thymocytes has demonstrated two transcripts of 2.9 and 2.1 kb, respectively, the shorter one being significantly more abundant. Both Ly-1 transcripts were clearly detected in total and nuclear thymic RNA (46). The less abundant 2.9 kb Ly-1 transcript, however, was detected mostly in the nuclear thymic RNA, suggesting that it probably represents a nuclear precursor transcript. In contrast, total RNA extracted from highly purified me^{V} splenic B cells as well as from me^{V} and NZB hybridomas (UN17-19, Z49, and Z51) all showed Ly-1 transcripts of 2.9 and 1.6 kb. It is significant to note that the 2.9 kb Ly-1 hybridoma transcript corresponds to the longer, less abundant thymic Ly-1 transcript (Fig. 1). The shorter, 1.6 kb Ly-1 transcript identified in me^{V}-enriched B cells and hybridomas can be explained by: (1) cross-hydridization of Ly-1 cDNA probe, obtained from a thymic library, with transcripts of a homologous gene, specifically expressed in B cells; (2) aberrant transcription; or (3) alternate splicing of a primary Ly-1 transcript or different transcription initiation/termination of the Ly-1 gene transcript related to either cell type (B versus T) or fusion event (hybridoma vs. thymocytes). These possibilities were investigated in S1 nuclease protection experiments.

RNA obtained from thymus, CH31LX, a B-cell lymphoma line which stains

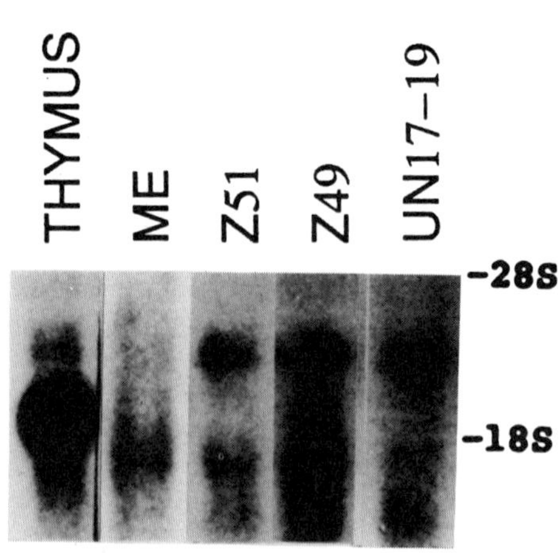

FIGURE 1 Northern blot of total RNA extracted from thymocytes, me^{V}-enriched B cells and Z51, Z49 (NZB), and UN17-19 (me^{V}) hybridomas hybridized with the Ly-1 cDNA probe.

brightly for Ly-1, two Ly-1$^+$ hybridomas (Z41 and UN40-9), and SP2/0 myeloma cells was analyzed in S1 nuclease protection experiments. As depicted in Figure 2, a protected fragment of 1.6 kb was observed for both thymic and CH31LX RNA, while in the case of both hybridomas analyzed, a protected fragment of 0.8 kb was observed. An additional protected fragment of 1.2 kb was observed in thymic RNA. These results clearly demonstrate that the Ly-1 transcripts previously detected in Northern analysis in thymus, CH31LX, and the two hybridomas tested are the products of the same gene. No protected fragments were observed with SP2/0 RNA (46).

C. Correlation of Ly-1 Gene Transcription and the Detection of Ly-1 Polypeptide in Hybridomas

In order to investigate the functionality of the Ly-1 hybridoma transcripts detected by Northern and S1 nuclease protection experiments, we carried out Western blot-

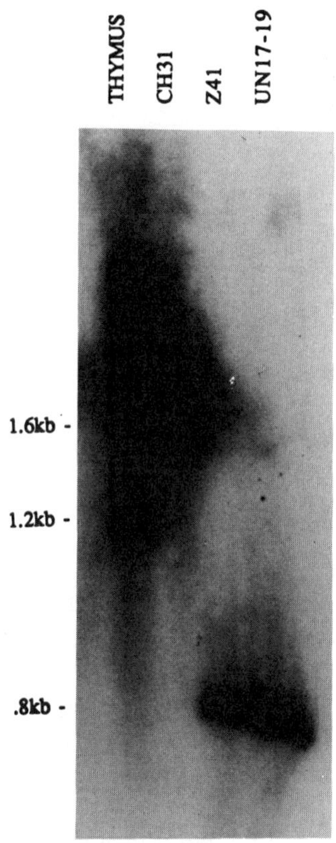

FIGURE 2 S1 nuclease protection. Two hundred ng Ly-1 cDNA insert was hybridized with 10 μg total RNA obtained from thymocytes, CH31LX lymphoma cells, and Z41 and UN17-19 hybridomas. The DNA-RNA heteroduplex was S1 digested, electrophoresed, transferred to nitrocellulose, and hybridized with the Ly-1 cDNA probe.

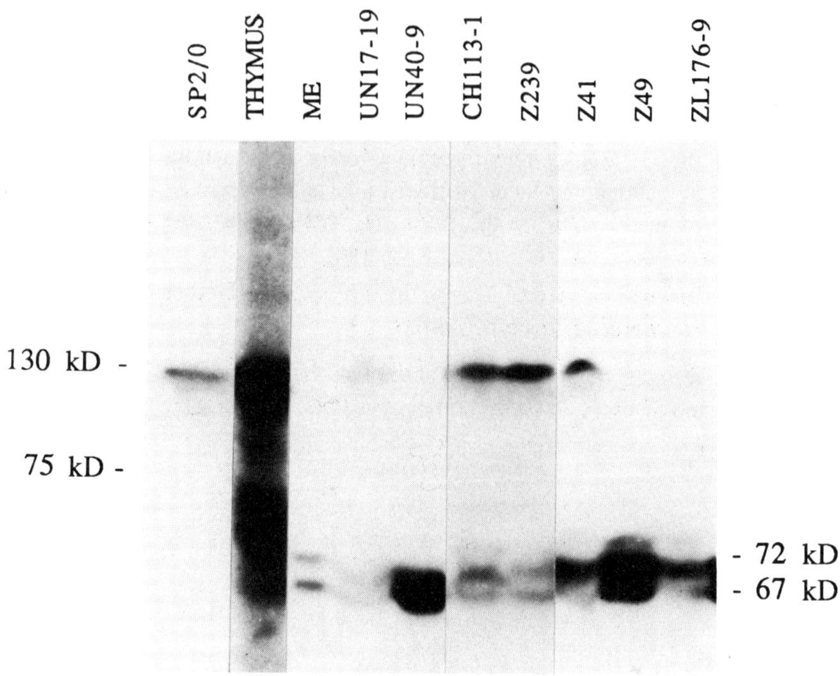

FIGURE 3 Western blot of cellular lysate obtained from SP2/0 myeloma cells, thymocytes, *me*^{V}-enriched B cells, and UN17-19, UN-40-9 (*me*^{V}), CH113-1 (C_3H/HeJ), Z239, Z41, Z49, and ZL176-9 (NZB) hybridomas. Cytoplasmic lysates were obtained under reducing conditions from 10^7 cells, electrophoresed under reducing conditions, transferred to DEAE membrane, and incubated with ^{125}I-labeled anti–Ly-1 monoclonal antibodies.

ting and immunofluorescence staining in a represenative number of hybridomas expressing Ly-1 transcripts and highly purified B cells isolated from *me*^{V} splenocytes.

The Western data presented in Figure 3 show that in the thymic lysate three bands of 67, 72, and 130 kD were observed, and in *me*^{V} B cell lysate only the bands of 67 and 72 kD reacted with anti-Ly-1 MAb. These two bands were also detected in all hybridomas studied. The band of 130 kD observed in thymus was also detected in some hybridomas. Duplicate blots incubated with an isotype-matched MAb (anti-FcR) did not reveal any of these bands. The 67 and 72 kD bands detected in our Western blotting analysis correlate with the previously described labeled material obtained from NP-40 extracts of murine thymocytes precipitated with specific anti–Ly-1 polyclonal antiserum (47). The 67 kD band detected in both Western and immunoprecipitation experiments corresponds to the mature Ly-1 gene product made up of 471 amino acid residues (37). The 72 kD band detected in our Western analysis and the 80 kD band previously detected by immunoprecipitation in thymocytes probably represent glycosilated forms or partially processed gene products.

The significance of the 130 kD band, which was detected in thymus, some of the hybridomas, as well as in SP2/0 lysates, is not clear. The presence of reducing agents in both the lysing and loading buffers formally excludes the possibility that the 130 kD band is a dimer of the 67 kD protein. Since this band was also observed in SP2/0 lysates, a myeloma line in which no Ly-1 transcripts were detected, and which is clearly negative by immunofluorescence, we conclude that the 130 kD polypeptide probably bears a cross-reactive epitope interacting with the rat anti–Ly-1 MAb.

Immunofluorescence staining with anti–Ly-1 and anti–Lyt-2 MAbs was also carried out on this group of Ly-1$^+$ hybridomas. The data illustrated in Figure 4 show a strong intracytoplasmic staining of all six hybridomas studied. Three of these six Ly-1$^+$ hybridomas studied exhibited a weak surface staining (ZL176-9, UN17-19, and UN40-9). The staining profile pattern of surface and intracytoplasmic immunofluorescence is identical to previous results obtained with NZB splenocytes (21).

In view of the surface versus intracytoplasmic immunofluorescence results, it is also apparent that in hybridomas, and probably B cells in general, the Ly-1 protein accumulates in the cytoplasm where it can be readily detected. Only a small fraction of the Ly-1 protein, however, probably becomes anchored on the membrane, which explains the characteristic "dull" surface staining seen in hybridomas and sorted B cells. A very likely explanation of this phenomenon is the generation of isoforms at the carboxy terminus in B and T cells, since the C-terminal region of the Ly-1 protein is involved in membrane anchoring. This process has recently been described for the human dystrophin gene (48). There are other examples indicating that the cytodifferentiation antigens identified with the same monoclonal antibodies can differ in T and B cells. Thus, while T200 antigen is of 200 kD in T cells, in B cells it has a size of 180 kD (49). The different size of Ly-1 transcript seen in B cells and hybridomas is probably due to alternate splicing or different initiation/termination of transcription. Alternative splicing of the mRNA coding for glucose-6-phosphate dehydrogenase in different tissues was described in human (50), and it was demonstrated that the secreted form of CD8 also arises from alternative splicing (51).

D. Expression of the Ly-1 Gene in 140 Hybridomas Producing Autoantibodies

Since we established a good correlation between the detection of hybridoma Ly-1 transcripts and polypeptides, we used Northern blot analysis in order to determine the frequency of hybridomas of the Ly-1$^+$ phenotype (Ly-1$^+$ hybridomas) in a large panel of 140 hybridomas producing autoantibodies derived from normal and autoimmune prone murine strains. Table 1 illustrates the strain of origin and the specificities of the autoAbs produced. A large fraction of the hybridomas

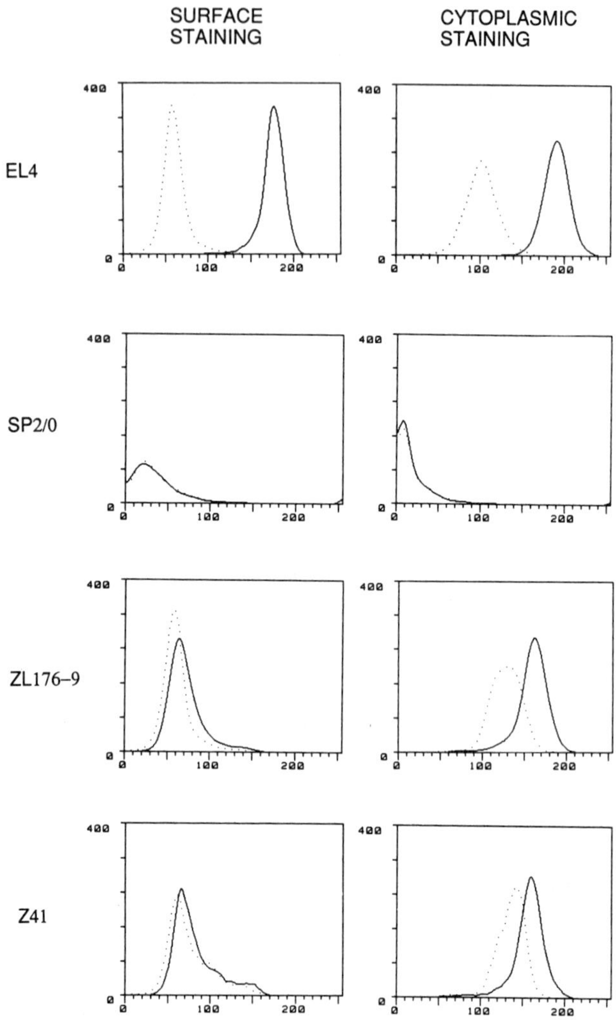

FIGURE 4 FACSCAN contours of surface (left panel) and cytoplasmic (right panel) immunofluorescence staining of EL4 (T-cell control), SP2/0, and UN17-19, UN40-9 (me^{V}), CH113-1 (C_3H/HeJ), Z41, Z49, and ZL176-9 (NZB) hybridomas. The solid line represents the staining profile with 53-7.5, the anti–Ly-1 reagent. The dotted line represents the staining profile with the isotype-matched 53-6.7 anti–Lyt-2 reagent.

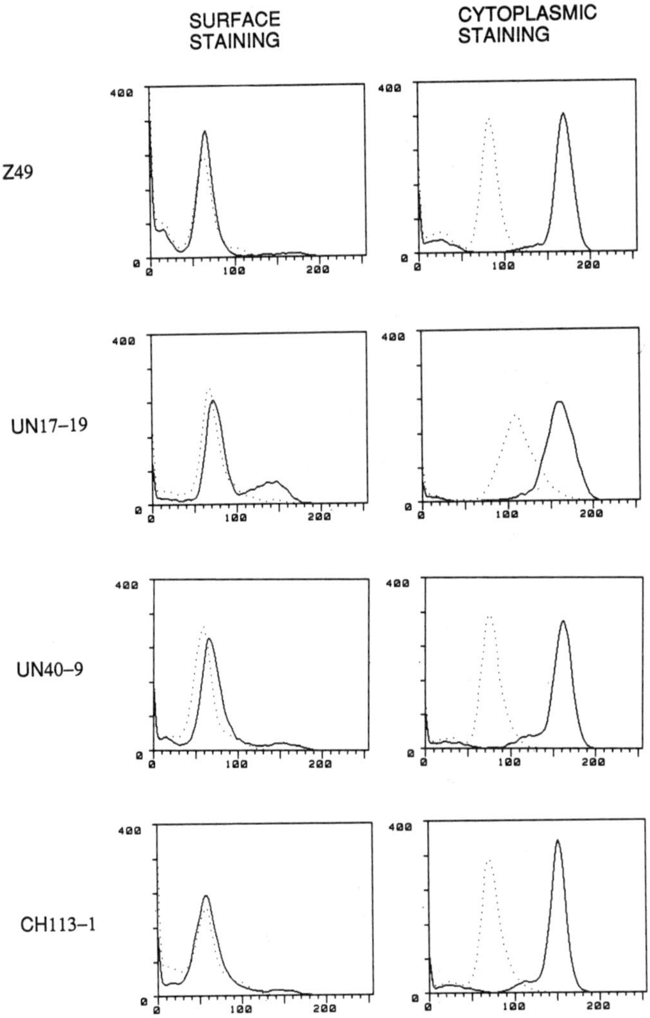

FIGURE 4 *(Continued)*

were obtained from strains prone to autoimmune disease such as NZB, me^V, and MRL/1pr. The hybridomas specific for collagen II (CII) were obtained from DBA/1J mice injected with CII, whereas those obtained from C_3H/HeJ originated from animals injected with anti-idiotypic antibodies (45,52). The BALB/c NL series of hybridomas were obtained from 1-month-old LPS-stimulated lymphocytes and were selected by screening with the V_HX24 probe. These hybridomas bind to polysaccharides such as levan, ACHO, and galactan and were

TABLE 1 Origin and Specificity of Hybridomas

MRL/1pr	MRL5-51, MRL55-23, MRL50-8, MRL55-18, GP75-9 (RF) M56 (Sm) FM35-4, 63-99-7 (DNA) GP88, GP138-10, GP99-5, GP75-9, GP133, GS13-1, GS11-1, GS4-1, H45-5, H16-5, H17-1, H4-2, H91-12, 63-86-7 (Multispecific)
DBA/1J	D3m, E10, C1, C1D2, A12, B1, D3 (CII)
B6-me^V	UN32-15 (IF) UN17-19 (RF) UN42-5, UN34-11 (Thy) UN55-5 (NA) UN59-9, UN37-5, UN40-9 (Multispecific)
C3H/HeJ	CH44-7, CH113-1, CH55-8 (DNA) CH154-1, CH24-10, CGS21-17 (Multispecific)
BALB/c	HB2 (DNA) HB8, HB9 (Microfibrils) CP8ED2 (Br-MRBC) NL103-3, NL119-3, NL121-6, NL127-2, NL104-1, NL105-10, NL124-1, NL126-4, NL112-9, NL113-6, NL122-5, NL110-6 (Polysaccharides) F4F5, F9, A7, F1B4 (Multispecific)
(CBA/N x BALB/c F_1	M15-1 (Myosin) M40-1, M34-5, M25-8, M25-9, F5-2, F30-4 (Multispecific) M16-3 (Unknown)
NZB (6-d old)	A2F9 (Actin) A1C10, A4G8, B15S3 (TNP) B8H5, B6F2 (DNA) B1E2, A9A7, A3D2, B13D4, B1F5, B10B9 (Multispecific)
NZB (1-mo old)	Z51, Z317 (TG) Z41, Z218ZK9A4-10 (DNA) Z49, Z39 (AchR) ZK4G3-8 (Br-MRBC) Z121, ZX25, Z14, ZK2H5-3, ZK2A7-3, ZK2A8-11, ZK5F11-3 (Multispecific) Z250, ZK244, ZK2A11-1, ZK9D9-1, Z239, ZK2H6-2, ZK9B9-8, ZK3G11-1, ZK8E8-1 (Unknown)
NZB (5-mo old)	N8G2 (Myosin) N5C5, N8F6, N10E9, Z8E5 (Multispecific)

(Continued)

TABLE 1 *Continued*

NZB (16-mo old)	ZL154-1 (H2b) ZL177-5 (RF) ZL173-6, ZL179-6, ZA1C7-5, ZA2B12-10, ZA3E3-12, ZA4A10-13, ZA4B7-2, ZA2G8-3, ZA3E5-12 (DNA) ZL37-9 (AchR, DNA) ZA4B8-2, ZA1B8-1, ZA1C7-12, ZO121-12, ZO55-3, ZO120-6 (Coombs) ZA2C2-6, ZL34-8, ZL37-14, ZA4C3-1 (Multispecific) ZA5C2-5, ZA5E4-8, ZA4A7-1, ZA1B8-1, ZA1E3-1, ZA3C4-2 (Unknown)

RF, rheumatoid factor; Sm, Smith antigen; CII, collagen type II; IF, intrinsic factor; Thy, thymocytes; NA, nuclear antigen; Br-MRBC, bromelain-treated mouse red blood cells; AchR, acetylcholine receptor; H2b, histone 2b; TG, thyroglobulin.

used as controls. Ly-1 transcripts were detected in 48 out of 140 hybridomas tested. No Ly-1 transcripts were detected in the BALB/c NL series of hybridomas. Figure 5 illustrates a Northern blot carried out with RNA extracted from a representative group of hybridomas obtained from adult BALB/c and NZB mice of various ages. The data presented in Table 2 show the strain distribution of the Ly-1$^+$ and Ly-1$^-$ hybridomas. Approximately one half of NZB and seven of eight *me*^{V} hybridomas express the Ly-1 gene, data in agreement with the high proportion of Ly-1 B cells previously reported in these strains (11,28). Only 6 out of 22 hybridomas obtained from 1-month-old MRL/1pr mice, 2 out of 19 obtained from BALB/c mice, and 1 out of 6 obtained from C_3H/HeJ mice was found to express the Ly-1 gene. Interestingly, one out of eight (CBA/N × BALB/c) F_1 hybridomas was found to express the Ly-1 gene. Prior studies have reported an inability to detect Ly-1 B cells in this strain by conventional surface immunofluorescence techniques.

The data depicted in Table 3 summarizes the Ly-1 phenotype and the fine specificities of the autoAbs produced in our panel of hybridomas. The most significant findings are that the majority of DNA-specific autoAbs are produced by hybridomas of the Ly-1$^+$ phenotype, whereas the majority of hybridomas producing RF and multispecific autoAbs are produced mostly by hybridomas of the Ly-1$^-$ phenotype. Despite the small sample size it should also be noted that hybridomas producing autoAbs specific for H_2b, IF, AchR, actin, thymocytes, and Br-MRBC all express the Ly-1 gene. On the other hand, none of the DBA/1J hybridomas producing CII-specific autoAbs and only one out of six NZB hybridomas producing Coombs autoAbs originate from the Ly-1$^+$ phenotypic B-cell subset. These two types of autoAbs are considered to be pathogenic.

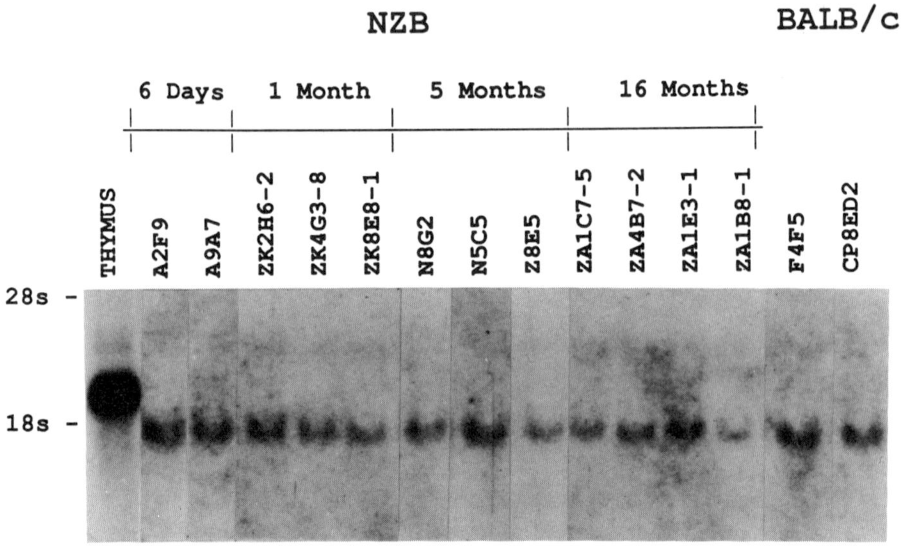

FIGURE 5 Northern blot of RNA extracted from representative BALB/c and NZB mice of various ages (6 days, 1, 5, and 16 months). The blots were hybridized with the Ly-1 cDNA probe.

Our data on Ly-1 hybridoma gene transcripts and the corresponding proteins detected with monoclonal anti–Ly-1 antibodies show that the identification of Ly-1 gene transcript is a valuable marker for the Ly-1 phenotypic assignment, taking into account the low density or even absence of the Ly-1 antigen on the surface of B cells. Using this criterion, we have shown that a significant proportion of autoAb-producing hybridomas are of the Ly-1$^+$ phenotype. This proportion is particularly high in hybridomas obtained from NZB and *me*^{V} mice, which is in agreement with prior data showing an increased proportion of this B-cell subset

TABLE 2 LY-1 Gene Expression in Hybridomas Obtained from Various Murine Strains

	NZB	MRL/ 1pr	DBA/1J	ME^V	C3H/ HeJ	BALB/c	(CBA/N x BALB/c)F_1
Ly-1$^+$	31	6	0	7	1	2	1
Ly-1$^-$	38	16	7	1	5	6	7
Total	69	22	7	8	6	8	8

TABLE 3 Expression of LY-1 Gene in Hybridomas Producing Autoantibodies of Various Specificities

	LY-1^+	LY-1^-	Total
DNA	11	9	20
RF	2	5	7
Sm	0	1	1
H2b	1	0	1
CII	0	7	7
IF	1	0	1
TG	1	1	2
NA	0	1	1
Br-MRBC	2	0	2
AchR	2	0	2
Microfibrils	0	2	2
Myosin	1	1	2
Actin	1	1	1
Thy	2	0	2
RBC (Coombs)	1	5	6
TNP	1	2	3
Polysaccharides	0	12	12
Multispecific	13	38	51
Total	39	83	

RF, rheumatoid factor; Sm, Smith antigen; H2b, histone 2b; CII, collagen type II; IF, intrinsic factor; TG, thyroglobulin; NA, nuclear antigen; Br-MRBC, bromelain-treated mouse red blood cells; AchR, acetylcholine receptor; Thy, Thymocytes.

in these autoimmune murine strains. Since we did not find a high frequency of Ly-1^+ hybridomas in other strains prone to autoimmune diseases such as MRL/1pr, we believe that the expansion and dominance of the Ly-1 B-cell subset is related to the characteristic genetic background of each murine strain and is not necessarily influenced by the presence of autoimmune manifestations. In this context, autoimmune diseases are clearly genetically multifactorial with the Ly-1 B cells playing a major role in the production of a restricted subset of autoAbs with distinct specificities such as DNA, RF, and multispecific. This in turn is probably a consequence of an apparent genetic restriction of a biased utilization of immunoglobulin V genes. The analysis of the V_H and V_K gene family utilization in our panel of hybridomas has demonstrated a biased usage of D-proximal V_H gene segments.

Our data clearly demonstrate that a high proportion of autoAbs specific for DNA, BR-MRBC, and thymocytes are produced by Ly-1 B cells, and a smaller fraction of hybridomas producing RF and multispecific autoAbs expressed the Ly-1 gene. This is surprising since the clones producing multispecific autoAbs, which represent a large fraction of the preimmune repertoire, were considered to belong to the Ly-1 B-cell subset. It is important to note that two types of pathogenic autoAbs, one group specific for CII and the second group represented by NZB hybridomas producing Coombs antibodies, are not produced by Ly-1^+ hybridomas.

Collectively, these results strongly suggest that non–organ-specific antibodies are produced by both Ly-1^+ and Ly-1^- B cells and that at least some pathogenic autoantibodies such as those specific for collagen II and erythrocytes are produced by Ly-1^- B cells.

REFERENCES

1. Boumsell, L., Bernard, A., and Dausset, J. 1978. Some chronic lymphocytic leukemia cells bearing surface immunoglobulins share determinants with T cells. *Eur. J. Immunol., 8*: 900.
2. Boumsell, L., Coppin, H., Dausset, J., and Bernard, A. 1980. An antigen shared by a human T cell subset and B cell chronic lymphocytic leukemia cells. Distribution on normal and malignant lymphoid cells. *J. Exp. Med., 152*: 229.
3. Wang, C. Y., Good, R. A., and Evans, R. L. 1980. Identification of a p69, 71 complex expressed on human T cells sharing determinants with B-type chronic lymphatic leukemic cells. *J. Exp. Med., 151*: 1539.
4. Royston, I., Majda, J. A., and Griffiths, J. C. 1980. Human T-cell antigens defined by monoclonal antibodies: the 65,000 dalton antigen of T cells (T65) is also found on chronic lymphocytic leukemia cells bearing surface immunoglobulins. *J. Immunol., 125*: 725.
5. Kamoun, M., Kadin, M. F., and Hansen, J. A. 1981. A novel human T cell antigen preferentially expressed on mature T cells and also on (B-type) chronic lymphatic leukemic cells. *J. Immunol., 127*: 987.
6. Knowles, D. M., Halper, J. P., and Wang, C. Y. 1983. Reactivity of monoclonal antibodies Leu-1 and Okt-1 with malignant human lymphoid cells. *Cancer, 52*: 1369.
7. Lanier, L. L., Lynes, M. A., Haughton, G., and Wettstein, P. 1978. Novel type of murine B-cell lymphoma. *Nature, 271*: 554.
8. Lanier, L. L., Warner, N. L., and Herzenberg, L. A. 1981. Expression of Lyt-1 antigen on certain murine B cell lymphomas. *J. Exp. Med., 153*: 998.
9. Lanier, L. L., Arnold, L. W., and Haughton, G. 1982. Transplantable B cell lymphomas in B10 H-2^aH-4^b p/Wts mice. *Immunogenetics, 16*: 367.
10. Slavin, S., and Strober, S. 1978. Spontaneous B-cell leukemia. *Nature, 272*: 624.
11. Hayakawa, K., Hardy, R. R., Parks, D. R., Herzenberg, L. A. 1983. The "Ly-1 B" cell subpopulation in normal, immunodefective, and autoimmune mice. *J. Exp. Med., 157*: 202.
12. Hayakawa, K., Hardy, R. R., Herzenberg, L. A. 1986. Peritoneal Ly-1 B cells: Genetic control, autoantibody production, increases lambda light chain expression. *Eur. J. Immunol., 16*: 450.
13. Mihara, M., Ohsugi, Y., Saito, K., Miyai, T., Togashi, M., Ono, S., Murakauri,

S., Dobashi, K., Hirayama, F., and T. Hamoka. 1988. Immunological abnormalities in NAB/NZWF1 mice: Thymus independence occurrence of B cell abnormalities and requirement for T cells in the development of autoimmune disease, as evidence by an analysis of the athymic nude individuals. *J. Immunol., 141*: 85.

14. Kaushik, A., Lim, A., Poncet, P., and Dighiero, G. 1988. Comparative analysis of natural antibody specificities among hybridomas originating from spleen and peritoneal cavity of adult NZB and Balb/c mice. *Scand. J. Immunol., 27*: 461.
15. Myama-Inaba, M., Kuma, S., Inaba, K., Iwai, H., Iasumizu, R., Muramatsu, S., Steinman, R. M., and Ikehara, S. 1988. Unusual phenotype of B cells in the thymus of normal mice. *J. Exp. Med., 168*: 811.
16. Braun, J. 1983. Spontaneous in vitro occurrence and long-term culture of murine lymphoblast cell lines. *J. Immunol., 130*: 2113.
17. Citri, Y., Braun, J., and Baltimore, D. 1987. Elevated myc expression and c-myc amplification in spontaneously occurring B lymphoid cell lines. *J. Exp. Med., 165*: 1188.
18. Hayakawa, K., Hardy, R. R., and Herzenberg, L. A. 1985. Progenitors of Ly-1 B cells are distinct from progenitors for other B cells. *J. Exp. Med., 161*: 1554.
19. Hayakawa, K., Hardy, R. R., Honda, M., Herzenberg, L. A., and Steinberg, A. D. 1984. Ly-1 B cells: Functionally distinct lymphocytes that secrete IgM autoantibodies. *Proc. Natl. Acad. Sci. USA, 81*: 2494.
20. Hayakawa, K., Ishii, R., Kishimoto, T., Herzenberg, L. A., and Hardy, R. R. 1987. Localization of Ly-1 B cells in the peritoneal cavity: Genetic control of frequency. In *New Horizons in Animal Models for Autoimmune Disease* (Kyogaku, M., and Wigzell, H., eds.). Academic Press, Tokyo.
21. Manohar, V., Brown, E., and Chused, T. M. 1982. Expression of Lyt-1 by a subset of B lymphocytes. *J. Immunol., 129*: 532.
22. Raveche, E. S., Alabaster, O., and Steinberg, A. D. 1981. Analysis of NZB hyperdiploid spleen cells. *J. Immunol., 126*: 154.
23. Raveche, E. S., Lalor, P., Stall, A., and Conroy, J. 1989. In vivo effects of hyperdiploid Ly-1^+ B cells of NZB origin. *J. Immunol., 141*(22): 4133.
24. Stall, A. M., Farinas, M. C., Tarlington, D. M., Lalor, P. A., Herzenberg, L. A., Strober, S., and Herzenberg, L. A. 1989. Ly-1 B cell clones similar to human CLL routinely develop in older normal mice and young NZB related animals. *Proc. Natl. Acad. Sci. USA, 85*: 7312.
25. Manny, N., Datta, S. K., and Schwartz, R. 1979. Synthesis of IgM by cells of NZB and SWR mice and their crosses. *J. Immunol., 122*: 1220.
26. Green, M. C., and Shultz, L. D. 1975. Motheaten and immunodeficient mutant of the mouse. Genetics and Pathology. *J. Hered., 66*: 250.
27. Shultz, L. D., Coman, D. R., and Sidman, C. L. 1984. "Viable motheaten" a new allele at the motheaten locus. Pathology. *Am. J. Pathology, 116*: 179.
28. Sidman, C. L., Shultz, L. D., Hardy, R. R., Hayakawa, K., and Herzenberg, L. A. 1986. Production of immunoglobulin isotypes by Ly-1^+ B cells in viable motheaten and normal mice. *Science, 232*: 1423.
29. Painter, C., Monestier, M., Chew, Sidman, C., and Bona, C. 1988. Specificities and V genes encoding monoclonal autoantibodies from viable motheaten mice. *J. Exp. Med., 167*: 1137.

30. Sidman, C. L., Shultz, L. D., and Evans, R. 1985. A serum derived molecule from autoimmune viable motheaten mice potentiates the action of a B cell maturation factor. *J. Immunol., 135*: 870.
31. Pages, J., and Bussard, A. 1975. Precommitment of normal mouse peritoneal cells by erythrocyte antigens in relation to autoantibody production. *Nature, 257*: 316.
32. Steele, E. J., and Cunningham, A. J. 1978. High proportion of Ig producing cells making autoantibody in normal mice. *Nature, 274*: 483.
33. Haughton, G., Arnold, L. W., and Mercolina, T. J. 1986. The CH series of murine B cell lymphomas: neoplastic analogues of Ly-1$^+$ normal B cells. *Immunol. Rev., 93*: 35.
34. Pennell, C. A., Arnold, L. W., and Haughton, G. 1985. Cross-reactive idiotypes and common antigen binding specificities expressed by a series of murine B-cell lymphomas; etiological implications. *Proc. Natl. Acad. Sci. USA, 82*: 3799.
35. Mercolino, T. J., Arnold, L. W., and Haughton, G. 1986. Phosphatidyl choline is recognized by a series of Ly-1$^+$ murine B-cell lymphomas specific for erythrocyte membranes. *J. Exp. Med., 163*: 155.
36. Jones, N. H., Clabby, M. L., Herzenberg, L. A., and Strominger, J. L. 1986. Isolation of complementary DNA clones encoding the human lymphocyte glycoprotein T$/Leu-1. *Nature, 323*: 346.
37. Huanng, H.-J. S., Jones, N. H., Strominger, J. L., and Herzenberg, L. A. 1987. Molecular cloning of Ly-1, a membrane glycoprotein of mouse T lymphocytes and a subset of B cells. *Proc. Natl. Acad. Sci. USA, 84*: 204.
38. Griffith, L. C., Schulman, H., and Tagawa, M. 1989. In vivo and in vitro phosphorylation of murine lymphocyte differentiation antigen CD5. *Biochem. Biophys. Res. Commun., 159*(2): 536.
39. Hollander, N., Pillemer, E., and Weissman, I. L. 1981. Effects of Lyt antibodies on T-cell functions: augmentation by anti-Lyt-1 as opposed to inhibition by anti-Lyt-2. *Proc. Natl. Acad. Sci. USA, 78*: 1148.
40. Nishimura, Y., Bierer, B. E., Jones, W. K., Strominger, J., and Burakoff, S. J. 1988. Expression and function of a CD5 cDNA in human and murine T cells. *18*: 747.
41. Umland, S. P., Go, N. F., Cupp, J. E., and Howard, M. 1989. Responses of B cells from autoimmune mice to IL-5. *J. Immunol., 142*: 1528.
42. Defrance, T., Vanbervliet, B., Durand, I., and Banchereau, J. 1989. Human interleukin 4 down-regulates the surface expression of CD5 on normal and leukemic B cells. *Eur. J. Immunol., 19*: 293.
43. Freedman, A. S., Freeman, G., Whitman, G., Segil, J., Daley, J., Levine, H., and Nadler, L. M. 1989. Expression and regulation of CD5 on in vitro activated human B cells. *Eur. J. Immunol., 19*: 849.
44. Ansar-Ahmed, S., Dauphinee, M. J., Montoya, A. I., and Talal, N. 1989. Estrogen induces normal murine CD5+ B cells to produce autoantibodies. *J. Immunol., 142*: 2647.
45. Bailey, N. C., Fidanza, V., Mayer, R., Mazza, G., Fougereau, M., and Bona, C. Activation of clones producing self reactive antibodies by foreign antigens anti-idiotype antibody carrying the internal image of the antigen. *J. Clin. Invest.*, (in press).
46. Mayer, R., Zaghouani, H., Usuba, O., and Bona, C. Ly-1 gene expression in murine hybridomas producing autoantibodies. *Autoimmunity* (in press).

47. Durda, P. J., Shapiro, C., and Gottlieb, P. D. 1978. Partial molecular characterization of the Ly1 alloantigen on mouse thymocytes. *J. Immunol., 120*: 53.
48. Feener, C. A., Koenig, M., and Kunkel, L. M. 1989. Alternative splicing of human dystrophin mRNA generates isoforms at the carboxy terminus. *Nature, 338*: 509.
49. Trowbidge, I. S., Ralph, P., and Bevan, J. 1975. Differences in the surface proteins of mouse B and T cells. *Proc. Natl. Acad. Sci. USA, 72*: 157.
50. Hirono, A., and Beutler, E. 1989. Alternative splicing of human glucose-6-phosphate dehydrogenase messenger RNA in different tissues. *J. Clin. Invest., 83*: 343.
51. Giblin, P., Ledbetter, J. A., and Kavathas, P. 1989. A secreted form of the human lymphocyte cell surface molecule CD5 arises from alternative splicing. *Proc. Natl. Acad. Sci. USA, 86*: 998.
52. Monestier, M., Manheimer-Lory, A., Bellon, B., Painter, C., and Bona, C. 1986. Shared idiotypes and restricted Vh genes characterize murine autoantibodies of various specificities. *J. Clin. Invest., 78*: 753.

5

The Primary Antibody Repertoire: The Somatic Genotype and Paratopic Phenotype of B-Cell Populations

Garnett Kelsoe
University of Maryland School of Medicine, Baltimore, Maryland

I. INTRODUCTION

The serum of normal mice contains readily detectable amounts of autoantibodies, usually of the IgM isotype (1–3). The antibodies react with a variety of self determinants including those associated with pathologic autoimmunity (2,4–8). Presumably, these IgM antibodies represent the products of unmutated B cells (9) activated by internal or cross-reactive incidental antigens. Thus it is apparent that the *Igh, Igκ*, and *Igλ* loci may encode self-reactive paratopes. Indeed, the frequency of autoreactive paratopes is considerable, representing a substantial fraction of the expressed antibody repertoire (2,10–14). As these reactivities may be detected even at very low concentrations of antibody (10^{-6}–10^{-9} M), it is reasonable to believe that naturally occurring autoantibodies are physiologically significant. Often, the affinity of such autoantibodies equals that of immunogen-induced primary antibodies (15,16).

Do self-reactive antibodies represent a special subset of the paratopic repertoire? Some studies have indicated that autoreactive paratopes are preferentialy encoded by some V_H gene families (5,17–19). In contrast, others have analyzed panels of autoreactive hybridomas or B cells from autoimmune mice and found unbiased use of V_H gene families (12,14,20–22). At this time, it remains unclear if these discrepancies result from methodologic or sampling differences or reflect specialization of some V_H families (or exons) for particular but not all autopecificities. Thus, the genetic relatedness between autoreactive paratopes and those specific for nonself determinants remains obscure.

In this chapter, I shall describe and define the antibody repertoire in two ways: (1) as the distribution of V_H and V_κ exons (families) expressed within the splenic B-cell population, and (2) as the sum of specific paratope frequencies. In this manner, the character of the specificity repertoire may be compared to the somatic genotype of B-cell populations. My colleagues and I have used such comparisons to investigate the nature of the primary antibody repertoire and to infer the modes of evoluton that have resulted in the present structure of the *Ig-V* loci. Two such questions are relevant to the present discussions: Has natural selection acted upon these loci to create specific paratopic repertoires, and if so, have the selecting antigens been internal or external? Answers to these questions are fundamental to an understanding of autoreactive antibody.

II. CONSTRUCTION OF THE PRIMARY ANTIBODY REPERTOIRE

Distinct elements, the V (variable), D (diversity), and J (joining) gene segments, participate in genomic rearrangements to form that portion of the active Ig H- (V_HDJ_H) and L-chain ($V_\kappa J_\kappa$; $V_\lambda J_\lambda$) genes encoding the variable regions of the antibody molecule (reviewed in Ref. 23). In mice these gene segments are dispersed within complex loci on chromosomes 12 (*Igh*), 5 (*Igκ*), and 16 (*Igλ*) as clusters of reiterated homologs (24–29). V_H and V_κ exons have been classified into homology families based upon sequence similarity. Generally, families are colocated, defining discrete regions within the locus; however, significant interspersion is known to exist among V_H families (25,26) and is expected for V_κ as well (P. Gearhart, personal communication).

Each V(D)J fusion exon contains three regions of extreme genetic variability that encode the complementary-determining regions (CDR) of the antibody's antigen-combining site (30). Two of these hypervariable regions are located within the V_H or V_κ segments, while the third is created by assembly at the V(D)J borders (23,30). Subsequent to the expression of the Ig H- and L-chain polypeptides, the antibody paratope is created by the pairing of the two chains bringing the six CDR into apposition (31). Here, the CDR residues participate in a blunt-ended surface of some 2 × 4 nm that will interact with antigen ligands (31).

Thus, prior to the introduction of antigen, the antibody repertoire depends on two mechanisms for the generation of paratopic diversity. First is the process of V(D)J fusion; these fusion exons are made diverse by the possibility of large numbers of distinct combinatorial associations and by random events that modify the V(D)J junction borders (23). Second is the association of the Ig H- and L-chain polypeptides. Any bias within the primary antibody repertoire, e.g., for determinants consistently associated with pathogens or against autoreactivity, must be established through these two processes.

III. AFFINITY OF PRIMARY ANTIBODIES

Discussion of the repertoire of antibody specificities is uninformative in the absence of a definition of what represents physiologically significant affinities for antigen. However, just what constitutes adequate affinity for paratope/antigen interactions is a point of debate (32). Traditionally, only antibodies expressing extremely high dissociation constants (10^{-8}–10^{-10} M) have been considered biologically important. Virtually without exception, such antibodies are the result of repeated immunizations.

In contrast, antibodies produced in the initial response to a variety of antigens possess affinities in the μM range (10^{-5}–10^{-7} M) (15,16,33–36). This affinity defines a demonstrable threshold ($\cong 10^{-5}$ M) for significant antibody/antigen interaction: Obviously affinities in this range are sufficient to induce B-cell proliferation and differentiation. Indeed, Manser and colleagues have shown that even lower affinities (10^{-4} M) may be sufficient to activate B lymphocytes (37). Thus, I shall consider antibody paratopes with affinities $\leq 10^{-5}$ M to be immunologically relevant.

It is now clear that virtually without exception, high affinity antibodies represent somatically mutated genes that have been selected by competition for antigens (reviewed in Ref. 38). Such genes arise from those of the unmutated primary or germline repertoire and may provide critical protective benefit (note, however, that not all antibody-producing vertebrates seem to possess the hypermutation mechanism (39), nor do T lymphocytes evidence mutation within the TCR (40). Nonetheless, somatically mutated Ig genes are not heritable and therefore evolutionarily irrelevant. Only study of the primary repertoire permits deductions to be made on the fundamental nature of the paratopic repertoire.

IV. SOMATIC GENOTYPE OF B-CELL POPULATIONS

A. Expression of V_H and $V\kappa$ Gene Families

Several laboratories have studied V_H and V_κ gene family use in fetal, neonatal, and adult mice by the analysis of hybridomas, in situ hybridization of single B cells or B-cell colonies (44–50), quantification of splenic mRNA, and screening of splenic cDNA libraries (41–53). With a single exception (44), these studies demonstrate that, in general, the frequencies at which V_H gene families are productively rearranged in adult mice is stoichiometric, that is, proportional to V_H family size (Table 1). In fetal or neonatal mice, however, J_H expression is biased

TABLE 1 V_H Gene Family Complexity and Expression in Adult C57BL/6 Mice[a]

V_H family	Complexity	Proportion (%) of V_H[b]	Expression (%) in spleen
7183	12	9	8
Q52	15	11	13
S107	4	3	2
X-24	2	1.5	1
V_H11	2	1.5	N.D.
36-60	5	4	N.D.
VGAM 3.8	5	4	N.D.
V_H12	1	0.7	N.D.
5606	10	7	8
V_H10	2	1.5	N.D.
3609	16	12	14
J558	62	46	45

[a]V_H complexities obtained from Ref. 26. V_H expression represents the analysis of $>6 \times 10^5 C\mu^+H$ B-cell colonies.

[b]Proportion calculated as: Complexity V_H family/Total V_H complexity.

for those V_H families (and individual exons) located in the 3′ region of the *Igh-V* locus. The expression of V_κ gene families is surprisingly different; neither is the expression of V_κ gene families in the adult mouse stoichiometric, nor is there bias for use of 3′ exons in the fetus or neonate (Table 2). Indeed, although expression of a significant fraction of V_κ gene families has been studied, no clear pattern of V_κ exon use has emerged.

My laboratory has investigated V_H and V_κ expression by the method of filter paper cloning of mitogen-reactive B lymphocytes (54). Briefly, suspensions of splenocytes are prepared and plated into sterile filter paper discs. Subsequently, media containing thymic feeder cells and a mitogen such as lipopolysaccharide (LPS) is added and the cells are cultured for 4–6 days at 37 °C in a humidified atmosphere of air enriched (5%) with CO_2. Under these conditions mitogen-reactive splenic B cells proliferate to form pure colonies of daughter cells imprisoned within the disc's woven cellulose fibers. As each colony represents the progeny of a single founder B lymphocyte, the technique is entirely analogous to the plating and growth of bacteria on agar. Colonies grow rapidly with cell-doubling times averaging 14 hours. By day 5 of culture, 40–60% of all colonies routinely contain in excess of 100 cells. At this time, discs are removed from culture and blotted onto antigen-coated nitrocellulose sheets to identify antigen-specific colonies (49,54,55) and/or fixed and hybridized with successive rounds of V_H-, V_κ-, or C-specific DNA probes (44,49,51,53,54).

Using this method, my colleagues and I have screened almost 10^6 individual B-cell colonies derived from several murine strains. Tables 1 and 2 summarize

TABLE 2 V_κ Gene Family Complexity and Expression in Adult C57BL/6 Mice[a]

V_κ family	Complexity[b]	Proportion (%) of V_κ[c]	Expression (%) in spleen
21	10	5	3
19	10	5	6
10	5	3	1
8	12	6	5
4	8	4	3
9	11	6	5
1	3	1.5	25
24	2	1	<0.5
22	7	4	4
2	5	2	2

[a]V_κ complexities obtained from Ref. 51 for the probes used to determine V_κ expression. V_κ expression represents the analysis of $> 4 \times 10^4 C\mu$ B-cell colonies.
[b]Reported V_κ complexities vary considerably (compare Refs. 27,28). The complexities obtained here agree well with those of D'Hoostelaere (27).
[c]Proportion calculated as: Complexitity of V_κ family/250 (estimated) Total V_κ.

the results of this extensive census for the C57BL/6 (*Igh*[b] and *Ig*κ^c) strain of mice. The 12 V_H gene families currently known comprise a total genomic complexity of ≅136 distinct hybridizing fragments. Using this value, the relative size or proportion of each V_H gene family may be calculated and compared with empirically derived frequencies for V_H gene family expression. Table 1 demonstrates that for the seven V_H gene families we have studied in detail, all are expressed at frequencies proportional to family size. The concordance between observed frequencies and the calculated proportional size of V_H families suggests that in the adult mouse virtually any V_H exon is equally likely to participate in productive rearrangements. Furthermore, the fit between the observed and calculated values is so precise—at least for the C57BL/6 strain—that one may predict V_H expression with a high degree of confidence simply by knowing V_H complexity.

Table 2 presents similar data for 10 V_κ gene families. V_κ gene families range in size from a few members (e.g., $V_\kappa 24$) to ≅10–15 homologs (e.g., $V_\kappa 8$). Analyses of genomic hybridizations with various specific V_κ probes have suggested a total genomic complexity of ≅250 elements (51). When this value is used to calculate proportional sizes for V_κ families, it is clear that no single family dominates as does J558 for V_H (Table 2). Furthermore, although in many cases V_κ family size and expression may correlate, there are at least two cases in which stoichiometric expressions not observed. The $V_\kappa 1$ and $V_\kappa 24$ gene families have similar genomic complexities (3 and 2, respectively) and yet are expressed differentially (Table 2). $V_\kappa 1$ expression dominates all other families, occurring in $\cong$25% of all splenic B cells. In contrast, $V_\kappa 24$ expression may be detected in only 0.3% of B lymphocytes, a 10^3-fold reduction. Thus, V_κ use frequencies cannot be predicted by the complexity of families but must be determined empirically.

B. Rates of V_H and V_κ Pairing

Following the independent rearrangement of the *Igh* and L-chain loci, the primary antibody repertoire depends upon the frequencies at which the various V_H and V_L exons pair. My colleagues and I have investigated this process (53) using two independent experimental strategies, in situ hybridizations of B cell colonies (see above), and the analysis of mRNA from mitogen-induced hybridoma clones. In these complementary experiments, we determined the frequencies of 25 V_H + V_κ gene family pairings to approximate the rates of individual exon pairing. Results from both kinds of experiments supported the same conclusion: The pairing of V_H and V_κ gene families was unbiased. Thus, observed frequencies for specific V_H + V_κ pairings could be predicted from the product of the *independent* V_H and V_κ frequencies (Table 3). For example, if V_H Q52 exons are expressed in some 13% of splenic B cells and the $V_\kappa 8$ family is present at a frequency of 5%, the observed frequency for cells expressing both V_H Q52 and $V_\kappa 8$ exons is ($0.13 \times 0.05 \cong$) 0.7%.

Should unbiased pairing of V_H and V_κ families prove true generally and extend to individual exons, the antibody repertoire as approximated by V_H + V_κ pairings may be calculated in a straightforward manner. (In principle, this process could include frequencies of $J_{H/L}$ and D in the product as well.) When this is done (Table 3), it becomes apparent that, with the exception of V_HJ558 + $V_\kappa 1$ pairings, V_H + V_κ pairs are distributed nearly uniformly in the adult C57BL/6 mouse.

V. ASSOCIATION OF PARATOPIC SPECIFICITY WITH V_H GENE FAMILY EXPRESSION

Often, one or a few V_H or V_L gene segments have been associated with specific immune responses; phosphorylcholine (PC) induces an antibody response in almost all strains of mice that nearly exclusively uses a single member of the V_H S107 gene family, V1 (56). This physiologic dominance plus the remarkable phylogenetic preservation of the S107 V_H gene family have lead to the speculation that these gene segments have been selected by evolution for optional reactivity to PC (56).

The motion of specialization of V gene segments (or families) for particular determinants predicts nonrandom associations between V gene family expression and paratopic specificity in the primary antibody repertoire. My laboratory has

TABLE 3 $V_V + V_\kappa$ Family Pairings Distribute Randomly in Adult C57BL/6 Mice

Family	V_HQ52 (12.5%)	V_HS107 (2.7%)	V_HX-24 (2.0%)	V_HJ558[a] (42.5%)
V_κ21 (2.6%)[b]	0.3%	<0.1%	<0.1%	1.2%
V_κ19 (6.1%)	0.7%	0.2%	0.1%	2.9%
V_κ8 (9.0%)	1.8%	0.3%	0.1%	4.2%
V_κ4 (3.3%)	0.4%	0.1%	<0.1%	1.5%
V_κ9 (5.1%)	0.6%	0.2%	0.1%	2.4%
V_κ1 (25.8%)	3.1%	0.5%	0.3%	12.1%
V_κ24 (0.3%)	<0.1%	<0.1%	<0.1%	0.1%

[a]Values in ( ) indicate the independent V_H frequency among $C\mu^+$ cells.
[b]Values in ( ) indicate the independent V_κ frequency among $C\mu^+$ or C_κ^+ cells.
Source: Ref. 53.

tested this prediction by determining the antibody specificity and V_H gene family expressed by LPS–induced colonies of murine splenic B cells (49). Briefly, filter paper discs bearing B-cell colonies were blotted onto nitrocellulose sheets coated with PC or hen egg lysozyme (HEL). Colonies that secreted antibody specific for the bound antigen left a "footprint" of adsorbed Ig. Subsequently, discs were fixed and hybridized to determine V_H and $C\mu$ expression. Footprints of bound antibody were identified by incubation of the washed nitrocellulose sheets with radioiodinated anti-mouse κ L-chain antibody followed by autoradiography. Finally, autoradiographs of the serial immunoblot and hybridizations were compared to identify V_H gene family expression among antigen-specific colonies.

The results of these experiments are summarized in Table 4. Note that stoichiometric expression of the V_HX-24, -S107, -Q52, and -J558 gene families occurred among both unselected and antigen-specific colonies. These findings suggest that in the primary antibody repertoire of adult C57BL/6 mice, similar paratopic specificities may be generated by all V_H gene families. Presumably, this great flexibility with respect to V_H:paratope associations is made possible by the great diversity of V_H plus ($DJ_H + V_LJ_L$) combinations available. It may be calculated that given the random associations of V-region genetic elements (see above), each V_H exon may participate in some ($10\ D \times 4J_H \times 250V_\kappa \times 4J_\kappa =$) 4×10^4 unique κ^+ antibody molecules. Given this degree of potential diversity, it is not surprising that each V_H family is capable of producing paratopes specific for many different (any?) antigenic determinants.

VI. PARATOPE FREQUENCIES IN THE PRIMARY REPERTOIRE

The expression of V_H and V_κ gene families and rates of specific $V_H + V_\kappa$ pairing in the adult C57BL/6 mouse are apparently stochastically driven processes

TABLE 4 V_H Family Expression Among Unselected and Antigen-Specific B-Cell Colonies

	V_H gene family expression (% of $C\mu^+$)			
	V_HX-24	V_HS107	V_HQ52	V_HJ558
Unselected colonies ($C\mu^+$)	1.1%	3.1%	9.7%	38.2%
PC-specific colonies ($PC^+/C\mu^+$)	1.2%	2.8%	9.7%	36.1%
HEL-specific colonies ($HEL^+/C\mu^+$)	2.2%	3.5%	10.0%	43.8%

Source: Ref. 49.

(see above). What is the derivative phenotype of these random genetic processes? Although the literature describing paratope frequencies in the antibody repertoire is extensive, until recently no predictions of paratope frequencies could be made—the frequencies of antigen-specific B cells were always determined empirically. However, it is now known that paratope frequencies are generally directly proportional to the molecular mass, or more specifically the surface area, of the (protein) antigen ligand (10,14,57). In an antibody repertoire based largely on stochastic processes, this result makes a great deal of sense.

Consider a protein antigen as a set of epitopes. Small, less complex proteins will possess fewer epitopes than large molecules. Should random genetic assembly and pairing of V(D)J fusion exons result in an antibody repertoire that is unbiased, i.e., the probability of paratope a = paratope b, c, d . . . etc., then the frequencies of paratopes (B-cell clones) specific for protein antigens will be determined solely by the size of the antigen. This conjecture has been verified using both B-cell colonies (57) and hybridomas (10,14). Interestingly, this predicted relationship is valid for both self (or self-homologous) proteins and for phylogenetically distant antigens. Indeed, the frequencies of murine B cells specific for murine, human, bovine, or chicken serum albumins are not statistically different (57). Also, paratope frequencies are not correlated to the degree of amino acid sequence disparity between antigens and their self protein homologs (14).

VII. CONCLUSIONS

The antibody repertoire is created by genetic processes that are largely controlled by stochastic events. This results in an antibody repertoire in adult mice that is apparently unbiased for any particular (set of) specificities. I have taken these findings to suggest that evolution has not acted to ensure the expression—or absence—of B cells necessarily reactive to foreign or self epitopes. Instead of specificity, diversity may be the character of the primary repertoire.

Given the highly pleiotropic nature of the phenotypes encoded by any single V gene segment (one V_H segment may participate in some 4×10^4 genetically distinct antibodies), this is not a surprising conclusion. It may be that the *Ig-V* loci have evolved largely independent of natural selection per se and instead have been shaped by neutral evolutionary forces (49).

In this context, there can be no genetic basis for the discrimination of self and not-self. Autoreactive antibody, any antibody, results from a kind of somatic genetic roulette. The pathologic sequelae of self-reactive antibodies must be controlled/prevented by higher order, physiologic mechanisms.

REFERENCES

1. Dighiero, G., P. Lymberi, J. C. Mazie, S. Rouyre, G. S. Butler-Brown, R. G. Whalen, and S. Avrameas. 1983. Murine hybridomas secreting natural monoclonal antibodies reacting with self antigens. *J. Immunol., 131*: 2267.
2. Prabhakar, B. S., J. Saegusa, T. Onodera, and F. L. Notkins. 1984. Lymphocytes capable of making monoclonal antibodies that react with multiple organs are a common feature of the normal B cell repertoire. *J. Immunol., 133*: 2815.
3. Portnoi, D., A. A. Freitas, D. Holmberg, A. Bandeira, and A. Coutinho. 1986. Immuno-competent autoreactive B lymphocytes are activated cycling cells in normal mice. *J. Exp. Med., 164*: 25.
4. Schwartz, R. S. 1986. Anti-DNA antibodies and the problem of autoimmunity. *Cell. Immunol., 99*: 38.
5. Trepicchio, W., and K. J. Barret. 1987. Eleven MRL *lpr/lpr* anti-DNA autoantibodies are encoded by genes from four V_H gene families: a potentially biased usage of V_H genes. *J. Immunol., 138*: 2323.
6. Manheimer-Lory, A. J., M. Monestier, B. Bellon, F. W. Alt, and C. A. Bona. 1986. Fine specificity, idiotype and nature of cloned heavy-chain variable region genes of murine monoclonal rheumatoid factor antibodies. *Proc. Natl. Acad. Sci. USA, 83*: 8293.
7. Schlomchik, M. J., A. Marshak-Rothstein, C. B. Wolfowica, T. L. Rothstein, and M. G. Weigert. 1987. The role of clonal selection and somatic immunity in autoimmunity. *Nature* (Lond.), *328*: 805.
8. Aguado, M. T., R. S. Balderas, R. L. Rubin, M. A. Suchosal, R. Kofler, B. K. Birshtein, D. S. Secher, F. J. Dixon, and A. N. Theofilopoulos. 1987. Specificity and molecular characteristics of monoclonal IgM rheumatoid factors from arthritic and non-arthritic mice. *J. Immunol., 139*: 1080.
9. Gearhart, P. J., N. D. Johnson, R. Douglas, and L. Hood. 1981. IgG antibodies to phosphorylcholine exhibit more diversity than their IgM counterparts. *Nature* (Lond.), *291*: 29.
10. Souroujon, M., M. E. White-Scharf, J. Andre-Schwartz, M. L. Gefter, and R. S. Schwartz. 1988. Preferential autoantibody reactivity of the preimmune B cell repertoire in normal mice. *J. Immunol., 140*: 4173.

11. Hartman, A. B., C. P. Mallet, J. Srinivasappa, B. S. Prabhakar, A. L. Notkins, and S. J. Smith-Gill. 1989. Organ reactive autoantibodies from non-immunized adult BALB/c mice are polyreactive and express non-biased V_H gene usage. *Molec. Immunol.*, *26*: 359.
12. Rousseau, P. G., C. P. Mallet, and S. J. Smith-Gill. 1989. A substantial proportion of the adult BALB/c available B cell repertoire consists of multireactive B cells. *Molec. Immunol.*, *26*: 993.
13. Srinivasappa, J., J. Seagusa, B. S. Prabhakar, M. K. Gentry, M. J. Buchmeier, T. J. Wiktor, H. Koprowski, M. B. A. Oldstone, and A. L. Notkins. 1986. Molecular mimicry: Frequency of reactivity of monoclonal antiviral antibodies with normal tissues. *J. Virol.*, *57*: 397.
14. Striebich, C. C., R. M. Miceli, D. H. Schulze, G. Kelsoe, and J. Cerny. 1990. Antigen-binding repertoire and IgH chain gene usage among B cell hybridomas from normal and autoimmune mice. *J. Immunol.* (in press).
15. Ternynck, T., and S. Avrameas. 1987. Murine natural monoclonal autoantibodies: A study of their polyspecificities and their affinities. *Immunol. Rev.*, *94*: 99.
16. Chua, M. M., S. H. Goodgal, and F. Karush. 1987. Germline affinity and germline variable-region genes in the B cell response. *J. Immunol.*, *138*: 1281.
17. Naparstek, Y., J. Andre-Schwartz, T. Manser, L. J. Wysocki, L. Breitman, B. D. Stollar, M. Gefter, and R. S. Schwartz. 1986. A single germline V_H gene segment encodes autoantibodies characteristic of systemic lupus erythematosis. *J. Exp. Med.*, *164*: 614.
18. Monestier, M., A. Manheimer-Lowry, B. Bellon, C. Painter, H. Dang, N. Talal, M. Zanetti, R. Schwartz, D. Pisetsky, R. Kuppers, N. Rose, J. Brochier, L. Keareskog, R. Holmdahl, B. Erlanger, F. Alt, and C. Bona. 1986. Shared idiotopes and restricted immunoglobulin variable region heavy chain genes characterize murine autoantibodies of various specificities. *J. Clin. Invest.*, *78*: 753.
19. Bona, C., K. N. Kasturi, R. Mayer, and V. Fidanza. 1988. V gene usage by autoantibodies and their polymorphism in autoimmune mice. *Autoimmunity*, *2*: 29.
20. Kofler, R., D. J. Noonan, D. E. Levy, M. C. Wilson, N. P. H. Moller, F. J. Dixon, and A. N. Theofilopoulos. 1985. Genetic elements used for a murine lupus anti-DNA autoantibody are closely related to those for antibodies to exogenous antigens. *J. Exp. Med.*, *161*: 805.
21. Eisenberg, R. A., S. Y. Craven, R. W. Warren, and P. L. Cohen. 1987. Stochastic control of anti-Sm autoantibodies in MRL-*lpr/lpr* mice. *J. Clin. Invest.*, *80*: 691.
22. Kastner, D. L., T. M. McIntyre, C. P. Mallett, A. B. Hartman, and A. D. Steinberg. 1989. Direct quantitative in situ hybridization studies of IgV_H utilization. A comparison between unstimulated B cells from autoimmune and normal mice. *J. Immunol.*, *143*: 2761.
23. Yancopoulos, G. D., and F. W. Alt. 1986. Regulation of the assembly and expression of variable-region genes. *Ann. Rev. Immunol.*, *4*: 339.
24. Brodeur, P. H., and R. Riblet. 1984. The immunoglobulin heavy chain variable region (Igh-V) locus in the mouse. I. One hundred Igh-V genes comprise seven families of homologous genes. *Eur. J. Immunol.*, *14*: 922.
25. Blankenstein, T., and U. Krawinkel. 1987. Immunoglobulin V_H region genes of the mouse are organized in overlapping clusters. *Eur. J. Immunol.*, *17*: 1351.

26. Brodeur, P., G. E. Osman, J. J. Mackle, and T. M. Lalor. 1988. The organization of the mouse Igh-V locus: Dispersion, interspersion, and the evaluation of V_H gene family clusters. *J. Exp. Med.*, *168*: 2261.
27. D'Hoostelaere, L. A., K. Hupi, B. Mock, C. Mallett, and M. Potter. 1988. The Igϰ L chain allelic groups among the Igϰ haplotypes and Igϰ crossover populations suggest a gene order. *J. Immunol.*, *141*: 652.
28. Kofler, R., M. A. Duchosal, and F. J. Dixon. 1989. Complexity, polymorphism, and connectivity of mouse Vϰ gene families. *Immunogenet.*, *29*: 65.
29. Miller, J., A. Bothwell, and U. Storb. 1981. Physical linkage of the constant region genes for immunoglobulins λ_I and λ_{III}. *Proc. Natl. Acad. Sci. USA*, *78*: 3829.
30. Milstein, C. 1985. From the structure of antibodies to the diversification of the immune response. *Eur. Mol. Biol. Organ. J.*, *4*: 1083.
31. Amit, A. G., R. A. Mariuzza, S. E. V. Phillips, and R. J. Poljak. 1986. Three-dimensional structure of an antigen-antibody complex at 2.8Å resolution. *Science* (Wash., D.C.), *233*: 747.
32. Conger, J. D., B. L. Pike, and G. J. V. Nossal. 1987. Clonal analysis of the anti-DNA repertoire of murine B lymphocytes. *Proc. Natl. Acad. Sci. USA*, *84*: 2931.
33. Rudikoff, S., M. Paulita, J. Humphrey, and M. Heller. 1984. Somatic diversification of immunoglobulins. *Proc. Natl. Acad. Sci. USA*, *81*: 2162.
34. McKean, D. M., K. Hupi, M. Bell, L. Staudt, W. Gerhard, and M. Weigert. 1984. Generation of antibody diversity in the immune response of BALB/c mice to influenza virus hemagglutinin. *Proc. Natl. Acad. Sci. USA*, *81*: 3180.
35. Wysocki, L., T. Manser, and M. Gefter. 1985. Somatic evoluton of variable region structures during an immune response. *Proc. Natl. Acad. Sci. USA*, *83*: 1847.
36. Griffiths, G. M., C. Berek, M. Kaartinen, and C. Milstein. 1987. Somatic mutation and maturation of the immune response to 2-phenyl oxazolone. *Nature* (Lond.), *312*: 271.
37. Fish, S., E. Zenowich, M. Fleming, and T. Manser. 1989. Molecular analysis of original antigenic sin I. Clonal selection, somatic mutation, and isotype switching during a memory B cell response. *J. Exp. Med.*, *170*: 1191.
38. Rajewsky, K., I. Forster, and A. Cumano. 1987. Evolutionary and somatic selection of the antibody repertoire in the mouse. *Science* (Wash., D.C.), *238*: 1088.
39. Litman, G. W., M. J. Shamblott, R. Haire, C. Amemiya, H. Nishikata, K. Hinds, F. Harding, R. Litman, and J. Varner. 1989. Evolution of immunoglobulin gene complexity. In *Progress in Immunology VII* (F. Melchers, E. D. Albert, H. von Boehmer, M. P. Dierich, L. DuPasquier, K. Eichmann, D. Gemsa, O. Gotze, J. R. Kalden, S. H. E. Kaufman, H. Kirchner, K. Resch, G. Riethmuller, A. Schimpl, C. Sorg, M. Steinmetz, H. Wagner, H. G. Zachau, eds.). Springer-Verlag, Berlin, Heidelberg, pp. 361–368.
40. Ikuta, K., T. Ogura, A. Shimizu, and T. Honjo. 1985. Low frequency of somatic mutation in beta-chain variable region genes of human T-cell receptors. *Proc. Natl. Acad. Sci. USA*, *82*: 7701.
41. Sheehan, K. M., and P. H. Brodeur. 1989. Molecular cloning of the primary IgH repertoire: A quantitative analysis of V_H gene usage in adult ice. *Eur. Molec. Biol. Organ. J.*, *8*: 2313.

42. Yancopoulos, G. D., S. N. Desiderio, M. Paskind, J. F. Kearney, D. Baltimore, and F. W. Alt. 1984. Preferential utilization of the most J_H- proximal V_H gene segments in pre-B cell lines. *Nature* (Lond.), *311*: 727.
43. Perlmutter, R. M., J. F. Kearney, S. P. Chang, and L. E. Hood. 1985. Developmentally controlled expression of V_H genes. *Science* (Wash., D.C.), *227*: 1597.
44. Wu, G., and C. Paige. 1986. V_H gene family utilization in colonies derived from B and pre-B cells detected by the RNA colony blot assay. *Eur. Molec. Biol. Organ. J.*, *5*: 3475.
45. Schulze, D. H., and G. Kelsoe. 1987. Genotypic analysis of B cell colonies by in situ hybridization. Stoichiometric expression of three V_H families in adult C57BL/6 and BALB/c mice. *J. Exp. Med.*, *166*: 163.
46. Malynn, B., J. Berman, G. Yancopoulos, C. Bona, and F. W. Alt. 1987. Expression of the immunoglobulin heavy chain variable gene repertoire. *Curr. Topics Microbiol. Immunol.*, *135*: 75.
47. Jeong, H. D., J. L. Komisar, E. Kraig, and J. M. Teale. 1988. Strain dependent expression of V_H gene families. *J. Immunol.*, *140*: 2436.
48. Jeong, H. D. and J. M. Teale. 1988. Comparison of the fetal and adult functional B cell repertoires by analysis of V_H gene family expression. *J. Exp. Med.*, *168*: 589.
49. Kelsoe, G., R. Miceli, J. Cerny, and D. H. Schulze. 1989. Mapping of antibody specificities to V_H gene families. *Immunogenet.*, *29*: 288.
50. Jeong, H. D., and J. M. Teale. 1989. V_H gene family repertoire of resting B cells. Preferential use of D-proximal families early in development may be due to distinct B cell subsets. *J. Immunol.*, *143*: 2752.
51. Kaushik, A., D. H. Schulze, C. Bona, and G. Kelsoe. 1989. Murine V_κ gene expression does not follow the V_H paradigm. *J. Exp. Med.*, *169*: 1859.
52. Teale, J. M., and E. G. Morris. 1989. Comparison of V_κ gene family expression in adult and fetal B cells. *J. Immunol.*, *143*: 2768.
53. Kaushik, A., D. H. Schulze, F. A. Bonilla, C. Bona, and G. Kelsoe. 1990. Stochastic pairing of $V_H + V_\kappa$ families occurs in polyclonally activated B cells. *Proc. Natl. Acad. Sci. USA* (in press).
54. Kelsoe, G. 1987. Cloning of mitogen- and antigen-reactive B lymphocytes on filter paper disks: Phenotypic and genotypic analysis of B cell colonies. *Methods. Enzymol.*, *150*: 287.
55. Kelsoe, G., and J. T. Stout. 1986. Cloning of mitogen- and antigen-reactive B lymphocytes on filter paper discs II. Paratope frequencies within the mitogen selected repertoire. *Cell. Immunol.*, *98*: 506.
56. Perlmutter, R. M., B. Berson, J. A. Griffin, and L. Hood. 1985. Diversity in the germline antibody repertoire. Molecular evolution of the T15 V_H gene family. *J. Exp. Med.*, *162*: 1989.
57. Kelsoe, G., and D. Farina. 1987. Is the antibody repertoire biased? In: *Evolution and Vertebrate Immunity. The Antigen-Receptor and MHC Gene Families* (G. Kelsoe and D. H. Schulze, eds.). University of Texas Press, Austin, pp. 163–174.

6

Characteristics of V Genes Encoding Murine Autoantibodies

Kuppuswamy N. Kasturi
Mount Sinai School of Medicine, New York, New York

I. INTRODUCTION

The recognition of an antigen by an antibody is a specific phenomenon. The binding specificity of an antibody is contributed by light as well as heavy polypeptide chains of the immunoglobulin molecule. Structurally, autoantibodies are similar to antibodies directed against nonself antigens. But the complexities surrounding their origin are not yet completely unraveled. Autoreactive B cells, T cells, and self-reactive antibodies against a variety of autoantigens are present in unimmunized animals as well as in healthy individuals (1–11). Such data, indeed, challenge the theory of clonal deletion during ontogeny and self-tolerance proposed by Burnet (12). To date, however, autoantibodies (autoAbs) directed against very specific antigens such as blood group antigens or polymorphic antigens of MHC have not been described. Therefore, a clonal deletion mechanism cannot be completely excluded at the present time. The picture emerging is that the clonal selection process operates along with peripheral regulation by a phenomenon involving either active suppression or inactivation of autoreactive clones (13–15) and idiotype anti-idiotype interactions (7,16–19). The initial repertoire of a highly connected set of B cells ("first circle") specialized in self-recognition appears to regulate the emergence of a "second circle" of B cells which are poorly connected with each other or with the cells of the first circle (20).

Hypergammaglobulinemia appears to be a consistent feature of many autoimmune disorders (21). Moreover, it is also known that the ratio of autoAb-secreting B cells to Ig-secreting B cells present in autoimmune animals is similar to those found in normal mice (11). These data suggest that autoimmune mice simply have a higher frequency of Ig-secreting cells. More recent data, however, indicate that, in autoimmune strains, with increasing age, a higher proportion of B cells secrete autoreactive Abs (22). Thus, the combination of polyclonal activation and antigen-specific stimulatory mechanisms appear to contribute to the production of autoantibodies (23–27).

Although not all autoAbs have been shown to be responsible for the disease state in which they are found, it has been clearly shown that at least some of the autoAbs contribute to the pathogenesis of the diseases in which they are found: autoimmune hemolytic anemia, insulin-resistant diabetes mellitus, Graves' disease, myasthenia gravis, and lupus nephritis (28–32). Often pathogenic autoAbs are somatically mutated and mostly IgG (33–35). They can be mono- or polyreactive (36–40). The vast amount of data accumulated during the past decade on genetic and structural analysis of such autoAbs has provided insight into the understanding of the basis of generation and specificity of AutoAbs. In this chapter, I will try to analyze current data on the molecular characteristics V genes encoding of autoantibodies and discuss their relevance to the generation and specificity of autoantibodies.

II. STRUCTURE AND ORGANIZATION OF MOUSE Ig GENES

A. Structure of Ig Gene

The immunoglobulin molecule is composed of two identical light and two heavy polypeptide chains (41). Each polypeptide chain is composed of a variable region and a constant region. The antigen-binding specificity resides in the variable region of the molecule (42). The constant region is involved in effector functions. The variable region of heavy and light chains can be divided into regions of conserved amino acid sequences known as framework regions (FRs) and regions of highly variable sequences referred to as hypervariable regions or complementarity-determining regions (CDRs) (43). The genes coding for heavy, kappa, and lambda light chains are located on separate murine chromosomes (12, 6, and 16, respectively).

1. Heavy Chains

There are several constant region genes encoding constant region domains of different heavy-chain isotypes (μ, δ, γ, ϵ, α) and subclasses. There are two or more constant region domains depending on the isotype. Each C-region domain is coded by a separate exon. 5′ to each C-region gene there is a switch sequence except for the δ gene segment. The complete V_H gene is assembled from three different gene segments which are located upstream of constant region gene cluster. A few kb upstream of the C genes, a set of four J_H segments is located (44). At 1–80 kb upstream of J_H is located a cluster of more than 12 D-region segments (45–47). A set of 100–1000 V_H segments are found further upstream of the D-region segments. The assembly of complete V_H involves two rearrangement events, namely D to J_H joining followed by V_H to DJ_H joining (46,48). Special conserved sequences which flank V_H, D, and J_H segments serve as rearrangement signals (49–52). Each comprises a palindromic heptamer immediately adjacent to the gene segment, separated by a spacer from a nonamer. The heptamer nonamer unit is found on the 3′ side of all V and D segments and the 5′ side of all D and J segments. The 3′ and 5′ forms are complementary inversions which can base pair with each other. The spacer length is either 12 or 23 bp. The "12/23" rule is that a segment with the 12 bp spacer can only combine with a segment having a 23 bp spacer (49–52). The rearrangement is brought about by a site-specific recombinase (53). The variable gene segment (V_H) contains about 98 amino acids, the diversity segment (D) encodes for 1–15 amino acids, and the joining segment (J_H) contains 12–17 amino acids. There are three CDRs and four FRs in heavy chains. The first two CDRs are coded by the V_H gene segment, while the third is coded by VDJ junctions and part of J_H. The first three FRs are coded by V_H gene segment and the last FR (FR4) is entirely coded by J_H.

2. *Light Chains*

A single gene segment codes for the constant domain of light chain. For the kappa (K) light chain, only one constant region gene segment is present, whereas there are four constant region gene segments (three are functional) that can code for lambda light-chain constant domain (54,55). In mouse, λ light-chain expression is rare (5%). The complete variable region of K or lambda is assembled from two DNA segments (51,52). A cluster of four functional (and one nonfunctional) J_K segments is located upstream of the C_K gene segment. Further upstream there is a large set of (200) V_K gene segments, each with a leader exon. In the case of λ light chain gene locus there are just three Vλ segments, each followed downstream by two J-C units (55,56). Assembly of light-chain V gene segments is also carried out by a mechanism similar to that seen in V_H gene assembly (51,52). The V_L segment codes for the first 95 amino acids of the light chain, and J_L codes for residues 96–108. The site at which V_L and J_L gene segments join may vary relative to the recognition sequences, and as a result an additional amino acid may be generated at the 96th position. The light-chain CDRs are similar to those of heavy chains except that CDR3 is less complex because a diversity segment is not involved in the formation of light chains (57). Kappa light-chain gene segments are rearranged first and only when such rearrangements are unproductive the lambda gene family is rearranged. Lambda-expressing cells generally show deletion of the C_K gene segment (58).

B. Organization of Ig V Genes

The number of V_H genes present in mouse is still uncertain. Southern blot analysis estimations put the number at 100 genes (59), while solution hybridizations estimate over 1000 genes (60). Based on nucleic acid sequence homology, the V_H segments have been classified into 12 distinct gene families. V_H genes with more than 80% homology are grouped under the same gene family (61–69). Each V_H gene family consists of 1–60 members. V_H families are organized mostly as nonoverlapping clusters (63–65), although both overlapping and interspersion of V_H gene segments from different families have been reported recently (61,66–69).

There are 50–200 V_K gene segments in the mouse. Based on amino acid and nucleic acid sequence homology, V_K genes are grouped into 28 families (70–73). Each V_K gene family consists of about 1–10 members. The V_K locus also shows interspersion of certain V_K gene families. The λ light-chain locus is composed of only three V genes (56). The order in which V_H and V_K gene families are known to be organized is shown in Figure 1.

C. Generation of Antibody Diversity

Antibody diversity is generated by several mechanisms which operate at multiple levels: (1) the random pairing or co-expression of heavy- and light-chain germline variable-region genes; (2) combinatorial association of different germline DNA segments contributing to the diversity of the variable regions of heavy and light chains (46,52); (3) combinatorial association of germline DNA segments of variable-region genes coupled with imprecise joining at the recombination sites (48); (4) gene conversion and recombination between members of multigene families (74,75); and (5) somatic mutation during ontogeny of B-cell lines (76–79).

D. V Gene Polymorphism

Abnormalities in the structure or organization of immunoglobulin genes may contribute to or be associated with autoimmune diseases. Restriction fragment length polymorphism (RFLP) analysis can reveal differences in the organization, duplication, conversion, deletion, and even point mutations of the genes in these loci. By such an analysis of germline DNA from autoimmune disease-prone strains, it would be theoretically possible to detect any alterations in the organization and structure or presence of a unique set of V genes.

Murine V_H genes are highly polymorphic (80). The most commonly observed variations are: (1) the presence of a V gene in one strain of mouse having no

A

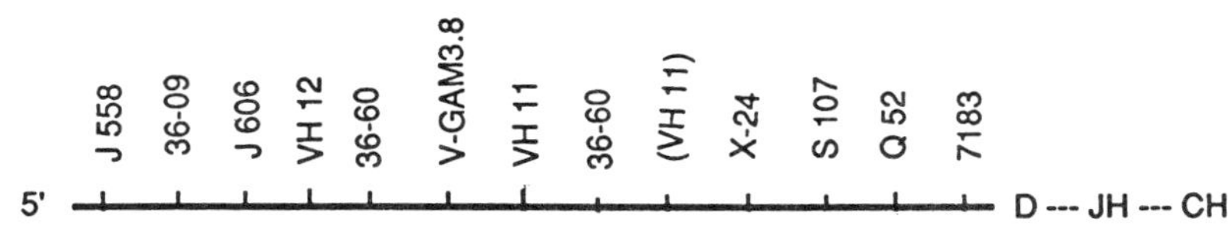

B

5' -($V_κ$11, $V_κ$24, $V_κ$9-$V_κ$26)-($V_κ$1, $V_κ$9)-($V_κ$4, $V_κ$8, $V_κ$10, $V_κ$12, $V_κ$13, $V_κ$19)-($V_κ$28, Rn7S)-$V_κ$23-($V_κ$21, $J_κ$ - $C_κ$)

FIGURE 1 Relative positions of V_H gene families (A) and V_K gene families (B). The relative order of V_H gene families is based on data from deletion mapping and RFLP analysis (61,67). The relative order of V_K gene families is based on data defined by RFLP analysis of recombinant populations and deletion mappings (72). The actual physical distances and orientations are not known.

obvious counterpart or allele in the second strain, i.e., the RFLP variation is related to the presence or absence of a locus (81,82), and (2) variation due to allelic differences between strains (63,83).

Using V_H gene-specific probes, Kofler and colleagues (84) analyzed germline DNA from autoimmune strains, their ancestors and normal IgH haplotype-matched strains and concluded that there are no significant RFLP differences in the V_H locus except in the Q52 gene family of NZB and NZW compared to AKR mice. The Ig V_H gene complex of the lupus-prone mice is essentially identical to that in related strains that are not lupus prone. Similar conclusions were drawn from several other independent studies (85–87) except for the minor polymorphic abnormalities observed in two V_H gene families, S107 and 36-09, of tightskin mice (85). It is possible, however, that subtle differences present in the regulatory sequences, not detectable by RFLP analysis, could contribute to the generation of autoantibodies in autoimmune strains. Theophilopoulos et al. have shown by sequence analysis that the IgH enhancer region of lupus strain BxSB and that of control strain BALB/c are, in fact, identical (88). A single nucleotide difference found in the MRL lpr/lpr IgH enhancer region resides outside the enhancer core region and most probably is not functionally relevant as determined by DNAse I footprinting and protein-binding studies (89,90). Other studies, by determining the sequence of V_H genes coding for autoantibodies, also indicate that they are encoded by structural or genetic elements closely related to or identical to those found in antibodies to foreign antigens in normal mice (73,84,91). A number of V_H gene families in human display little or no polymorphism (92). Dijak et al., using oligonucleotide probes specific for framework region sequences, however, have identified the presence of allelic variations in certain V_H gene families (93). But no significant difference could be detected by RFLP analysis of V_H genes in SLE patients compared to controls and siblings (94).

The organization and complexity of V_K genes in mouse is less well defined than the V_H locus. Based on amino acid similarity up to the first invariant tryptophan at position 35, mouse K light chains have been classified into 28 groups (71,73). These protein groups correspond to nonoverlapping V_K gene families. Initially, it was thought that V_K genes are not polymorphic. But studies by peptide mapping (95), isoelectrofocusing (96,97), RFLP analysis (72,98), idiotype (99–101), and sequence analysis (101,102) have demonstrated that a complex polymorphism exists. Mapping and assessment of the complexity of the V_K gene families (72) as well as RFLP analysis of several autoimmune and nonautoimmune control mouse strains using a number of V_K gene probes have been reported recently (81,82,103). There are differences in the complexities of V_K genes observed by different investigators. This might relate to the variability in the stringency conditions as well as the differences in the probes used in hybridizations.

The RFLP analysis of a number of autoimmune and normal strains with V_K

gene probes indicates that polymorphisms of V_K genes is greater than that found for V_H genes in mice (81,82). However, RFLPs unique for autoimmune-prone mouse strains, as compared to strains with matched haplotypes, are limited. Significant differences were noted only in NZB and tightskin mouse strains (Fig. 2). The RFLP pattern of NZB, whose origin is uncertain, is different from that of C57BL/6 but resembles closely the pattern of C58 (82). The genetic elements encoding anti-DNA antibodies in NZB were also found to be identical or related to those encoding antibodies to foreign antigens in nonautoimmune mice (73). The polymorphism observed in the V_K9 gene of *me*^{V} mice (Fig. 2) also does not appear to be related to the coding sequence of the V gene segments since three V_K9 gene sequences of *me*^{V} mice autoantibodies compared were found to be identical to those from nonautoimmune strains of mice (179). Comparison of various V_K haplotypes suggests occurrence of recombinations within V_K gene families (82).

III. V GENE USAGE

A. Expression of V Gene Families in Neonatal and Adult Murine B Cells

Little is known, at present, regarding the expression of various V gene families and events leading to specific V_H and V_K gene pairing during B-cell development. Such information could provide insights into the nature of the molecular mechanisms that might be involved in the generation of the V gene repertoire for foreign as well as self-antigens. Recent studies using B-cell colony assays of adult mice spleen cells (104,105) and the analysis of hybridomas derived from LPS-activated spleen cells (106) revealed that V_H gene families are utilized randomly, the family representation being proportional to the family size, with no detectable bias. However, a comparative analysis of V_H gene utilization patterns in neonatal liver cells and unstimulated or polyclonally activated spleen cells indicates that the process of rearranging V_H genes and forming the V_H repertoire in early B-cell development is position dependent, nonrandom, and biased towards utilization of J_H-proximal V_H segments. This process is modified in a strain specific manner in peripheral B lineage cells (107,109). It has been postulated that the differences seen in V_H expression reflects developmentally regulated changes in the accessibility of V_H locus to the recombination process (110). However, the preferential rearrangement of 3′ germline V_H genes in neonatal B cells does not appear to influence the antigen-specific repertoire at that stage of development. Indeed, studies have shown that the same germline V_H and V_K genes and the same frequency of V_H:V_K pairing are seen during the neonatal antibody response to nonself antigens as are found during the primary response in adults (111).

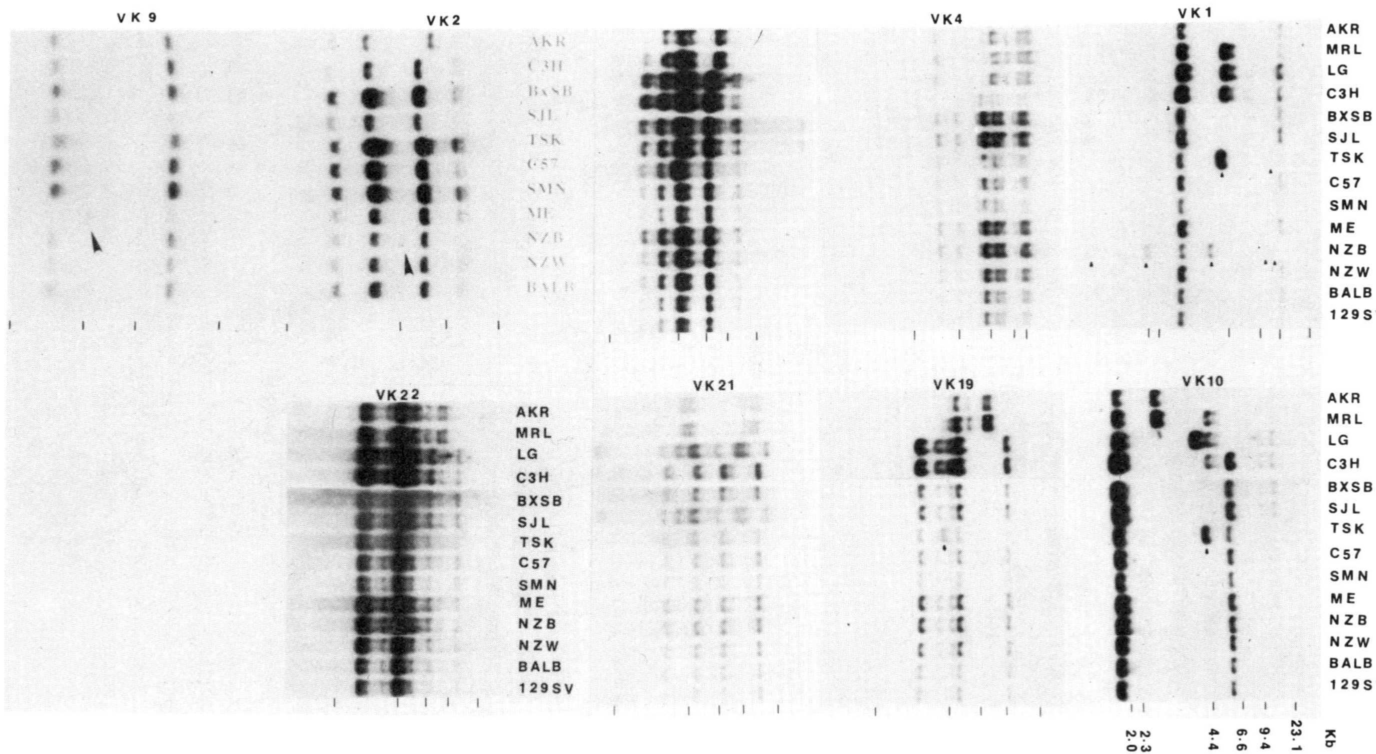

FIGURE 2 Southern blot hybridizations of Hind III digested liver genomic DNA from 14 mouse strains. Polymorphic differences are indicated by arrows. V_K gene probes used in hybridizations are described in Refs. 91 and 95.

By contrast, utilization of V_K genes appear to be rather random and not position dependent in neonatal spleen cells, pre-B-cell lines, or fetal liver cells. The V_K genes across the entire locus are used without bias (112,113). Moreover, no correlation has been found between orientation of the locus and the frequency of a particular V_K gene rearrangement. Furthermore, V_K gene expression does not appear to be related to genomic complexity either in neonatal or adult spleen cells. V_K gene expression is more heterogeneous, and some overexpression of certain V_K gene families has been observed. For instance, V_K1 and V_K9 gene families are expressed up to 40 and 25% in neonatal spleen cells and 25 and 5%, respectively, in adult spleen cells.

B. Utilization of V Genes by Autoantibodies

Antibodies specific for haptens and polysaccharides are encoded by genes derived from a restricted pool of V gene families, and in certain situations even restricted V_H:V_K pairings have been observed (114,119). On the other hand, antibodies specific for protein antigens are coded by genes from a broad spectrum of V gene families (120,121).

The antiself response may be essentially unrestricted. But genetic restriction may exist among autoantibodies of a given specificity. This appears to be related to the structural requirement for the specificity. Such a restriction might also arise due either to the involvement of a particular subset of B cells or to a positive selection driven by antigen in a polyclonally activated population (33–35,122).

A number of studies relating to the utilization of V genes by hybridomas derived from autoreactive B cells indicate that J_H proximal V_H gene families are used frequently (Table 1). For instance, rheumatoid factor (RF) autoantibodies and anti-DNA autoantibodies of MRL Ipr/Ipr mice and normal strains utilize V_H genes primarily from the V_H 36-60 gene family (86,123,124). A large number of autoantibodies with other specificities were also found to utilize genes from the Q52 and V_H7183 families (36). Further, hybridomas selected for 7183 V_H gene expression also appear to produce self-reactive antibodies at a higher frequency (8). Again, no significant difference could be seen between normal and autoimmune strains in the usage of V_H 7183 by autoantibodies (91). Restrictive use of genetic elements has been observed only among anti-BrRBC (bromelain-treated RBC) autoantibodies. In a study, all six autoantibodies, derived from CBA and NZB mice analyzed by mRNA sequencing, were found to use the same V_H (V_H11) and same V_K (V_K9) in germline configuration (125).

However, several other studies have noted the absence of any bias in the utilization of V_H genes, as in the case of autoantibodies derived from *me*^{V} mice (126) and RF autoantibodies (127). Furthermore, there is not enough evidence to show that 3′ V_H gene families such as 7183 genes are used less frequently in response to exogenous antigenic stimuli than any other family of comparable size. In

TABLE 1 Utilization of V_H Genes by Autoantibodies

Autoantibody specificity	No. of hybridomas tested	V_H gene family expressed							
		J558	36-09	J606	36-60	S107	X-24	Q52	7183
TG & TSH	19	5	—	1	—	—	—	1	12
RF	68	38	—	2	6	—	—	3	19
Collagen II	14	6	1	—	2	—	2	1	2
DNA	25	11	1	—	2	2	—	1	8
Sm	10	3	—	—	—	1	1	—	5
Multispecific	25	9	1	4	—	1	—	4	6
Total	161	72	3	7	10	4	3	10	52

Source: Refs. 8, 103, 122, 124.

fact, a slight overrepresentation of 7183 genes has been described in the adult murine B-cell repertoire (128).

In the case of V_K genes, we found preferential use of V_K1, V_K4, V_K8, V_K10, and V_K19 gene families by autoantibodies specific for RF, DNA, Sm, TG, collagen, as well as several multispecific autoantibodies (Table 2). Preferential or biased used of these V_K genes is related neither to the complexity nor to the position of the V genes in the V_K locus. There were also reports indicating the preferential use of V_K1, V_K8, V_K12, and V_K19 among RF autoantibodies derived from BALB/c and 128SV mice which were injected with polysaccharides or protein antigens (129). The anti-DNA autoantibodies derived from MRL-Ipr/Ipr and (NZBxW)F_1 mice also demonstrate preferential use of V_K1 and V_K19 genes (91,130). Similarly, a disproportionate usage of V_KII and V_KIII genes among human RF autoantibodies has also been observed (131,132).

IV. ORIGIN AND SPECIFICITY OF AUTOANTIBODIES

A. Origin

The origin of autoantibodies still remains a subject of controversy and numerous hypotheses have been postulated. Some of the most important are presented here.

Autoreactive B-cell clones, not eliminated during ontogeny, are prevented from expansion by suppressor regulatory mechanism (13). Autoantibodies are, therefore, produced only in minute quantities in normal individuals. Failure of the suppressor mechanism, however, could lead to expansion of the existing autoreactive clones.

A pool of autoreactive B cells normally present in healthy individuals may be expanded or activated by either polyclonal activators, such as LPS, produced by infectious agents (25,133), or by cross-reactive foreign antigens (7,134,135), or due to perturbations in idiotype anti-idiotype network (134,145–147).

TABLE 2 Utilization of V_K Genes by Autoantibodies

Autoantibody specificity	No. of hybridomas tested	V_K gene family expressed											
		1	2	4	8	9	10	19	21	22	23	24	NI
RF	68	8	0	6	10	0	5	19	6	1	2	6	5
DNA	16	3	0	2	1	0	0	1	0	1	0	1	7
Sm	7	3	0	1	2	0	0	1	0	0	0	0	1
TG	11	1	0	1	1	0	3	2	0	0	0	0	1
Collagen II	13	1	0	0	0	1	4	0	0	2	0	0	5
Multispecific	33	9	0	4	2	1	6	2	0	4	0	0	7
Total	138	25	0	14	16	2	18	25	6	8	2	7	26

Source: Refs. 91, 103, 122.

The concept of cross-reactivity between self and nonself epitopes is supported by the demonstration of the presence of polyspecific natural autoantibodies (6,136,137), and the existence of apparent structural homology between a wide variety of nonself antigens and autoantigens: the proliferative response of T cells from rheumatoid arthritis patients to a conserved 65 kD heat shock protein from *M. tuberculosis* (138); the binding of anti-*Klebsiella* polysaccharide antibodies to DNA (134); the presence of homology between gp110 of EBV and the hypervariable regions of DR1 and DR4 molecules in arthritis (139); the presence of homology between toposiomerase I and a hexapeptide of retroviral P^{30gag} protein recognized by antitopoisomerase I antibodies present in scleroderma patients (140); the presence of antibodies against a 70 kD RNP, sharing homology with another P^{30gag} protein, in patients with SLE and mixed connective tissue disease (141) and the presence of cross-reactive antibodies to MBP and measles virus in multiple sclerosis (142). Experimental studies also indicate that indeed such cross-reactive clones can be activated by immunization with cross-reactive foreign antigens (see for review Ref. 103).

Affinity maturation of the antibody response to foreign antigens can also provide the opportunity for the production of autoantibodies by nonautoreactive B cells. A single point mutation in an antiphosphocholine antibody encoded by V_H S107 converts it into an autoantibody reacting with dsDNA (143,144).

Finally, perturbations of the idiotype anti-idiotype network can result in the activation of autoreactive B-cell clones which are otherwise silent. Antibodies against several foreign antigens share idiotopes (16/6 Id, IdX, or Id62) with autoantibodies (134,145,146). Immunization with such foreign antigens or infections can activate autoreactive clones sharing these idiotopes (134). Antiacetylcholine receptor antibodies and α1-3 dextran antibodies in human and mice show idiotypic connectivity (147), as do anti-DNA antibodies found in SLE which share 16/6 idiotype (148). Similarly, anti-Id antibodies carrying the internal image of self-antigens such as insulin and TSH can contribute to the induction of insulin-resistant diabetes (30,31), or Graves' disease (32). Anti-idiotype antibodies of epibody nature exhibiting binding activity to self antigens could also play an important role in the induction of autoantibodies (149).

Recent studies suggest that Ly-1^+ B cells ($CD5^+$ B cells in human) contribute in a disproportional manner to the production of naturally occurring autoantibodies (150–153). $CD5^+$ B cells represent 10–25% of circulating and splenic B lymphocytes (153), whereas Ly-1^+ B cells constitute only 1–2% of spleen cells in mice. But the major proportion of B lymphocytes of peritoneal cavity in mice are Ly-1^+ B cells (150). By cell transfer experiments, it has been shown that Ly-1^+ B cells persist over a long period of time in the immune system without any somatic mutations occurring in the V regions (154). This is consistent with the fact that somatic mutations have not been found in autoantibodies derived from Ly-1^+ B cells (154,155,179).

B. Specificity of Autoantibodies

Multispecific autoantibodies generally exhibit low intrinsic affinity to a variety of self and exogenous antigens (8,129,151,156), though some polyspecific natural autoantibodies have been shown to exhibit high affinity to several antigens including DNA (157). Polyspecific antibodies are directed against easily accessible autoantigens as well as hidden self antigens or cryptic membrane epitopes (158,159). Whether the polyspecific antibodies were polyclonal (isolated by affinity chromatography from serum) or monoclonal (obtained from spleen cell hybridomas of unimmunized mice), they cross-reacted with several structurally unrelated antigens such as DNA, myosin, actin, tubulin, and spectrin (6,160). Such polyreactive autoantibodies are found in a number of autoimmune diseases. Some of them were found to be pathogenic and exhibited cross-reactive idiotypes. Activation of such clones may be related to idiotypic cross-reactivity or antigenic cross-reactivity. For instance, various SLE autoantibodies react with DNA, phospholipids, constant region of IgG, and cytoskeletal antigens (161). These polyspecific antibodies may, perhaps, have a positive role in cleansing the organism of self and nonself products, preventing immune response against self-mimicking determinants present on foreign antigens (162–164). Conversely, they may enhance host immune reactions to foreign antigens and participate in idiotype network regulation.

Recent studies suggest that polyreactive antibodies with similar patterns of autoreactivity can be encoded by entirely different genetic elements. Two such NAAbs described react with actin, tubulin, myosin, DNA, and α fetoprotein (156). They are encoded by J_H-proximal unmutated germline V_H genes from 36-60 and Q52 gene families and germline V_K genes from V_K19 and V_K8 gene families. The binding site appears to extend beyond CDRs in such polyspecific antibodies.

FR2 and FR3 regions of the V_K genes used by anti-IgG rheumatoid factor antibodies also appear to be involved in the specific interactions (129). Similarities or differences in charge distribution on the Fab surface can also account for such immunologic cross-reactivity (165). Such antigen antibody interactions can also be enhanced following cooperative or confromational changes in either the antigen or antibody molecules (166).

By contrast monospecific autoantibodies exhibit high affinity and may belong to IgM, IgG, or IgA isotype. The best known example of a monoreactive IgM autoantibody is that of anti-BrRBC specific natural autoantibodies (125,155). These autoantibodies appear to be produced by Ly-1^+ B cells and are encoded by germline V genes similar to IgM rheumatoid factor antibodies and anti-DNA antibodies (167,168). A high degree of genetic restriction as well as specific V_H:V_K pairing has been observed in anti-BrRBC autoantibodies while IgM RFs and anti-DNA autoantibodies are genetically unrestricted. The latter antibodies were found to use a wide variety of V genes similar to the preimmune anti-DNA antibody repertoire (33,91). In human, these autoantibodies were found to be genetically more restricted (73,169–171), though they were also encoded by dissimilar V_H genes (172). The genetic diversity of anti-DNA antibodies seems to agree with the observation that anti-DNA autoantibodies recognize a number of different epitopes (168).

IgG type anti-IgG rheumatoid factor autoantibodies appear to be of monoclonal or oligoclonal origin in MRL-lpr/lpr mice (34). In contrast to IgM autoantibodies, these antibodies show a high rate of somatic mutations in hypervariable regions, characteristic of an immunoglobulin receptor–dependent selection or activation process. Such a nonrandom pattern of somatic mutations has been found in multiple clones comparable to the response elicited by exogenous antigens following secondary antigenic simulation (173–175). Similarly, IgG type anti-DNA antibodies found in MRL-lpr/lpr mice are also derived from multiple clones and exhibit a high degree of nonrandom somatic variations (35). Such mutations are particularly associated with the introduction of specific residues such as arginine and dsDNA specificity. Three-dimensional structural analysis and computer modeling studies of two anti-DNA antibodies from lupus mice, indeed, show the presence of a cleft in the antibody-combining site rich in arginine and tyrosine residues that can accommodate a stretch of poly(dT) or SSDNA (176). The V_H segments coding for these antibodies belong to two different V_H gene families but had a unique and similar combination of D segments and J_H sequences suggesting a common recognition site for antigen or for idiotypic regulation of the heavy chain. Further, a number of studies also indicate that certain anti-idiotypic antibodies recognize a majority of anti-DNA antibodies from normal and autoimmune individuals (177). The idiotypic relatedness of anti-DNA antibodies does not correlate with the usage of any particular V gene family since diverse V genes are used (35,73). It is unlikely that internal images of anti-DNA autoantibodies play a role in the activation of autoreactive B-cell clones because of the heterogenous nature of the binding specificities of these antibodies (178). Sharing of idiotopes could be related to the recurrent motifs rich in arginine residues (176). Thus the forbidden gene products are derived from several unrelated gene families and are not disease specific.

V. CONCLUSION

Few or no polymorphic differences have been observed in V_H or V_K locus between autoimmune disease-prone strains and haplotype-matched controls. Autoantibodies are encoded by structural and genetic elements similar to those used by antibodies to nonself antigens. The J_H proximal V_H genes are more frequently used by autoantibodies both in autoimmune and nonautoimmune mice. In contrast, no position-dependent usage of V_K genes by autoantibodies is seen. However, certain V_K gene families (V_K1, V_K4, V_K10, and V_K19) are more frequently used by autoantibodies. This bias does not appear to be related to the complexity of the particular V_K locus. In autoimmune mice, the initial broad autoreactive B-cell repertoire producing somatically unmutated IgM autoantibodies tends to become at later stages more specific for a related set of autoantigens. The refinement of specificity is often associated with class switch, clonal restriction, and somatic mutation correlating with the onset of the disease. Sharing of conserved sequences or cross-reactive idiotopes is commonly seen among autoantibodies. The mechanism of specific or preferential activation of B-cell subpopulations producing autoantibodies could be due to autoantigen-driven or cross-reactive nonself antigen–stimulated mechanism or to perturbation of the anti-idiotype network by idiotypic mimicry.

ACKNOWLEDGMENTS

I wish to thank Dr. Thomas M. Fasy for reviewing the manuscript and Ms. Anita Spingarn for her skillful secretarial help.

REFERENCES

1. Karsenti, E., B. Guilbert, M. Bornens, and S. Avrameas. 1977. Antibodies to tubulin in normal nonimmunized animals. *Proc. Natl. Acad. Sci. USA.*, *74*: 3997–4001.
2. Sawada, S., and N. Talal. 1979. Characteristics of *in vitro* production of antibodies to DNA in normal and autoimmune mice. *J. Immunol.*, *122*: 2309–2315.
3. Avrameas, S., B. Guilbert, and G. Dighiero. 1981. Natural antibodies against tubulin, actin, myoglobulin, thryoglobulin, fetuin, albumin and transferrin are present in normal human sera and monoclonal immunoglobulins from multiple myeloma and Waldenstrom's macroglobulinaemia may express similar antibody specificities. *Ann. Immunol.* (Inst. Pasteur), *132c*: 231–236.

4. Lutz, H. V., and G. Wipf. 1982. Naturally occurring autoantibodies to skeletal proteins from human red blood cells. *J. Immunol.*, *128*: 1695–1699.
5. Fish, F., and M. Ziff. 1982. The *in vitro* and *in vivo* induction of anti-double stranded DNA antibodies in normal and autoimmune mice. *J. Immunol.*, *128*: 409–417.
6. Dighiero, G., P. Lymberi, J. C. Mazie, S. Rouvy, G. S. Butler-Brown, R. G. Whalen, and S. Avrameas. 1983. Murine hybridomas secreting natural monoclonal antibodies reacting with self antigens. *J. Immunol.*, *131*: 2267–2272.
7. Lymberi, P., Dighiero, G., Ternynck, T., and S. Avrameas. 1985. A high incidence of cross-reactive idiotypes among murine natural autoantibodies. *Eur. J. Immunol.*, *15*: 702–707.
8. Bellon, B., A. Lory-Manheimer, M. Monestier, T. Moran, A. Dimitriu-Bona, F. Alt, and C. Bona. 1987. High frequency of autoantibodies bearing cross-reactive idiotope among hybridomas using V 7183 genes prepared from normal and autoimmune strains. *J. Clin. Invest.*, *79*: 1044–1053.
9. Dighiero, G., A. Kaushik, P. Poncet, and X. R. Ge. 1987. Origin and significance of autoantibodies. *Concepts Immunopathol.*, *4*: 42–76.
10. Logtenberg, T., A. Kroon, F. H. J. Gmeling-Meyling, and R. E. Ballieux. 1987. Analysis of human tonsil B cell repertoire by somatic hybridization: occurrence of both mono-specific and multi-specific autoantibody secreting cells. *Eur. J. Immunol.*, *17*: 855–859.
11. Klinman, D. M, and A. D. Steinberg. 1987. Similar *in vivo* expansion of B cells from normal DBA/2 and autoimmune NZB mice in xid recipients. *J. Immunol.*, *139*: 2284–2289.
12. Burnet, F. M. 1959. *The Clonal Selection Theory of Acquired Immunity*. Cambridge University Press.
13. Cunningham, A. J. 1976. Self tolerance maintained by active suppressor mechanisms. *Transplant. Rev.*, *31*:23–43.
14. Nossal, G. J. V. 1983. Cellular mechanisms of immunologic tolerance. *Ann. Rev. Immunol.*, *1*: 33–62.
15. Shoenfeld, Y., and R. S. Schwartz. 1984. Immunologic and genetic factors in autoimmune diseases. *New Engl. J. Med.*, *311*: 1019–1029.
16. Jerne, N. K. 1974. Toward a network theory of immune system. *Ann. Immunol.* (Inst. Pasteur), *125c*: 373–389.
17. Bona, C., K. E. Stein, R. Lieberman, and W. E. Paul. 1979. Direct and indirect suppression induced by anti-idiotype antibody in the inulin-bacterial levan antigenic system. *Mol. Immunol.*, *16*: 1093–1101.
18. Holmberg, D., S. Forsgren, L. Forni, F. Ivars, and A. Coutinho. 1984. Idiotypic determinants of natural IgM antibodies that resemble self Ia antigens. *Proc. Natl. Acad. Sci. USA*, *81*: 3175–3179.
19. Kearney, J. F., and M. Vakil. 1986. Idiotype directed interactions during ontogeny play a major role in the establishment of the adult B cell repertoire. *Immunol. Rev.*, *94*: 39–49.
20. Fougereau, M., and C. Schiff. 1988. Breaking the first cycle. *Immunol. Reviews*, *105*: 69–84.
21. Theofilopoulos, A. N., D. L. Shawler, R. A. Eisenberg, and F. J. Dixon. 1980.

Splenic immunoglobulin secreting cells and their regulation in autoimmune mice. *J. Exp. Med., 151*: 446–466.

22. Klinman, D. M., R. A. Eisenberg, and A. D. Steinberg. 1990. Development of the autoimmune B cell repertoire in MRL-lpr/lpr mice. *J. Immunol., 144*: 506–511.
23. Izui, S., P. J. McConahey, A. N. Theofilopoulos, and F. J. Dixon. 1979. Association of circulating retroviral gp70 anti-gp70 immune complexes with murine systemic lupus erythromatosus. *J. Exp. Med., 149*: 1099–1116.
24. Hang, L., M. T. Aguado, F. J. Dixon, and A. N. Theofilopoulos. 1985. Induction of severe autoimmune disease in normal mice by simultaneous action of multiple immuno-modulators. *J. Ex. Med., 161*: 423–434.
25. Dziarski, R. 1982. Preferential induction of autoantibody secretion in polyclonal activation by peptidoglycan and lipopolysaccharide. I. *In vitro* studies. *J. Immunol., 128*: 1018–1025.
26. Dziarski, R. 1988. Autoimmunity: Polyclonal activation or antigen activation. *Immunol. Today, 9*: 340–342.
27. Klinman, D. M., Y. Ishigatsubo, and A. D. Steinberg. 1988. Acquisition and maturation of expressed B cell repertoire in normal and autoimmune mice. *J. Immunol., 141*: 801–806.
28. Datta, S. K., H. Patel, and D. Berry. 1987. Induction of a cationic shift in IgG anti-DNA autoantibodies—Role of T helper cells with classical and novel phenotypes in murine models of lupus nephritis. J. Exp. Med., 165: 1252–1268.
29. Madaio, M. P., J. Carlson, J. Cataldo, A. Ucci, P. Migliorini, and O. Pankewycz. 1987. Murine monoclonal anti-DNA antibodies bind directly to glomerular antigens and form immune deposits. *J. Immunol., 138*: 2883–2889.
30. Sege, K., and P. A. Paterson. 1978. Use of anti-idiotypic antibodies as cell surface receptor probes. *Proc. Natl. Acad. Sci. USA, 75*: 2443–2447.
31. Marion, R., D. Elias, B. M. deLongh, G. J. Bruining, J. J. van Rood, Y. Schechter, and T. R. Cohen. 1983. Autoantibodies to the insulin receptor in juvenile onset insulin dependent diabetes. *Nature, 303*: 817–818.
32. Farid, N. R., Briones-Urbina, and M. Nazruil Islam. 1982. Biological activity of anti-thyrotrophin anti-idiotypic antibody. *J. Cell Biochem., 19*: 305–313.
33. Shlomchik, M. J., A. H. Aucoin, D. S. Pisetsky, and M. G. Weigert. 1987. Structure and function of anti-DNA autoantibodies derived from a single autoimmune mouse. *Proc. Natl. Acad. Sci. USA, 84*: 9150–9154.
34. Shlomchik, M. J., A. Marshak-Rothstein, C. B. Wolfowicz, T. L. Rothstein, and M. G. Weigert. 1987. The role of clonal selection and somatic mutation in autoimmunity. *Nature, 328*: 805–809.
35. Shlomchik, M., M. Masulli, H. Shan, M. Z. Radic, D. Pisetsky, A. Marshak-Rothstein, and M. Weigart. 1990. Anti-DNA antibodies from autoimmune mice arise by clonal expansion and somatic mutation. *J. Exp. Med., 171*: 265–297.
36. Monestier, M., A. Manheimer-Lory, B. Bellon, C. Painter, H. Dang, N. Talal, M. Zanetti, R. Schwartz, D. Pisetsky, R. Kuppers, N. Rose, J. Brochier, L. Kareskog, R. Holmdahl, B. Erlanger, F. W. Alt, and C. Bona. 1986. Shared idiotype and restricted immunoglobulin variable region heavy chain genes characterize murine autoantibodies of various specificities. *J. Clin. Invest., 78*: 753–759.

37. Theofilopoulos, A. N., R. S. Balderas, L. Hang, and F. J. Dixon. 1983. Monoclonal IgM rheumatoid factors derived from arthritic MRL/lpr-lpr mice. *J. Exp. Med.*, *158*: 901-919.
38. Schwartz, J. A., S. K. Datta, Y. Shoenfeld, D. A. Isenberg, B. D. Stollar, and R. S. Schwartz. 1984. Binding of cytoskeletal proteins by monoclonal anti-DNA lupus antibodies. *Clin. Immunol. Immunopathol.*, *31*: 261–271.
39. Pisetsky, D. S., S. O. Hoch, C. L. Klatt, M. A. O'Donnell, and J. D. Keene. 1985. Specificity and idiotypic analysis of a monoclonal anti-Sm antibody with anti-DNA activity. *J. Immunol.*, *135*: 4080–4085.
40. Rubin, R. L., R. S. Balderas, E. M. Tan, F. J. Dixon, and A. N. Theofilopoulos. 1984. Multiple autoantigen binding capabilities of mouse monoclonal antibodies selected for rheumatoid factor activity. *J. Exp. Med.*, *159*: 1429–1440.
41. Gally, J. A., and G. M. Edelman. 1972. The genetic control of immunoglobulin synthesis. *Ann. Rev. Genetics, 6*: 1–46.
42. Segal, D. M., E. A. Padlan, G. H. Cohen, S. Rudikoff, M. Potter, and D. R. Davies. 1974. The three dimensional structure of a phosphonylcholine binding mouse immunoglobulin Fab and the nature of the antigen binding site. *Proc. Natl. Acad. Sci. USA, 71*: 4298–4302.
43. Wu, T. T., and E. A. Kabat. 1970. An analysis of the sequences of the variable regions of Bence-Jones proteins and myeloma light chains and their implications for antibody complementarity. *J. Exp. Med.*, *132*: 211–240.
44. Shimizu, A., N. Takahashi, Y. Yaoita, and T. Honjo. 1982. Organization of the constant region gene family of the mouse immunoglobulin heavy chain. *Cell, 28*: 499–506.
45. Kurosawa, Y., and S. Tonegawa. 1982. Organization, structure and assembly of immunoglobulin heavy chain diversity DNA segments. *J. Exp. Med.*, *155*: 201–218.
46. Tonegawa, S. 1983. Somatic generation of antibody diversity. *Nature, 302*: 575–581.
47. Wood, C., and S. Tonegawa. 1983. Diversity and joining segments of mouse IgH genes are closely linked and in the same orientation. *Proc. Natl. Acad. Sci. USA, 80*: 3030–3034.
48. Alt, F. W., G. D. Yancopoulos, T. K. Blackwell, C. Wood, E. Thomas, M. Boss, R. Coltman, N. Rosenberg, S. Tonegawa, and D. Baltimore. 1984. Ordered rearrangement of immunoglobulin heavy chain variable region segments. *EMBO J.*, *3*: 1209–1219.
49. Early, P., H. Huang, M. Davis, K. Calame, and L. Hood. 1980. An immunoglobulin heavy chain variable region gene is generated from three separate segments of DNA:V_H, D and J_H. *Cell, 19*: 981-992.
50. Sakano, H., R. Maki, Y. Kurosawa, W. Roeder, and S. Tonegawa. 1980. Two types of somatic recombinations are necessary for the generation of complete immunoglobulin heavy chain genes. *Nature, 286*: 676–683.
51. Max, E. E., J. G. Seidman, and P. Leder. 1979. Sequences of five potential recombination sites encoded close to an immunoglobulin K constant region gene. *Proc. Natl. Acad. Sci. USA, 76*: 3450–3454.
52. Sakano, H., K. Huppi, G. Heinrich, and S. Tonegawa. 1979. Sequences at somatic recombination sites of immunoglobulin light-chain genes. *Nature, 280*: 288–294.

53. Alt, F. W., and D. Baltimore. 1982. Joining of immunoglobulin heavy chain gene segments: Implications from a chromosome with evidence of three D-JH fusions. *Proc. Natl. Acad. Sci. USA, 79*: 4118–4122.
54. Blomberg, B., A. Traunecker, H. Eisen, and S. Tonegawa. 1981. Organization of four mouse lambda light chain immunoglobulin genes. *Proc. Natl. Acad. Sci. USA, 78*: 3765–3769.
55. Miller, J., A. Bothwell, and U. Storb. 1981. Physical linkage of the constant region genes for immunoglobulins lambda I and lambda III. *Proc. Natl. Acad. Sci. USA, 78*: 3829–3833.
56. Dildrop, R., A. Gause, W. Muller, and K. Rajewsky. 1987. A new V gene expressed in lambda-2 light chains of the mouse. *Eur. J. Immunol., 17*: 731–734.
57. Yancopoulos, G. D., and F. W. Alt. 1986. The regulation of variable region gene assembly. *Ann. Rev. Immunol., 4*: 339.
58. Hieter, P. A., S. J. Korsmeyer, T. A. Waldman, and P. Leder. 1981. Human immunoglobulin kappa light chain genes are deleted or rearranged in producing B cells. *Nature, 290*: 368–372.
59. Brodeur, P. H., and R. Riblet. 1984. The immunoglobulin heavy chain variable region (Igh-V) locus in the mouse. I. One hundred Igh-genes comprise seven families of homologous genes. *Eur. J. Immunol., 14*: 922–930.
60. Livant, D., C. Blatt, and L. Hood. 1986. One heavy chain variable region gene segment subfamily in Balb/c mouse contains 500-1000 or more members. *Cell, 47*: 461–470.
61. Brodeur, P. H., G. E. Osman, J. J. Mackle, and T. M. Lalor. 1988. Organization of the mouse Igh-V locus Dispersion, interspersion and the evolution of V_H gene family clusters. *J. Exp. Med., 168*: 2261–2278.
62. Kofler, R. 1988. A new murine Ig V_H gene family. *J. Immunol., 140*: 4031–4034.
63. Bothwell, A. L. M., M. Paskind, A. Reth, T. Imanishi-Kari, K. Rajewsky, and D. Baltimore. 1981. Heavy chain variable region contribution to the Npb family of antibodies: Somatic mutation evident in a 2 variable region. *Cell, 24*: 625–637.
64. Kemp, D. J., B. Tyler, O. Bernard, N. Gough, S. Gerondakis, J. M. Adams, and S. Cory. 1981. Organization of genes and spacers within the mouse immunoglobulin V_H locus. *J. Mol. Appl. Genet., 1*: 245.
65. Loh, D. Y., A. L. M. Bothwell, M. White-Scharf, T. Imanishi-Kari, and D. Baltimore. 1983. Molecular basis of a mouse strain-specific anti-hapten response. *Cell, 33*: 85–93.
66. Reth, M., S. Jackson, and F. W. Alt. 1986. VDJ formation and DJ replacement during pre-B differentiation: a non-random usage of gene segments. *EMBO J., 5*: 2131–2138.
67. Pennel, C. A., K. M. Shecham, P. H. Brodeur, and S. H. Clarke. 1989. Organization and expression of V_H gene families preferentially expressed by Ly-1^+ (CD5) B cells. *Eur. J. Immunol., 19*: 2115–2121.
68. Blankenstein, T., and V. Krawinkel. 1987. Immunoglobulin V_H region genes of the mouse are organized in overlapping clusters. *Eur. J. Immunol., 17*: 1351–1357.
69. Christoph, T., and V. Krawinkel. 1989. Physical linkage of variable diversity and joining gene segments in the immunoglobulin heavy chain locus of the mouse. *Eur. J. Immunol., 19*: 1521–1523.

70. Cory, S. B., M. Tyler, and J. M. Adams. 1981. Sets of immunoglobulin V genes homologous to ten cloned V sequences implications for the number of germline V genes. *J. Mol. Appl. Genet.*, *1*: 103–116.
71. Potter, M., J. B. Newell, S. Rudikoff, and E. Haber. 1982. Classification of mouse V groups based on partial amino-acid sequence to the first invariant-tryptophan: Impact of 14 new sequences from IgG myeloma proteins. *Mol. Immunol.*, *19*: 1619–1630.
72. D'Hoostelaere, L., K. Huppi, B. Mock, C. Mallett, D. Gibson, J. Hilgers, and M. Poter. 1988. The organization of the immunoglobulin kappa locus in mice. *Curr. Top. Microbiol. Immunol.*, *137*: 116.
73. Kofler, R., R. Strohal, R. S. Balderas, M. E. Johnson, D. J. Noonan, M. A. Duchosal, F. J. Dixon, and A. N. Theofilopoulos. 1988. Immunoglobulin K light chain variable gene complex organization and immunoglobulin genes encoding anti-DNA autoantibodies in lupus mice. *J. Clin. Invest.*, *82*: 852–860.
74. Clarke, S. H., J. L. Claflin, and S. Rudikoff. 1982. Polymorphisms in immunoglobulin heavy chains suggesting gene conversions. *Proc. Natl. Acad. Sci. USA*, *79*: 3280–3284.
75. Krawinkel, U., G. Zaebelein, M. Bruggmann, A. Radbruch, and K. Rajewsky. 1983. Recombination between antibody heavy chain variable region genes: Evidence for gene conversion. *Proc. Natl. Acad. Sci. USA*, *80*: 4997–5001.
76. Secher, D. S., C. Milestein, and K. Adatugbo. 1977. Somatic mutants and antibody diversity. *Immunol. Rev.*, *36*: 51–72.
77. Selsing, E., and U. Storb. 1981. Somatic mutation of immunoglobulin light chain variable region genes. *Cell*, *25*: 45–58.
78. Gearhart, P. J., N. D. Johnson, R. Douglas, and L. Hood. 1981. IgG antibodies to phosphorylcholine exhibit more diversity than their IgM counterparts. *Nature*, *291*: 29–34.
79. Manser, T. 1989. Evolution of antibody structure during the immune response: The differentiative potential of a single B lymphocyte. *J. Exp. Med.*, *170*: 1211–1230.
80. Rothbun, G. A., J. D. Capra, and P. W. Tucker. 1987. Organization of murine immunoglobulin V complex in the inbred stains. *EMBO J.*, *6*: 2931–2937.
81. Kasturi, K., M. Monestier, R. Mayer, and C. Bona. 1988. Biased usage of certain V_K gene families by autoantibodies and their polymorphism in autoimmune mice. *Molec. Immunol.*, *25*: 213–219.
82. Kofler, R., M. A. Duchosal, and F. J. Dixon. 1989. Complexity, polymorphism and connectivity of mouse V gene families. *Immunogenetics*, *29*: 65–74.
83. Siekevitz, M., B. Y. Huang, and M. L. Gefter. 1983. The genetic basis of antibody production: A single heavy chain variable region gene encodes all molecules bearing the dominant anti-arsonate idiotype in the strain A mouse. *Eur. J. Immunol.*, *13*: 123–132.
84. Kofler, R., D. J. Noonan, D. E. Levy, M. C. Wilson, N. P. H. Moller, F. J. Dixon, and A. N. Theofilopoulos. Genetic elements used for a murine lupus anti-DNA autoantibody are closely related to those code for antibodies to exogenous antigen. *J. Exp. Med.*, *161*: 805–815.
85. Bona, C., K. N. Kasturi, R. Mayer, and V. Fidanza. 1988. V genes usage by autoantibodies and their polymorphism in autoimmune mice. *Autoimmunity*, *2*: 29–53.

86. Painter, C., M. Monestier, B. Bonin, and C. A. Bona. 1986. Functional and molecular studies of V genes expressed in autoantibodies. *Immunol. Rev., 94*: 75–98.
87. Trepicchio, W., Jr., and K. J. Barrett. 1987. Eleven MRL/lpr/lpr anti-DNA autoantibodies are encoded by genes from four V gene famiies: a potentially biased usage of V genes. *J. Immunol., 138*: 2323–2331.
88. Theofilopoulos, A. N., R. Kofker, D. J. Noonan, P. Singer, and F. J. Dixon. 1986. Molecular aspects of murine systemic lupus erythematosus. *Springer Semin. Immunopathol., 9*: 121–142.
89. Augereau, P., and P. Chambon. 1986. The mouse immunoglobulin heavy chain enhancer: Effect on transcription *in vitro* and binding of proteins present in HeLa and lymphoid B cell extracts. *EMBO J., 5*: 1791–1797.
90. Sen, R., and D. Baltimore. 1986. Multiple nuclear factors interact with the immunoglobulin enhancer sequences. *Cell, 46*: 705–716.
91. Kofler, R., F. J. Dixon, and A. N. Theofilopoulos. 1987. The genetic origin of autoantibodies. *Immunol. Today, 8*: 374–379.
92. Sanz, I., P. Kally, C. Williams, S. Scholl, P. Tucker, and J. D. Capra. 1989. The smaller human V_H gene families display remarkably little polymorphism. *EMBO J., 8*: 3741–3748.
93. Dijk, K. W. V., H. W. Schroeder, R. M. Perlmutter, and E. C. B. Milner. 1989. Heterogenity in the human IgV_H locus. *J. Immunol., 142*: 2547–2554.
94. Zouali, M., M. P. Madaio, R. T. Canoso, and B. D. Stollar. 1989. Restriction fragment analysis of the V locus in human lupus. *Eur. J. Immunol., 19*: 1757–1760.
95. Edelman, G. M., and P. D. Gottlieb. 1970. A genetic marker in the variable region of light chains of mouse immunoglobulin. *Proc. Natl. Acad. Sci. USA, 67*: 1192–1199.
96. Gibson, D. M., and S. J. Maclean. 1979. Ef2: A new Ly-3-linked light chain marker expressed in normal mouse serum immunoglobulin. *J. Exp. Med., 149*: 1477–1486.
97. Gibson, D. M. 1984. Evidence for 65 electrophoretically distinct groups of light chains in Balb/c and NZB myeloma. *Mol. Immunol., 21*: 421–432.
98. Huppi, K., E. Jouvin-Marche, C. Scott, M. Potter, and M. Weigert. 1985. Genetic polymorphism at the K chain locus in mice: Comparison of restriction enzyme hybridization fragments of variable and constant region genes. *Immunogenetics, 21*: 445–447.
99. Laskin, J. A., A. Gray, A. Nisoff, N. R. Klinman, and P. D. Gottlieb. 1977. Segregation at a locus determining an immunoglobulin genetic marker for the light chain variable region affects inheritance of expression of an idiotype. *Proc. Natl. Acad. Sci. USA, 74*: 4600–4604.
100. Claflin, J. L. 1976. Genetic marker in the variable region of kappa chains of mouse anti-phosphorylcholine antibodies. *Eur. J. Immunol., 6*: 666–668.
101. Goldrick, M. M., R. T. Boyd, P. D. Ponath, S. Y. Lou, and P. D. Gottlieb. 1985. Molecular genetic analysis of the V_K ser group associated with two mouse light chain genetic markers. *J. Exp. Med., 162*: 713–728.
102. Lazure, C., W. T. Hum, and D. M. Gibson. 1981. Sequence diversity within a subgroup of mouse immunoglobulin kappa chains controlled by the Igk-Ef2 locus. *J. Exp. Med., 154*: 146–155.

103. Bona, C. A. 1988. V genes encoding autoantibodies: Molecular and phenotypic characteristics, *Ann. Rev. Immunol.*, *6*: 327–358.

104. Wu, G., and C. Paige. 1986. V_H gene family utilization in colonies derived from B and pre-B cells detected by the RNA colony blot assay. *EMBO J.*, *5*: 3475–3481.

105. Schulze, D. H., and G. Kelsoe. 1987. Genotypic analysis of B cell colonies by in situ hybridization. Stoichiometric expression of three V_H families in adult C57 BL/6 and Balb/c mice. *J. Exp. Med.*, *166*: 163.

106. Dildrop, R., V. Krawinkel, E. Winter, and K. Rajewski. 1985. V_H gene expression in murine lipopolysaccharide blasts distributes over nine known V_H gene groups and may be random. *Eur. J. Immunol.*, *15*: 1154–1156.

107. Yancopoulos, G., D. S. V. Desiderio, M. Paskind, J. F. Kearney, D. Baltimore, and F. W. Alt. 1984. Preferential utilization of the most J_H proximal V_H gene segments in pre-B cell lines. *Nature*, *311*: 727–733.

108. Perlmutter, R. M., J. F. Kearney, S. P. Chang, and L. E. Hood. 1985. Developmentally controlled expression of Ig V_H genes. *Science*, *227*: 1597–1600.

109. Jeong, H. D., and J. M. Teale. 1988. Comparison of the fetal and adult functional B cell repertoires by analysis of V_H gene family expression. *J. Exp. Med.*, *168*: 589-603.

110. Yancopoulos, G. D., B. A. Malynn, and F. W. Alt. 1988. Developmentally regulated and strain specific expression of murine V_H gene families. *J. Exp. Med.*, *168*: 417–435.

111. Borriero, L., C. Giorgetti, G. Smith, D. Landry, E. Selsing, E. Zhukovsky, and J. L. Press. 1990. Neonatal and adult primary B cells use the same germ-line V_H and V_K genes in their (T.G)-A-L specific repertoire. *J. Immunol.*, *144*: 583–592.

112. Kaushik, A., D. H. Schulze, C. Bona, and G. Kelsoe. 1989. Murine V_K gene expression does not follow the V paradigm. *J. Ex. Med.*, *169*: 1859–1864.

113. Lawler, A. M., J. F. Kearney, M. Kuehl, and P. J. Gearhart. 1989. Early arrangements of genes encoding murine immunoglobulin K chains, unlike genes encoding heavy chains, use variable gene segments dispersed throughout the locus. *Proc. Natl. Acad. Sci. USA*, *86*: 6744–6747.

114. Ollo, R., C. Auffray, J. L. Sikorar, and F. Rugeon. 1981. Mouse heavy chain variable regions: nucleotide sequence of germ-line V_H gene segment. *Nucleic Acid Res.*, *9*: 4099–4109.

115. LeGrain, P., J. Rocea-Serra, A. Moulin, M. Fougereau, and G. Buttin. 1985. A single V_H-gene associated with a variety of D and J_H segments encodes for a large family of ABPC-48 related antibodies induced by antiidiotypic immunization. *Mol. Immunol.*, *22*: 437–443.

116. Rudikoff, S., M. Paulita, J. Pumphrey, E. Mulhinski, and M. Potter. 1983. Galactan binding antibodies: Diversity and structure of idiotypes. *J. Exp. Med.*, *158*: 1385–1400.

117. Borden, P., and E. A. Kabat. 1987. Nucleotide sequence of the cDNAs encoding the variable region heavy and light chains of myeloma protein specific for the terminal non-reducing end of (I-6) dextran. *Proc. Natl. Acad. Sci. USA*, *84*: 2440–2443.

118. Matsuda, T., and E. A. Kabat. 1989. Variable region cDNA sequence and antigen binding specificity of mouse monoclonal antibodies to isomaltosyl oligosaccharides coupled to proteins. *J. Immunol.*, *142*: 863–870.

119. Kimura, H., E. S. Buescher, E. D. Ball, and D. M. Marcus. 1989. Restricted usage of V_H and V_K genes by murine monoclonal antibodies against 3 fucosyllactosamine. *Eur. J. Immunol., 19*: 1741–1746.
120. Smith Gill, S. J., C. R. Mainhart, T. B. Lavoie, S. Rudikoff, and M. Potter. 1984. V_L, V_H expression by monoclonal antibodies recognizing avian lysozyme. *J. Immunol., 132*: 963–967.
121. Smith Gill, S. J., P. A. Hamel, T. B. Lavoie, and K. J. Dorrington. 1987. Contributions of immunoglobulin heavy and light chains to antibody specificity for lysozyme and two haptens. *J. Immunol., 139*: 4135–4144.
122. Manheimer-Lory, A. J., M. Monestier, B. Bellon, F. W. Alt, and C. A. Bona. 1986. Fine specificity, idiotypy and nature of cloned V_H genes of murine monoclonal rheumatoid factor antibodies. *Proc. Natl. Acad. Sci. USA, 83*: 8293–8297.
123. Klinman, D. M., R. A. Eisenberg, and A. D. Steinberg. 1990. Development of the autoimmune B cell repertoire in MRL-lpr/lpr mice. *J. Immunol., 144*: 506–511.
124. Arant, S. E., J. A. Griffin, and W. J. Koopman. 1986. V_H gene expression is restricted in anti-IgG antibodies from MRL autoimmune mice. *J. Exp. Med., 164*: 1286–1300.
125. Reininger, L., A. Kaushik, S. Izui, and J. C. Jaton. 1988. A member of a new V_H gene family encodes antibromelainized mouse red blood cell autoantibodies. *Eur. J. Immunol., 18*: 1521–1526.
126. Painter, C. J., M. Monestier, A. Chew, A. Dimitriu-Bona, K. Kasturi, C. Bailey, V. E. Scott, C. L. Sidman, and C. A. Bona. 1988. Specificities and V genes encoding monoclonal autoantibodies from viable motheaten mice. *J. Exp. Med., 167*: 1137–1153.
127. Duchosal, M. A., R. Kofler, R. S. Balderas, M. T. Aguado, F. J. Dixon, and A. N. Theofilopoulos. 1989. Genetic diversity of murine rheumatoid factors. *J. Immunol., 142*: 1737–1742.
128. Lawler, A. M., P. S. Lin, and P. J. Gearhart. 1987. Adult B cell repertoire is biased toward two heavy chain variable region genes that rearrange frequently in fetal pre-B cells. *Proc. Natl. Acad. Sci. USA, 84*: 2454–2458.
129. Shlomchik, M. J., D. Nemazee, V. Sato, J. Van Snick, D. Carson, and M. G. Weigert. 1986. Variable region sequences of murine IgM anti-IgG monoclonal autoantibodies rheumatoid factors: A structural explanation for the high frequency of IgM anti-IgG B cells. *J. Exp. Med., 164*: 407–427.
130. Marion, T. N., A. L. M. Bothwell, and C. A. Janeway, Jr. 1987. Molecular analysis of heavy chain variable region genes that encode the shared DNA 3 idiotype among murine nucleic acid autoantibodies. *Fed. Proc., 46*: 487.
131. Adams, D. D. 1983. *Autoimmune Mechanisms in Autoimmune Endocrine Diseases*. Wiley, New York.
132. Goni, F., P. P. Chen, B. Pon-Estel, D. A. Carson, and B. Frangione. 1985. Sequence similarities and cross-idiotypic specificity of L chains among human monoclonal IgMk with anti-globulin activity. *J. Immunol., 135*: 4073–4079.
133. Dehoratius, R. J., and R. P. Messner. 1975. Lymphocytotoxic antibodies in family members of patients with systemic lupus erythematosus. *J. Clin. Invest., 55*: 1254–1258.

134. Naparstek, Y., D. Duggen, A. Schattner, M. P. Madaio, F. Goni, B. Frangione, D. Stollar, E. A. Kabat, and R. S. Schwartz. 1985. Immunochemical similarities between monoclonal antibacterial waldenstrom's macroglobulins and monoclonal anti-DNA lupus autoantibodies. *J. Exp. Med., 161*: 1525–1538.
135. Shoenfeld, Y., and D. Isenberg. 1988. Mycobacteria and autoimmunity. *Immunol. Today, 9*: 178–182.
136. Avrameas, S., G. Dighiero, P. Lymberi, and B. Guilbert. 1983. Studies on natural antibodies and autoantibodies. *Ann. Immunol.* (Inst. Pasteur), *134D*: 103–113.
137. Cairns, E., J. St. Germain, and D. A. Bell. 1985. The *in vitro* production of anti-DNA antibody by cultured peripheral blood or tonsillar lymphoid cells from normal donors and SLE patients. *J. Immunol., 135*: 3839–3844.
138. Van Eden, W., J. E. R. Thole, R. Van Der Zee, A. Noodzij, J. D. A. Van Embden, E. J. Hensen, and I. R. Cohen. 1988. Cloning of the mycobacterial epitope recognized by T lymphocytes in adjuvant arthritis. *Nature, 331*: 171–172.
139. Roudier, J., G. Rhodes, J. Peterson, J. H. Vaughan, D. A. Carson. 1988. Hypothesis, the Epstein-Barr virus glycoprotein gp110, a molecular link between HLA DR2, HLA DR1 and rheumatoid arthritis. *Scand. J. Immunol., 27*: 367–372.
140. Maul, G. G., S. A. Jimenez, E. Riggs, and Z. Kokula. 1989. Determination of an epitope of the diffuse systemic sclerosis marker antigen, DNA topoisomerase I: Sequence similarity with retroviral P^{30gag} protein suggests a possible cause for autoimmunity in systemic sclerosis. *Proc. Natl. Acad. Sci. USA, 86*: 8492–8496.
141. Query, C. C., and J. D. Keene. 1987. A human autoimmune protein associated with U1 RNA contains a region of homology that is cross-reactive with a retroviral p^{30gag} antigen. *Cell, 51*: 211–220.
142. Richert, J. R., C. A. Reuben Burnside, G. E. Deibler, and M. W. Kies. 1988. Peptide specificities of myelin basic protein reactive human T cell clones. *Neurol., 38*: 739–742.
143. Diamond, B., and M. D. Scharff. 1984. Somatic mutation of the T15 heavy chain gene gives rise to an antibody with autoantibody specificity. *Proc. Natl. Acad. Sci. USA, 81*: 5841–5844.
144. Giusti, A. M., N. C. Chien, D. J. Zack, S. V. Shin, and M. D. Schraff. 1987. Somatic diversification of S107 from an anti-phosphocholine to an anti-DNA autoantibody is due to a single base change in its heavy chain variable region. *Proc. Natl. Acad. Sci. USA, 84*: 2926–2930.
145. Zanetti, M., J. Rogers, and A. H. Katz. 1984. Induction of autoantibodies to thyroglobulin by anti-idiotype antibodies. *J. Immunol., 133*: 240–243.
146. Monestier, M., B. Bonin, P. Migliorinini, H. Dang, S. Datta, R. Kuppers, N. Rose, P. Maurer, N. Talal, and C. Bona. 1987. Autoantibodies of various specificities encoded by genes from V J558 family bind to foreign antigens and share idiotopes of antibodies specific for self and foreign antigens. *J. Exp. Med., 166*: 1109–1124.
147. Vakil, M., and J. F. Kearney. 1988. Regulatory influences of neonatal multispecific antibodies on developing B cell repertoire. *Int. Rev. Immunol., 3*: 117–131.
148. Madaio, M. P., A. Schattner, M. Schattner, and R. S. Schwartz. 1986. Lupus serum and normal human serum contain anti-DNA antibodies with the same idiotypic marker. *J. Immunol., 137*: 2535–2540.

149. Bona, C. A., C. Y. Yang, H. Kohler, and M. Monestier. 1986. Epibody: The image of network created by a single antibody. *Immunol. Rev.*, *90*: 115-128.
150. Hayakawa, K., R. R. Hardy, M. Honda, L. A. Herzenberg, A. D. Steinberg, and L. A. Herzenberg. 1984. Ly1-B cells: Functionally distinct lymphocytes that secrete IgM autoantibodies, *Proc. Natl. Acad. Sci. USA*, *81*: 2494–2498.
151. Casali, P., G. Inghirami, M. Kamura, T. F. Davies, and A. L. Notkins. 1986. Human monoclonals from antigen-specific selection of lymphocytes and transformation by EBV. *Science*, *234*: 476–479.
152. Casali, P., B. S. Prabhakar, and A. L. Notkins. 1988. Characterization of multireactive autoantibodies and identification of Leu1+ B lymphocytes as cells making self and exogenous molecules. *Int. Rev. Immunol.*, *3*: 17–45.
153. Casali, P., and A. L. Notkins. 1989. CD5+ B lymphocytes, polyreactive antibodies and the human B-cell repertoire. *Immunol. Today*, *10*: 364–368.
154. Forster, I., H. Gu, and K. Rajewsky. 1988. Germline antibody V regions as determinants of clonal persistence and malignant growth in the B cell compartment. *EMBO J.*, *7*: 3693-3703.
155. Reninger, L., P. Ollier, P. Poncet, A. Kaushik, and J. C. Jaton. 1987. Novel V genes encode virtually identical variable regions of six murine monoclonal anti-bromelain-treated red blood cell autoantibodies. *J. Immunol.*, *138*: 316–323.
156. Naparstek, Y., J. Andre-Schwartz, T. Manser, L. J. Wysocki, L. Breitman, B. D. Stollar, M. Gefter, and R. S. Schwartz. 1986. A single germline V_H gene segment of normal A/J mice encodes autoantibodies characteristic of systemic lupus erythematosus. *J. Exp. Med.*, *164*: 614-626.
157. Ternynck, T., and S. Avrameas. 1986. Murine natural monoclonal autoantibodies: A study of their polyspecificities and their affinities. *Immunol. Rev.*, *94*: 99–112.
158. Lutz, H. V., R. Flepp, and G. Wipf. 1984. Naturally occurring autoantibodies to exoplasmic and cryptic regions of band 3 protein: The major integral membrane protein of human red blood cells. *J. Immunol.*, *133*: 2610-2618.
159. Kaushik, A., P. Poncet, and A. Bussard. 1986. Autoantibodies against bromelainized mouse erythrocyte: Strain distribution of idiotype expression and relative peritoneal cell activity. *Cell. Immunol.*, *102*: 323-334.
160. Klinman, D. M., S. Banks, A. Hartman, A. D. Steinberg. 1988. Natural murine autoantibodies and conventional antibodies exhibit similar degree of antigenic cross-reactivity. *J. Clin. Invest.*, *82*: 652–657.
161. Schwartz, R. S. 1988. Polyvalent anti-DNA autoantibodies: Immunochemical and biologicval significance. *Int. Rev. Immunol.*, *3*: 97–115.
162. Grabar, P. 1975. Autoantibodies and immunological theories: An analytical review. *Clin. Immunol. and Immunopathol.*, *4*: 453–466.
163. Garbar, P. 1983. Autoantibodies and physiological role of immunoglobulins. *Immunol. Today*, *14*: 337.
164. Cohen, I. R., and A. Cooke. 1986. Natural autoantibodies might prevent autoimmune disease. *Immunol. Today*, *7*: 363–364.
165. Baccala, R., Quang, V., B. Guilbert, T. Ternynck, and S. Avrameas. 1989. Two murine natural polyreactive autoantibodies are encoded by non-mutated germline genes. *Proc. Natl. Acad. Sci. USA*, *86*: 4624–4628.

166. Strickland, F. M., J. T. Gleason, and J. Cerny. 1987. Re-expression of a T15 idiotope on variant immunoglobulins after the binding of another anti idiotypic antibody. *J. Immunol.*, *138*: 3868–3872.
167. Theofilopoulos, A. N., R. S. Balderas, L. Hang, and F. J. Dixon. 1983. Monoclonal IgM rheumatoid factors derived from arthritic MRL/Mp-lpr/lpr mice. *J. Exp. Med.*, *158*: 901–919.
168. Pollard, K. M., J. E. Jones, E. M. Tan, A. N. Theofilopoulos, F. J. Dixon, and R. L. Rubin. 1986. Polynucleotide specificities of murine monoclonal anti-DNA antibodies. *Clin. Immunol. Immunopathol.*, *40*: 197–208.
169. Conger, J. D., B. L. Pike, and G. J. V. Nossal. 1987. Clonal analysis of the anti-DNA repertoire of murine B lymphocytes. *Proc. Natl. Acad. Sci. USA*, *94*: 2931–2935.
170. Souroujon, M., M. E. White-Scharf, A. Schwartz, L. M. Gefter, and R. S. Schwartz. 1988. Preferential autoantibody reactivity of preimmune B cell repertoire in normal mice. *J. Immunol.*, *140*: 4173–4179.
171. Atkinson, P. M., G. W. Lampman, B. C. Furie, Y. Naparstek, R. S. Schwartz, B. D. Stollar, and B. Furie. 1985. Homology of the NH2-terminal amino-acid sequences of the heavy and light chains of human monoclonal lupus autoantibodies containing the dominant 16/6 idiotype. *J. Clin. Invest.*, *75*: 1138–1143.
172. Dersimonian, H., R. S. Schwartz, K. J. Barnett, and B. D. Stollar. 1987. Relationship of human variable region heavy chain germ-line genes to genes encoding anti-DNA autoantibodies. *J. Immunol.*, *139*: 2496–2501.
173. Clarke, S. H., K. Huppi, D. Ruezinsky, L. Staudt, W. Gerhard, and M. Weigert. 1985. Inter and intra-clonal diversity in the antibody response to influenza hemagglutinin. *J. Ex. Med.*, *161*: 687–704.
174. Caton, A. J., G. G. Brownlee, L. M. Staudt, and W. Gerhard. 1986. Structural and functional implications of a restricted antibody response to a defined antigenic region on the influenza virus hemagglutinin. *EMBO J.*, *5*: 1577–1587.
175. Siekevitz, M., C. Kocks, K. Rajewsky, and R. Dildrop. 1987. Analysis of somatic mutation and class switching in naive and memory B cells generating adoptive primary and secondary responses. *Cell*, *48*: 757–770.
176. Eilat, D., D. M. Webster, and A. R. Rees. 1988. V-region sequences of anti-DNA and anti-RNA autoantibodies from NZB/NZW F1 mice. *J. Immunol.*, *141*: 1745–1753.
177. Madaio, M. P., A. Schattner, M. Shattner, and R. S. Schwartz. 1986. Lupus serum and normal human serum contain anti DNA antibodies with the same idiotypic marker. *J. Immunol.*, *137*: 2535–2540.
178. Andrezejewski, C., J. Rauch, E. Lafer, B. D. Stollar, and R. S. Schwartz. 1981. Antigen binding diversity and idiotypic cross-reactive among hybridoma autoantibodies to DNA. *J. Immunol.*, *126*: 226–231.
179. Kasturi, K. N., R. Mayer, C. A. Bona, V. G. Scott, and C. L. Sidman. 1990, Germline genes encode viable molteaten mouse autoantibodies against thymocytes and red blood cells. *J. Immunol.* *145*, 2304–2311.

7

Immunoglobulin Variable Gene Expression in Human Autoantibodies

J. H. van Es, M. E. M. Schutte, S. B. Ebeling, F. H. J. Gmelig-Meyling, and T. Logtenberg
University Hospital Utrecht, Utrecht, The Netherlands

I. INTRODUCTION

Probably the most impressive characteristic of the immune system is its ability to recognize and interact with a virtually unlimited variety of foreign antigens while simultaneously maintaining a state of nonresponsiveness towards self antigens. For a long time, lack of responsiveness to the body's own constituents was believed to depend on the physical or functional elimination of self-reactive lymphocytes. However, the concepts of clonal deletion and clonal anergy have come under severe attack in recent years. Lymphocytes reactive with self antigens are now believed to be present in all healthy individuals and may, according to current views, even be in a nonresting state.

Most immunologists accept that there are no structural differences between foreign and self antigens that could account for the immune system's capacity to discriminate between self and nonself. The central enigma is obvious: How does the immune system generate its enormous recognition potential, necessary for the elimination of a large number of foreign antigens, while simultaneously preventing the generation of harmful responses against self antigens? The clue to this question may be found by studying the processes that govern the generation of the B- and T-cell receptor repertoires from germline-encoded elements (the preimmune repertoire) and the subsequent utilization of these repertoires in normal and autoimmune responses.

We will summarize current data concerning the organization and expression of the DNA elements that encode the immunoglobulin receptor on human B cells. Particularly, we will focus on the expression of the immunoglobulin heavy- and light-chain variable-region genes expressed in the preimmune B-cell repertoire and in human autoantibodies derived from healthy individuals and patients with autoimmune disease.

II. ORGANIZATION OF THE HUMAN IMMUNOGLOBULIN V_H LOCUS

The antigen-binding region of immunoglobulin heavy (H) and light (L) chains are assembled from three (VDJ) or respectively two (VJ) germline DNA elements: V(ariable), D(iversity), and J(oining) segments (1). During precursor B-cell differentiation, these gene segments are somatically recombined to form a functional complex. The combinatorial assortment of the various elements present in the germline, the variability generated at the junctions, and somatic mutations all contribute to the diversification of the antibody repertoire (reviewed in Ref. 2).

The human V_H locus on chromosome 14 contains 100–200 gene segments that have been grouped into six families (denoted V_H1 to V_H6) that range in size from one member (V_H6) to at least 25 members (V_H3). The V_H6 gene segment is positioned at the 3′ end of the locus, 77 kb on the 5′ side of the cluster of J_H minigenes (3–5). Members of the other families are interspersed over the entire 2000 kb locus.

Several approaches have been taken to investigate polymorphisms of the human V_H locus. Direct cloning and sequencing of members of the smaller V_H gene families (V_H4, V_H5, and V_H6) from different individuals revealed remarkably little polymorphism (6,7). In addition, some members of the V_H3 gene family have been repeatedly cloned from the germline or from the expressed V_H repertoire of unrelated individuals (3,8–13). In contrast, studies employing V_H-specific oligonucleotide probes indicate that some members of the V_H3 gene family may be highly polymorphic, whereas other members are remarkably well conserved (14–16). Based on these observations, it is likely that at least a number of individual V_H elements belonging to different families are extremely well conserved in the outbred human population. The strong conservation of these elements in the germline may be indicative of an as yet unknown important physiologic role of the antibody variable region encoded by these V_H genes.

III. EXPRESSION OF VARIABLE REGION GENES DURING HUMAN B-CELL ONTOGENY

The frequency of utilization of V_H gene family members during B-cell ontogeny has been studied in various ways. Analysis of a collection of 15 cDNA clones from 130-day-old human fetal liver revealed usage of a restricted set of V_H elements derived from the large V_H3 family (13). These elements are closely related to the V_H segments expressed in developing murine B-lineage cells. This limited choice of V_H elements was interpreted as reflecting a developmentally ordered process of V_H gene utilization in humans. We have assayed the V_H gene families expressed by individual members of a collection of 187 monoclonal, IgM-secreting Epstein-Barr virus (EBV)–transformed cell lines derived from adult peripheral blood and 19-week-old fetal liver and spleen. We did not detect significant differences in frequencies of V_H gene utilization in fetal and adult tissue-derived collections. In both collections, the frequency of V_H gene family utilization correlated roughly with the complexity of the family (Table 1) (17), indicating that the repertoire is randomized in B lymphocytes that are the target for EBV transformation. Importantly, this analysis does not permit detection of qualitative differences between the collections of V_H genes expressed from multimembered families. For instance, although the frequency of V_H3 gene family usage may be the same by analysis in Northern blotting, adult and fetal collections might utilize different members of this family.

In another approach, we assayed the relative utilization of V_H gene families in fetal liver and spleen and in adult peripheral blood (18). This type of study permits the assessment of the total amount of V_H gene family–specific mRNA relative to the total amount of μ message in these tissues (19). Thus, in contrast to the study of IgM-secreting cell lines, this type of analysis includes mRNA derived from more immature B-lineage cells. Again, the V_H3 family appeared to be equally represented in the fetal and adult repertoires. On the other hand, these experiments revealed that the most J_H-proximal V_H6 gene was more abundantly expressed in fetal liver than in adult peripheral blood lymphocytes. Taken together, these results suggest that in humans, just as in mice (2), an initially position-dependent repertoire is generated during B-cell ontogeny but that this repertoire is normalized in mature B lymphocytes.

IV. NATURAL AND PATHOGENIC AUTOANTIBODIES

A central question in the pathogenesis of systemic autoimmune diseases such as systemic lupus erythematosus (SLE) is the origin of autoantibodies present in the sera of the patients. Several mechanisms have been proposed to explain the generation of such pathogenic autoantibodies. They may arise through polyclonal B-cell activation, resulting in the overproduction of antibodies, including

TABLE 1 Frequency of V_H Gene Utilization in Human EBV-Transformed Cell Lines and in CLL B-Cells[a]

	EBV cell lines				
	adult (n = 97)	fetal (n = 90)	CD5+ (n = 12)	CLL (n = 24)	Complexity no. of bands (%)
V_H1	15	20	8	<5	20–25 (33)
V_H2	<5	<5	8	<5	5–10 (11)
V_H3	60	60	16	15	25–30 (40)
V_H4	20	10	34	50	6–10 (11)
V_H5	5	<5	26	20	2–3 (4)
V_H6	<5	<5	8	15	1 (1)

[a]Data are presented as the percentage of the total number of cell lines in a given collection that hybridizes to a V_H gene family-specific probe. Complexity is defined as the number of V_H-hybridizing bands on a Southern blot (4).
n = number of samples analyzed.

autoantibodies (20). This model denies a role for (auto)antigen in the induction of the autoimmune response and predicts the existence of a polyclonally activated population of B cells, expressing unmutated or randomly mutated V-region genes. This hypothesis is consistent with the B-cell hyperactivity seen in patients with active SLE. Alternatively, pathogenic autoantibodies may arise after antigenic stimulation of a limited set of B cells. In this scenario, (auto)antigens may initially activate an oligoclonal population of B cells, which, through the process of somatic mutation and (auto)antigen selection, results in expansion of B cells that produce highly specific autoantibodies (29). Finally, pathogenic autoantibodies may arise after an initial polyclonal activation of B cells, followed by a process of (auto)antigen induction and selection (21,22). Recently, it has been shown that autoantibodies are not uniquely present in the sera of patients with autoimmune disease. Naturally occurring autoantibodies are found in the sera of all healthy individuals. They are predominantly of the IgM class and often cross-react with a number of structurally unrelated, auto- and xenoantigens (reviewed in Ref. 23). This particular property has earned them the label "polyreactive antibodies." Natural autoantibodies are not deleterious to the individual and thus seem to be functionally different from pathogenic autoantibodies associated with autoimmune disease. The biological role of natural autoantibodies is unclear, as is their relationship with pathogenic autoantibodies; isotype (24), charge (25), and affinity (26) have been implicated to explain the difference between these two types of autoantibodies. Currently, much research is aimed at elucidating the genetic and structural basis of both natural and pathogenic autoantibodies.

V. V_H GENE EXPRESSION IN HUMAN AUTOANTIBODIES

Several questions related to the mechanisms that are involved in the generation of natural and pathogenic human autoantibodies can be addressed by molecular genetic analysis of the V_H and V_L genes expressed in these two types of autoantibodies. These questions are: (1) may the germline contain coding information for autoantibodies and, if so, (2) is this coding information present in the germline of every individual; (3) do autoantibodies utilize the whole repertoire of available germline V elements or, alternatively, is there a restricted set of "autoantibody" V genes, possibly located at the 3′ end of the V_H locus; (4) what is the relationship between pathogenic and natural autoantibodies at the level of the expressed V regions; and (5) is the structure of the V_H and V_L elements in pathogenic autoantibodies indicative of polyclonal or antigen-driven responses? Several attempts have been made to address some of these questions in humans.

The presence of natural autoantibodies in preimmune sera of all individuals suggested that the gene segments encoding natural autoantibodies are normal constituents of the germline repertoire of V genes. In humans, direct evidence for this hypothesis came from nucleotide sequence analysis of the V gene elements expressed in autoantibodies secreted by hybridomas or EBV-transformed cell lines derived from normal adult or fetal tissues (6,9,10). In a number of independent cases, members of the V_H3 and V_H6 gene families, expressed in IgM autoantibodies with binding characteristics reminiscent of those diagnostic for SLE (anti-DNA and anti-Sm), were found to share 100% nucleotide sequence homology with previously cloned germline V_H genes of unrelated individuals.

In an attempt to correlate autoantibody reactivity with expression of certain V_H gene families, we have analyzed V_H gene utilization in a collection of nearly 200 monoclonal, IgM-secreting EBV-transformed cell lines, derived from adult peripheral blood and 19-week-old fetal liver and spleen. In addition, we have studied the antibodies secreted by these cell lines for reactivity against a panel of 24 (auto)antigens (6). There was no obvious correlation between antigen-binding patterns and expression of V_H segments from families 1–5. Again, this type of analysis does not reveal correlations between the expression of single members of a multigene family such as V_H3 and autoantibody reactivity. In contrast, it was noted that antibodies encoded by the most J_H-proximal V_H6 gene segment all bound to single-stranded DNA and, in addition, displayed various binding activities with other polynucleotides, cardiolipin, cytochrome *C*, and lysozyme (Table 2) (6). Such polyreactivity is a characteristic of some anti-DNA autoantibodies of both murine and human origin (27). These specificities were found to be encoded by the V_H6 gene, because the activity was found in multiple independent antibodies in which the light chain varied with respect to isotype and V_K subgroup (Table 2). Sequence analysis revealed that both germline and somatically mutated V_H6 genes (analyzed in fetal tissue– or blood lymphocyte–derived cell

TABLE 2 Origin, Isotype, and Antigen-Binding Pattern of V_H6-Expressing Cell Lines Derived from Healthy Subjects[a]

Clone	Origin	Isotype	ssDNA	nDNA	Card	Cyt c	Hel
A10	adult PB	IgM,K	+	+	+	−	+
A431	adult PB	IgM,L	+	+	+	+	−
L16	130 d FL	IgM,L	+	−	+	−	−
ML1	130 d FS	IgM,K	+	−	−	−	−

[a]Clones A10 and A431 were derived from different individuals. PB, peripheral blood; FL, fetal liver; FS, fetal spleen; K, kappa light chain; L, lambda light chain; Card, cardiolipin; Hel, hen egg lysozyme; Cyt c, cytochrome c.

lines, respectively) were expressed in these autoantibodies (Fig. 1). The pattern and extent of replacement mutations in A431 and A10 V_H regions suggested that these mutations were selected over multiple lymphocytic generations, characteristic of memory B cells (28). It is notable that the A10 and A431 antibodies bind to native DNA, a property not displayed by antibodies that express the germline V_H6 segments. This property may derive from the mutations and/or from light chains of these antibodies.

```
     1
GATACCACCGGAGAAATTGTGTTGACGCAGTCTCCAGGCACCCTGTCTTTGTCTCCAGGG  HIC
............................................................  T14

                     I--------------CDR1----------------I
GAAAGAGCCACCCTCTCCTGCAGGGCCAGTCAGAGTGTTAGCAGCAGCTACTTAGCCTGG  HIC
........................................C......G............  T14

                                          I---------CDR2----
TACCAGCAGAAACCTGGCCAGGCTCCCAGGCTCCTCATCTATGGTGCATCCAGCAGGGCC  HIC
...........G....C...........................................  T14

--I
ACTGGCATCCCAGACAGGTTCAGTGGCAGTGGGTCTGGGACAGACTTCACTCTCACCATC  HIC
............................................................  T14

                                        I------CDR3---------
AGCAGACTGGAGCCTGAAGATTTTGCAGTGTATTACTGTCAGCAGTATGGTAGCTCACCT  HIC
....................................................A.......  T14

-----------------JK1-------------------I------CK------
TGGACGTTCGGCCAAGGGACCAAGGTGGAAATCAAACGAACTGTGGCTGCACCA        HIC
......................................................        T14
```

FIGURE 1 Amino acid sequence comparison of the CDR1 and CDR2 regions of expressed V_H6 genes. The single-letter amino acid code is used. Dashes indicate identity with the sequence of cell line L16.

To further delineate the role of V_H6-encoded autoantibodies in B-cell ontogeny and in autoimmune disease, we developed a monoclonal antibody (MAb 4.89) that specifically recognizes antibodies that utilize the germline V_H6 gene segment (J. H. van Es et al., unpublished). This monoclonal antibody was used to analyze the supernatants of monoclonal, IgM-secreting, EBV-transformed B-cell lines derived from adult peripheral blood, cordblood and fetal tissues, and serum samples from neonates and healthy individuals and from patients with SLE for the presence of germline V_H6-encoded antibodies. The results of these experiments are summarized in Table 3. Supernatants from a small but significant percentage of fetal and neonatal EBV-transformed cell lines were found to react with MAb 4.89, whereas no reactivity was found in the supernatants of adult EBV-transformed B-cell lines. This result was consistent with our previous finding that V_H6-expressing cell lines derived from adult tissues showed evidence of somatic mutations, whereas V_H6-positive fetal tissue–derived cell lines were in germline configuration (Fig. 2). Moreover, sera from neonates but not from adults (whether healthy or diseases) showed reactivity with MAb 4.89. Together, these results indicate that B cells expressing germline V_H6 gene segments are present at a higher proportion in the fetal and neonatal B-cell repertoire than in the adult repertoire. These neonatal V_H6-expressing B cells are presumably in an activated state and secrete autoantibodies that contribute to the pool of natural autoantibodies in cordblood sera. Whether these antibodies are the precursors of pathogenic autoantibodies present in the sera of patients with SLE remains to be determined. In this context, it is noteworthy that the monoclonal autoantibody A10 (Table 2) bears an idiotype (16/6) associated with both natural and pathogenic autoantibodies (30, F. Young, unpublished).

Taken together, these results clearly show that natural autoantibodies from healthy individuals can be encoded by germline V_H genes. A number of these

TABLE 3 Presence of Germline V_H6-Encoded Antibodies in the Supernatant of EBV-Transformed B-Cell Lines[a]

	EBV cell lines	Serum
Fetal	5 (n = 241)	ND
Neonatal	5 (n = 270)	5 (n = 5)
Adult		
healthy individuals	0 (n = 320)	0 (n = 5)
SLE patients	0 (n = 141)	0 (n = 5)

[a]From different time points in the ontogeny (fetal, neonatal, adult) and in serum samples from healthy individuals (neonates and adults) and patients with SLE using a germline V_H6-specific MAb (MAb 4.89).

ND = not done.

n = number of samples analyzed.

```
                   CDR1                          CDR2
L16    .....SVS |SNSAAW| NWI.....EWL |GRTYYRSKWYNDYAVS| VKS.....
ML1    .....--- |------| ---.....--- |----------------| ---.....
A10    .....--- |-L----| ---.....--- |-----K----------| ---.....
A431   .....--- |----F-| ---.....--- |---------NTN----| ---.....
```

FIGURE 2 Comparison of the nucleotide sequence of the expressed V_KIIIb gene segment of an IgG anti-ssDNA antibody (T14) to the prototypic germline V_KIIIb gene expressed in the malignant B cells of a patient with CLL (HIC) (11). Dots indicate nucleotide identity. CDR, complementarity-determining region.

V_H regions are extremely well-conserved in the outbred human population. In addition, evidence for somatic mutations was found in the V_H6 gene segments encoding some of these natural autoantibodies. The question whether natural autoantibodies utilize a restricted set of V_H gene segments, possibly located at the 3′ end of the human V_H locus, cannot be answered at this time. More sequence data from V_H genes expressed in natural autoantibodies and a more detailed map of the human V_H locus are needed.

VI. V_L GENE EXPRESSION IN HUMAN AUTOANTIBODIES

Much of our knowledge of V_L gene expression in autoantibodies comes from a series of elegant experiments by Carson and colleagues on rheumatoid factors (RF). They developed a monoclonal anti-idiotypic antibody against a cryoglubulin with RF activity. In subsequent experiments, it was demonstrated that this monoclonal antibody 17.109 reacted with nearly 50% of human IgM paraproteins with RF activity, but not with IgM paraproteins without such a specificity, or substantially with normal pooled immunoglobulin or circulating B lymphocytes from normal adults (reviewed in Ref. 31). In addition, in 25% of patients with chronic lymphocytic leukemia (CLL) expressing kappa light chains, the malignant cells expressed the 17.109 idiotype (32). The structural basis of the 17.109 idiotype was shown to reside in the second and third complementary determining regions (CDRs) of a V_K gene segment belonging to the V_KIIIb subgroup. A germline V_KIIIb gene segment cloned from a placental library was shown to be identical or highly homologous to the V_K genes expressed in 17.109 positive CLL cells (32). Furthermore, this V_KIIIb gene segment appears to be well conserved in the human population. Because of its marked association with IgM autoantibodies with RF activity, this V_K gene has been designated V_K-RF. Although frequently expressed in CLL and in cryoglobulins with rheumatoid factor activity, its relationship with the rheumatoid factors found in patients with rheumatoid arthritis is unclear (33).

We recently cloned the expressed V_K light-chain gene from an EBV-transformed cell line (clone T14) derived from an SLE patient secreting an IgG anti-ssDNA autoantibody (37). The nucleotide sequence of this light chain showed >98.5% homology with the prototypic V_K-RF germline gene (Fig. 2). Strikingly, comparison of the CDR2 and CDR3 regions involved in expression of the 17.109 idiotype revealed only a single nucleotide difference in CDR2. To our knowledge, this is the first demonstration of the expression of V_K-RF in an IgG "pathogenic" autoantibody.

VII. THE CD5$^+$ B-CELL POPULATION: AUTOANTIBODIES AND V_H GENES

The CD5 (Leu-1) antigen was originally defined as a 67 kD glycoprotein expressed on all T cells. Subsequently, it was shown to be present on the malignant B cells in chronic lymphocytic leukemia (CLL). Furthermore, CD5 B cells are relatively abundant in early ontogeny and comprise a discrete subset of B cells in adult peripheral blood (reviewed in Ref. 34). Human CD5$^+$ B lymphocytes may represent an early stage in the ontogeny of mature B cells or, alternatively, may constitute a separate B-cell lineage, as has been suggested for the mouse equivalent of CD5$^+$ (Ly-1$^+$) B cells (35).

Analysis of the antibodies secreted by purified CD5$^+$ B cells from healthy individuals after in vitro stimulation with polyclonal B-cell activators revealed their capacity to bind to the autoantigens IgG (RF activity) and ssDNA (36,38). Subsequent analyses at the clonal level showed that in fact most of the CD5$^+$ B lymphocytes from healthy individuals, in contrast to CD5$^-$ B lymphocytes, secrete polyreactive antibodies, i.e., antibodies that bind to a number of unrelated antigens including self and foreign antigens (39). Moreover, polyreactive antibodies were detected after in vitro polyclonal activation of malignant CD5$^+$ B cells from patients with CLL (40). Furthermore, the rheumatoid factors produced by CD5$^+$ B cells from patients with rheumatoid arthritis were found to secrete both low-affinity polyreactive and high-affinity monoreactive rheumatoid factors (41), suggesting that the CD5$^+$ B cell may be involved in the production of pathogenic autoantibodies in this group of patients. In both normal and leukemic cells, polyreactive antibodies are predominantly of the IgM class, although other isotypes are present as well (40,42).

The presence of polyreactive antibodies in preimmune sera suggests that at least a portion of the CD5$^+$ B cells are activated and secrete Ig. The function of these naturally occurring polyreactive antibodies is presently unclear. A variety of stimuli, including viral and bacterial infections and deliberate immunizations with exogenous antigens, result in increased serum levels of polyreactive antibodies.

Several groups have studied frequencies of V_H gene families expressed in normal and malignant CD5$^+$ B cells. Initially, a member of the small V_H5 gene family was reported to be preferentially expressed in the malignant B cells of patients with CLL (42). This member was mapped to the 3′ end of the human V_H locus. We found an unexpectedly high frequency of expression of members of the V_H4, V_H5, and V_H6 gene families in human CLL cells (Table 1) (17). This held particularly for the V_H5 and V_H6 gene families, which together contain <5% of the known V_H genes, but accounted for nearly 40% of V_H gene expression in CLL cells. Similar patterns of restricted V_H gene utilization were demonstrated in a small panel of CD5-expressing EBV-transformed cell lines derived from healthy individuals (Table 1) (M.E.M. Schutte, *Eur. J. Immunol.* 1991, in press). Indeed, some but not all of these $CD5^+$ B-cell lines secrete polyreactive autoantibodies.

VIII. CONCLUSIONS

Current research on the origin of pathogenic and natural autoantibodies focuses on the V_H and V_L gene elements that are expressed in these two populations of autoantibodies. In a number of cases, it has been shown that germline V genes can encode IgM autoantibodies. Some of these V genes appear to be extremely well conserved in the human population, indicating a strong evolutionary pressure to preserve these elements. The physiologic role of these autoantibodies is unclear, as is their relationship with pathogenic autoantibodies. With the advancement of human monoclonal antibody technique, it has now become possible to investigate the antibody variable regions of pathogenic autoantibodies derived from patients with autoimmune disease. Comparison of these data with the accumulating body of data on V regions expressed in B-cell ontogeny, in different B-cell populations and in natural autoantibodies, will contribute to a better understanding of the processes involved in the generation of autoimmune disease.

ACKNOWLEDGMENTS

This work was supported by grants no. 900-507-113 and 9000-507-128 of The Netherlands Organization for the Advancement of Pure Research (NWO). T. L. is a fellow of the Royal Dutch Academy of Arts and Sciences.

REFERENCES

1. Tonegawa, S. 1983. Somatic generation of antibody diversity. *Nature, 302*: 575.
2. Alt, F. W., T. K. Blackwell, and G. D. Yancopoulos. 1987. Development of the primary antibody repertoire. *Science, 238*: 1097.
3. Berman, J. E., S. J. Mellis, R. Pollock, C. L. Smith, H. Suh, B. Heinke, C. Kowal, U. Surti, L. Chess, C. R. Cantor, and F. W. Alt. 1988. Content and organization

of the human Ig V_H locus: definition of three new V_H families and linkage to the Ig CH locus. *EMBO J.* *7*: 727.

4. Schroeder, H. W., M. A. Walter, M. H. Hofker, A. Ebens, K. W. van Dijk, L. C. Liao, D. W. Fox, E. C. B. Milner, and R. M. Perlmutter. 1988. Physical linkage of a human immunoglobulin heavy chain variable region gene segment to diversity and joining region elements. *Proc. Natl. Acad. Sci. USA, 85*: 8196.
5. Buluwela, L., and T. H. Rabbits. 1988. A V_H gene is located within 95 kb of the human immunoglobulin heavy chain constant region genes. *Eur. J. Immunol., 18*: 1843.
6. Logtenberg, T., F. M. Young, J. H. van Es, F. H. J. Gmelig Meyling, J. E. Bermann, and F. W. Alt. 1989. Autoantibodies encoded by the most JH-proximal human immunoglobulin heavy chain variable region gene. *J. Exp. Med., 170*: 1347.
7. Sanz, I., P. Kelley, C. Williams, S. Scholl, P. Tucker, and J. D. Capra. 1989. The smaller human V_H gene families display remarkably little polymorphism. *EMBO J., 8*: 3741.
8. Dermimonian, H., R. S. Schwartz, K. J. Barrett, and B. D. Stollar. 1987. Relationship of human variable region heavy chain germ-line genes to genes encoding anti-DNA autoantibodies. *J. Immunol., 139*: 2496.
9. Sanz, I., H. Dang, M. Takei, N. Talal, and J. D. Capra. 1989. V_H sequence of a human anti-Sm autoantibody. Evidence that autoantibodies can be unmutated copies of germline genes. *J. Immunol., 142*: 883.
10. Cairns, E., P. C. Kwong, V. Misener, P. Ip, D. A. Bell, and K. Siminovitch. 1989. Analysis of variable region genes encoding a human anti-DNA antibody of normal origin. *J. Immunol., 143*: 685.
11. Kipps, T. J., E. Tomhave, L. F. Pratt, S. Duffy, P. J. Chen, and D. A. Carson. 1989. Developmentally restricted immunoglobulin heavy chain variable region gene expressed at high frequency in chronic lymphocytic leukemia. *Proc. Natl. Acad. Sci. USA, 86*: 5913.
12. Matthyssens, G., and T. H. Rabbitts. 1980. Structure and multiplicity of genes for the human immunoglobulin heavy chain variable region. *Proc. Natl. Acad. Sci. USA, 77*: 6561.
13. Schroeder, Jr., H. W., J. L. Hillson, and R. M. Perlmutter. 1987. Early restriction of the human antibody repertoire. *Science, 338*: 791.
14. Willems van Dijk, K., H. W. Schroeder, R. M. Perlmutter, and E. C. B. Milner. 1989. Heterogeneity of the human Ig V_H locus. *J. Immunol., 142*: 2547.
15. Souroujon, M. C., D. B. Rubinstein, R. S. Schwartz, and K. J. Barrett. 1989. Polymorphisms in human H chain V region genes from the V_HIII gene family. *J. Immunol., 143*: 706.
16. Walter, M. A., P. S. Linsley, and D. W. Cox. 1987. ApaI polymorphism of a human immunoglobulin V_H3 subclass locus. *Nucleic Acids Research, 15*: 4697.
17. Logtenberg, T., M. E. M. Schutte, G. Inghirami, J. E. Berman, F. H. J. Gmelig Meyling, R. A. Insel, D. M. Knowles, and F. W. Alt. 1989. Immunoglobulin V_H gene expression in human B cell lines and tumors: Biased V_H gene expression in chronic lymphocytic leukemia. *International Immunology, 1*: 362.
18. Logtenberg, T., J. E. Berman, and F. W. Alt. 1990. Organization and expression of human V_H genes. In *Molecular Biology and Autoimmune Disease*.

19. Yancopoulos, G. D., B. A. Malynn, and F. W. Alt. 1988. Developmentally regulated and strain-specific expression of murine V_H gene families. *J. Exp. Med., 168*: 417.
20. Theophilopoulos, A. N., and F. J. Dixon. 1985. Murine models of systemic lupus erythematosus. *Adv. Immunol., 37*: 269.
21. Dziarski, R. 1988. Autoimmunity: Polyclonal activation or antigen induction. *Immunol. Today, 9*: 340.
22. Klinman, D. M., Y. Ishigatsubo, and A. D. Steinberg. 1988. Aquisition and maturation of expressed B cell repertoire in normal and autoimmune mice. *J. Immunol., 141*: 801.
23. Avrameas, S., B. Guilbert, W. Manaha, P. Matsiota, and T. Ternynck. 1988. Recognition of self and non-self constituents by polyspecific autoreceptors. *Int. Rev. Immunol., 3*: 1.
24. Schur, P. H., M. Monroe, and N. Rothfield. 1972. The τG subclass of antinuclear and antinucleic acid antibodies. *Arthritis Rheum., 25*: 174.
25. Ebling, F., and B. Hahn. 1980. Restricted subpopulations of DNA antibodies in kidneys of mice with systemic lupus. *Arthritis Rheum., 23*: 392.
26. Winfield, J. B., I. Faiferman, and D. Koffler. 1977. Avidity of anti-DNA antibodies in serum and IgG glomerular eluates in patients with systemic lupus erythematosus. Association of high avidity anti-native DNA antibody with glomerulo-nephritis. *J. Clin. Invest., 59*: 90.
27. Schwartz, R. S., and B. D. Stollar. 1985. Origins of anti-DNA autoantibodies. *J. Clin. Invest., 75*: 321.
28. Kocks, C., and K. Rajewski. 1989. Stable expression and somatic hypermutation of antibody V regions in B-cell developmental pathways. *Ann. Rev. Immunol., 7*: 537.
29. Schlomchik, M. J., A. H. Aucoin, D. S. Pisetsky, and M. G. Weigert. 1987. Structure and function of anti-DNA autoantibodies derived from a single autoimmune mouse. *Proc. Natl. Acad. Sci. USA, 84*: 9150.
30. Schoenfeld, Y., D. A. Isenberg, J. Rauch, M. P. Madaio, B. D. Stollar, and R. S. Schwartz. 1983. Idiotypic crossreactions of monoclonal human lupus autoantibodies. *J. Exp. Med., 158*: 718.
31. Carson, D. A., P. P. Chen, R. I. Fox, T. J. Kipps, F. Jirik, R. D. Goldfien, G. Silverman, V. Radoux, and S. Fong. 1987. Rheumatoid factors and immune networks. *Ann. Rev. Immunol., 5*: 109.
32. Kipps, T. J., S. Fong, E. Tomhave, P. P. Chen, R. D. Goldfien, and D. A. Carson. 1987. High-frequency expression of a conserved K light chain variable region gene in chronic lymphocytic leukemia. *Proc. Natl. Acad. Sci. USA, 84*: 2916.
33. Radoux, V., P. P. Chen, J. A. Sorge, and D. A. Carson. 1986. A conserved human germline V_K gene directly encodes rheumatoid factor light chains. *J. Exp. Med., 164*: 2119.
34. Hayakawa, K., and R. R. Hardy. 1988. Normal, autoimmune and malignant $CD5^+$ B cells: the Ly-1 B cell lineage. *Ann. Rev. Immunol., 6*: 197.
35. Herzenberg, L. A., A. M. Stall, P. A. Lalor, C. Sidman, W. A. Moore, and D. R. Parks. 1986. The Ly-1 B cell lineage. *Immunol. Rev., 93*: 81.
36. Hardy, R. R., K. Kayakawa, M. Shimizu, K. Yamasaki, and T. Kishimoto. 1987. Rheumatoid factor secretion from human Leu-1^+ B cells. *Science, 236*: 81.

37. van Es, J. H., F. H. J. Gmelig-Meyling, W. R. M. van de Akker, H. Aanstoot, R. M. W. M. Derksen, and T. Loglenberg. 1991. Somatic mutations in the variable regions of a human IgG anti-double-stranded DNA autoantibody suggest a role for antigen in the induction of SLE. *J. Exp. Med. 173*:461.
38. Casali, P., S. E. Burastero, M. Nakamura, G. Inghirami, and A. L. Notkins. 1987. Human lymphocytes making rheumatoid factor and antibody to ssDNA belong to $Leu1^+$ B cell-subset. *Science, 236*: 77.
39. Nakamura, M., S. E. Burastero, A. L. Notkins, and P. Casali. 1988. Human monoclonal rheumatoid factor-like antibodies from CD5 $(Leu\text{-}1)^+$ B cells are polyreactive. *J. Immunol., 140*: 4180.
40. Sthoeger, Z. M., M. Wakai, D. B. Tse, V. P. Viniciguerra, S. L. Allen, D. R. Budman, S. M. Lichtman, P. Schulman, L. R. Weiselberg, and N. Chiorazzi. 1989. Production of autoantibodies by CD5-expressing B lymphocytes from patients with chronic lymphocytic leukemia. *J. Exp. Med., 169*: 255.
41. Burastero, S. E., P. Casali, R. L. Wilder, and A. L. Notkins. 1988. Monoreactive high affinity and polyreactive low affinity rheumatoid factors are produced by $CD5^+$ B cells from patients with rheumatoid arthritis. *J. Exp. Med., 168*: 1979.
42. Casali, P., and A. L. Notkins. 1989. Probing the human B cell repertoire with Epstein-Barr virus: Polyreactive antibodies and $CD5^+$ lymphocytes. *Ann. Rev. Immunol., 7*: 513.
43. Humphries, C. G., A. Chen, W. A. Kuziel, J. D. Capra, F. R. Blattner, and P. W. Tucker. 1988. A new human immunoglobulin V_H family preferentially rearranged in immature B cell tumors. *Nature, 331*: 791.

8

Pathogenic Anti-DNA Autoantibodies and Pathogenic Autoantibody-Inducing T Cells

Syamal K. Datta, Sumati Rajagopalan, Theresa L. O'Keefe, Shibnath Ghatak, and Thereza Imanishi-Kari
Tufts–New England Medical Center, Boston, Massachusetts

I. INTRODUCTION

Systemic lupus erythematosus (SLE) is the prototypic *systemic* autoimmune disease characterized by a spontaneous production of autoantibodies to DNA. Although the primary antigens that trigger the autoimmune response in SLE are unknown, the anti-DNA autoantibodies play a major role in the pathogenesis of glomerulonephritis and other lesions of this disease (1,2). On the other hand, B cells of normal individuals and even normal fetal or newborn mice frequently produce antibodies that bind DNA (3–5). These types of antibodies are called *natural* autoantibodies. It is not clear if the *pathogenic* autoantibodies of SLE originate from natural autoantibodies, but they are certainly different from the latter in quality. Before we take up these issues, we shall discuss the significance of natural autoantibodies, particularly in the context of SLE.

II. NATURAL AUTOANTIBODIES, CD5$^+$ CELLS, AND POLYCLONAL B-CELL HYPERACTIVITY

Natural autoantibodies are IgM in class, and they are multispecific, cross-reacting with several autoantigens as well as exogenous antigens of common pathogenic microbes (3–5). An entire class of CD5$^+$ B lymphocytes (ly-1$^+$ in mice, Leu-1$^+$ in man) normally seems to be involved in making these natural autoantibodies (6–8). The natural autoantibodies usually have a weak affinity for autoantigens. Indeed, in certain cases the cross-reactivity of these antibodies for the autoantigens can be demonstrated only by using solid phase assays with very high, unphysiologic concentrations of the ligands (9,10). These observations suggest that natural autoantibodies may not be primarily directed against autoantigens. But the initial clue regarding the nature of these autoantibodies came from idiotypic analysis. The cross-reactive idiotypic (CRI) markers of certain IgM class anti-DNA antibodies were found to be shared by naturally occurring antibodies that were widely expressed in normal mice and humans, but the majority of those normal antibodies did not bind DNA (4,11,12). Such widely conserved public idiotypes are usually found in antibodies directed against common pathogens, and they can be shared by parallel sets of antibodies with differing specificities (11,13–15).

Following this clue, it was soon demonstrated that the variable regions of the IgM anti-DNA autoantibodies are encoded by unmutated germline genes, and they are closely related to antibodies with conserved germline idiotypes that are specific for common environmental pathogens (16–22). Indeed, these types of anti-DNA autoantibodies are not nephritogenic even when they are present at very high levels in serum, for instance in patients with monoclonal gammopathies or in normal mice injected with large doses of these autoantibodies (17,21,23,24). In SLE, due to polyclonal B-cell hyperactivity, high levels of natural anti-DNA autoantibodies are found to coexist with pathogenic autoantibodies. The conserved idiotypic markers of such natural autoantibodies can also be detected in the renal lesions of lupus, but again by using direct binding assays with very high concentrations of anti-idiotypic reagents (25). Moreover, the nature of the antibodies in the glomerular deposits that happen to share these idiotypic determinants has not been investigated. Those antibodies could have been secondarily deposited in preexisting renal lesions. Natural anti-DNA autoantibodies are known to share idiotypes with rheumatoid factors (22), and circulating rheumatoid factors can bind to the immune complexes deposited in the renal lesions of lupus nephritis (2). Thus, it is not clear whether the natural anti-DNA antibodies evolve into pathogenic autoantibodies. Indeed, the specificities of certain natural autoantibodies can be quite distinct from pathogenic autoantibodies. For instance, the Ly-1 B cells of both the autoimmune New Zealand Black (NZB) and normal mice produce a natural antierythrocyte antibody. This autoantibody binds to trimethylammonium groups in phosphatidyl choline determinants buried in the membranes of red cells, which can be exposed by limiting proteolysis with bromelain (26,27). This IgM autoantibody against bromelain-treated red cells is found in all mouse strains, and it probably helps in the removal of damaged or senescent red cells. This type of natural autoantibody is probably also directed against environmental pathogens, since phosphatidyl choline determinants are present in their membranes. By contrast, the pathogenic autoantibody responsible for autoimmune hemolytic anemia in NZB ice is IgG in isotype, its production is T-cell dependent, and it is specific for a glycoprotein exposed on the surface of autologous red cells (26,28). Recent studies have shown that the V genes encoding the natural anti-red cell autoantibodies can be different from those encoding the pathogenic anti-red cell autoantibodies (29,30). Another important feature of the Ly-1 B-cell–derived natural antierythrocyte autoantibodies is that they do not undergo somatic mutation, even after the B cells producing them have been expanded by hyperimmunization with the relevant antigens (27). By contrast, the variable regions of pathogenic autoantibodies show evidence of somatic mutation, as we shall describe later. Furthermore, genetic studies with the NZB crosses indicated that the mechanisms specific for the production of pathogenic autoantibodies are distinct from the Ly-1 B-cell hyperactivity in the NZB mice that result in excessive production of nonpathogenic (natural) autoantibodies (31–33). Indeed, the inheritance and expression of each type of pathogenic autoantibody can be independent of the other in NZB crosses. For instance, the nephritis-prone (NZB × SWR)F_1 mice uniformly produce pathogenic anti-DNA autoantibodies but not the pathogenic antierythrocyte autoantibodies that are characteristically expressed by their NZB parents (33). By contrast, (NZB × NZC)F_1 mice uniformly produce pathogenic (Coombs positive) antierythrocyte autoantibodies, but they rarely develop nephritis (34). Therefore, a generalized polyclonal B-cell abnormality is not the sole underlying mechanism of SLE since the autoimmune *disease* is not transmitted as one package. Discrete abnormalities specific for the regulation of each family of pathogenic autoantibody producing B cells appear to be operating in this disease.

III. PATHOGENIC ANTI-DNA AUTOANTIBODIES IN A MURINE MODEL OF LUPUS NEPHRITIS

The origins and nature of pathogenic anti-DNA autoantibodies were investigated in the NZB × SWR model of lupus nephritis. The NZB mice uniformly develop autoimmune hemolytic anemia, whereas lupus nephritis occurs rarely in this strain, an incidence of only 1% at 1 year of age. By contrast, when the autoimmune NZB mice are crossed with the normal SWR strain, 100% of the SNF_1 progeny die of accelerated lupus nephritis (33,35). The serum levels of anti-DNA autoantibodies are comparable in the NZB parental strain and the SNF_1 hybrids. However, the SNF_1 mice produce a select population of anti-DNA autoantibodies that are qualitatively different from the nonpathogenic anti-DNA antibodies produced by the NZB parents (36–38). Analysis of the autoantibodies eluted from the renal lesions of over 100 SNF_1 kidneys at different stages of nephritis revealed that the pathogenic autoantibodies that are predominantly deposited in the SNF_1 kidneys at the *initial* stages of nephritis are all IgG in isotype and are highly cationic in charge. By contrast, the anti-DNA autoantibodies produced by NZB mice are predominantly IgM in class and the rare IgG antibodies produced by these mice are all anionic in charge. In addition, these highly cationic, pathogenic autoantibodies of SNF_1 mice share a cross-reactive idiotype (CRI) called $Id^{LN}F_1$ (Idiotypes-Lupus Nephritis-F_1). The majority of monoclonal anti-DNA autoantibodies (MAbs) derived from different SNF_1 animals with nephritis also have antigenic specificity patterns, isotypes, cationic charge characteristics, and the $Id^{LN}F_1$ marker like the autoantibodies eluted from their renal lesions (36–38). These idiotypic relationships of the anti-DNA MAbs with the autoantibodies in the renal lesions of SNF_1 mice were determined by competition immunoassays in solution using highly diluted and specific anti-idiotypic reagents (37,38). Moreover, the $Id^{LN}F_1$-positive cationic anti-DNA MAbs produce typical lupus-like glomerular deposits and proteinuria when administered into young preautoimmune SNF_1 mice, but $Id^{LN}F_1$-negative anionic or neutral autoantibodies fail to do so. The pathogenic role of the highly cationic IgG anti-DNA autoantibodies in the SNF_1 mice is also supported by other studies. The onset of glomerulonephritis in several strains of lupus mice is accompanied by the production of this particular type of autoantibodies (38,40). B cells of the autoimmune NZB mice, which rarely develop nephritis, fail to produce IgG anti-DNA antibodies with cationic charge even upon polyclonal stimulation (39,41). Furthermore, IgG anti-DNA antibodies and immune complexes with cationic charge from persistent immune deposits in glomeruli when injected into normal mice, whereas anionic (or neutral) antibodies and immune complexes do not (24,42,43). And a minute population of cationic antibodies can mediate the glomerular deposition of immune complexes that are mainly composed of anionic or neutral antibodies (44). Thus, deposition of immune complexes containing cationic anti-DNA autoantibodies may initiate the renal lesions of SLE, which may then be followed by the deposition of neutral or anionic autoantibodies (38). This nephritogenic potential of cationic anti-DNA antibodies or cationic immune complexes probably arises from their affinity for the negatively charged proteoglycans that form anionic sites in the glomerular basement membranes (45,46).

The $Id^{LN}F_1$ positive antiDNA MAbs of SNF_1 mice encompass two major subfamilies called Id564 and Id612. The Id512 family consist of anti-DNA antibodies that bear Ig heavy-chain constant region (IgCH) allotype of either the NZB or the SWR parent, whereas the Id564 family consists of anti-DNA autoantibodies bearing the IgCH allotype of the SWR parent only, indicating their origin from the normal SWR strain (36–38). Indeed, the NZB parental strain lacks the V_H genes that encode the Id564 family of pathogenic autoantibodies (47). Moreover, all of anti-DNA MAbs belonging to the Id564 family are highly cationic in charge, and most of them are IgG2b in isotype with strong complement-fixing properties (36,37). So far, we have sequenced the variable regions of nine cationic anti-DNA MAbs that are representative of the Id564 family of pathogenic autoantibodies (48). Although derived from different SNF_1 animals, these pathogenic anti-DNA autoantibodies have highly homologous Leader-V_H sequences (Fig. 1A), which could explain their idiotypic cross-reactions. Moreover, the V_H regions of these autoantibodies contain numerous basic amino acid substitutions which are probably responsible for their cationic charge (36,48). The Leader-V_H sequences of these cationic autoantibodies are also closely related to that of a germline gene called VH23, which belongs to a family of genes encoding anti-NP antibodies in C57BL/6 mice (48). However, the Id564 family of anti-DNA autoantibodies did not arise from those anti-NP germline genes (47). These nine pathogenic autoantibodies of SNF_1 mice are produced by three clonally related sets of hybridomas, since the members of each set have almost identical V_H-D-J_H and V_κ-J_κ junctional sequences and identical rearrangements of their nonproductive immunoglobulin alleles (48) (Fig. 1). These results indicate that select clones of B cells producing these pathogenic autoantibodies are expanded in SNF_1 mice. As mentioned above, the $Id^{LN}F_1$-positive, pathogenic autoantibodies of SNF_1 mice have the antibody heavy-chain constant-region allotype of either the autoimmune NZB or the normal SWR parent, indicating their origins from genes contributed by the parental strains. Yet the levels of antibodies sharing the $Id^{LN}F_1$ marker increases markedly with age in the serum of only the nephritis-prone SNF_1 mice; they are not detectable in the serum of the parental strains. Thus select populations of pathogenic anti-DNA autoantibodies that are "dormant" in the normal SWR and the autoimmune NZB parents become expanded in the SNF_1 progeny (36–38,47,48). Similar idiotypic restriction of anti-DNA autoantibodies has also been detected in the NZB × NZW)F_1 model of lupus nephritis (49).

Evidence for an oligoclonal expansion of IgG autoantibody producing B cells was also found in other lupus strains, although the relationship of those autoantibodies to disease was not determined (50,51). Indeed, C57BL/6-*lpr* mice which do not develop rheumatoid arthritis produce IgG class rheumatoid factors with characteristics similar to those of the arthritis-prone MRL-*lpr* mice (2,50). Moreover, when a larger sample of IgG autoantibodies from lupus mice were examined, they were found to be more diverse (52,53). Nevertheless, idiotypic restriction, somatic mutation, and clonal expression of IgG autoantibody-producing B cells do occur in SLE (38,48,50). The implications of these results is that unlike natural autoantibodies, the pathognomonic autoantibodies of SLE are generated from an antigen-driven secondary immune response. However, there is no evidence for an altered or a cross-reactive antigen triggering SLE. Indeed, SLE cannot be induced by deliberate immunization with DNA. The antibodies that are induced by immunization with DNA are in fact quite different from the polyspecific autoantibodies produced spontaneously in SLE (54). Furthermore, in the graft-versus-host reaction, B cells of normal mice produce pathogenic lupus autoantibodies against unmodified autologous antigens (55,56). The cross-reactive

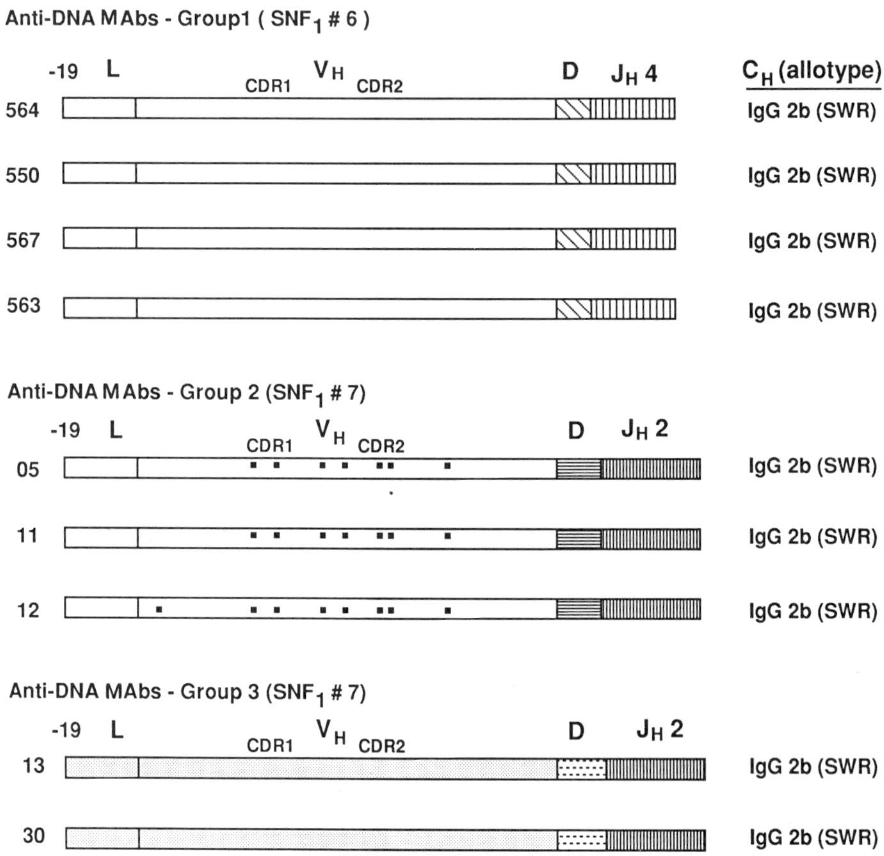

(a)

FIGURE 1 Schematic representation of variable region sequences of the Id564 family of cationic anti-DNA autoantibodies (MAbs). a) Heavy-chain sequences: The group 1 MAbs, derived from SNF_1 mouse #6, have identical Leader (L), V_H-D-J_H, and junctional sequences. The group 2 MAbs, although derived from a different SNF_1 animal #7, are 96% homologous to group 1 in their L-V_H sequences, except for seven replacement substitutions (small squares) and five silent substitutions (now shown). These MAbs use different D and J_H genes than group 1. The group 2 MAbs again have identical L-V_H-D-J_H and junctional sequences except for MAb 12, which has an additional silent (not shown) and a replacement substitution. The L-V_H sequence of the clonally related group 3 MAbs (derived from SNF_1 #7) are 84% homologous to the other groups, but their D segment is different from the previous set of anti-DNA MAbs. The group 1 MAbs bind to ssDNA

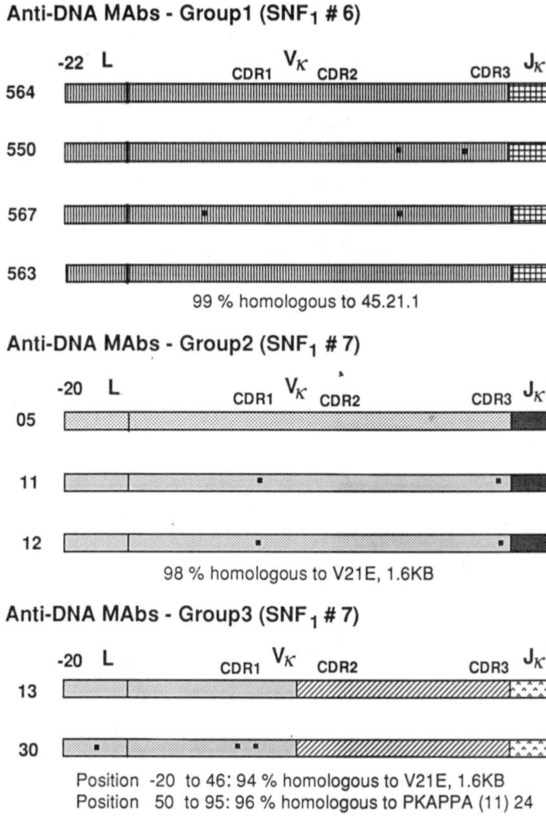

(b)

FIGURE 1 *(continued)*
and poly (I), whereas the group 2 and 3 MAbs bind ssDNA, dsDNA, and poly (dT) (36–38,48). b) Light-chain sequences: The V_κ sequences of each set of MAbs, unlike their V_H sequences, are quite different. The V_κ sequence of group 1 MAbs is 99% homologous to a germline V_κ gene called 45.21.1, that of group 2 MAbs is 98% homologous to another germline V_κ called V21E-1.6KB, and the group 3 MAbs are recombinants with 94% homology up to position 46 with V21E-1.6KB and 96% homology from position 50–95 with the germline PKAPPA (11) 24 gene (48). Each set of MAbs are clonally related, but within group 1, MAb 550 and 567 differ from 564 and 563 by two residues in V_κ, and the latter two MAbs differ by a silent substitution (not shown) (48). In group 2, MAbs 11 and 12 differ from 05 by two replacement and a silent substitution. In group 3, the MAb 30 differs from 13 by three nucleotide exchanges.

idiotypes shared by the pathogenic autoantibodies, such as $Id^{LN}F_1$, might be the target for the expansion of pathogenic autoantibody producing B cells in SLE.

The studies with the NZB × SWR model so far demonstrated that the pathogenic anti-DNA autoantibodies are a restricted population that have distinct idiotypic markers as well as unusual immunochemical and structural properties. Furthermore, the immunoregulatory and genetic mechanisms that mediate the expansion of such a select population of pathogenic autoantibodies in SNF_1 mice are also distinct from the defects in the NZB parents that result in excessive production of nonpathogenic (natural) anti-DNA antibodies.

IV. PATHOGENIC ANTI-DNA AUTOANTIBODY-INDUCING T CELLS

In the SNF_1 mice, certain T-helper (Th) cell subsets are responsible for inducing the production of the $Id^{LN}F_1$-positive, cationic IgG anti-DNA antibodies, and these Th subsets appear just before the onset of lupus nephritis (39,41). One set of these Th cells have the classical $CD4^+/CD8^-$ helper phenotype, whereas the other set of Th cells possess an unusual $CD4^-/CD8^-$ (double-negative) phenotype. IL-2–dependent, pathogenic antoantibody-inducing Th-cell lines with either of these phenotypes can be derived from nephritic SNF_1 mice (41).

A. $CD4^+$ Autoantibody-Inducing Th Cells and Complementation of T-Cell Receptor and MHC Genes

The $CD4^+$ Th-cell lines of SNF_1 mice are "autoreactive," i.e., they proliferate spontaneously in response to irradiated, syngeneic spleen cells (APC), and the proliferative response can be blocked by MAbs to appropriate MHC class II antigens (41). Remarkably, not all of the $CD4^+$ "autoreactive" Th lines are equal in pathogenic autoantibody-inducing capability. The $CD4^+$ Th lines of SNF_1 mice that preferentially respond to unique F_1-hybrid-MHC determinants have a significantly greater ability to augment the production of pathogenic anti-DNA antibodies in contrast to other autoreactive SNF_1 Th-cell lines that preferentially respond to one of the parental (NZB) MHC determinants (41). Moreover, the pathogenic autoantibody-inducing help of the Th lines is selective since they markedly augment the production of cationic IgG antibodies to ssDNA and dsDNA but not total polyclonal IgG (41). The preferential autoreactivity of the pathogenic autoantibody-inducing Th lines to unique F_1-hybrid-Ia determinants is consistent with the observation that in NZB × SWR backcross and F_2 mice, only the progeny that inherit the heterozygous I-A genotype develop severe and accelerated lupus nephritis (57). The hybrid Ia molecules expressed in the SNF_1 mice could selectively trigger the autoreactive T cells that induce pathogenic autoantibodies. The "autoreactive" $CD4^+$ Th cells could actually be responding to some endoenous epitope such as those present in $Id^{LN}F_1$, and such autoantigens could be presented in an immunogenic form by the F_1-hybrid-Ia molecules. The F_1-hybrid-Ia molecules could also affect the thymic elimination/selection process that deletes autoreactive T-cell clones early in ontogeny (58–60). Indeed, heterozygosity of MHC class II genes is also associated with lupus nephritis in the (NZB × NZW)F_1 model (61,62). Moreover, an expanded population of $CD4^+$, autoreactive T cells have been found in several strains of lupus mice (63–68).

The other important component for the autoreactive T-cell response is, of course, the T-cell receptor (TCR) expressed by the Th cells. It is significant that the SWR parents of the NZB × SWR crosses, although normal, have deleted about 50% of TCR Vβ gene families (69) (Fig. 2). Complementation of those TCR genes from the NZB parent could allow the generation of the pathogenic autoantibody-inducing Th cells in the SNF_1 mice. Indeed, inheritance of heterozygous TCR Vβ genes is associated with accelerated glomerulonephritis in NZB × SWR crosses (57), and many of the pathogenic autoantibody-inducing, $CD4^+$ Th-cell lines of SNF_1 mice do utilize the TCR Vβ genes that are lacking in the SWR but are contributed by the NZB parents (70). Heterozygosity of TCR Vβ genotype is also associated with high levels of IgG anti-DNA autoantibody production in the (NZB × NZW)F_1 model (71).

B. Double-Negative Autoantibody-Inducing Th Cells and Forbidden T-Cell Receptors

In addition to the $CD4^+$ Th subset, a population of double-negative Th cells that selectively augment the production of pathogenic autoantibodies are also expanded in the nephritic SNF_1 mice and several other lupus strains (39,41). These $CD4^-/CD8^-$ cells are Thy-1^+, express CD3 molecules of the TCR, and a proportion of them also express the Ly-5 (B220) antigen (39,41). A similar population of double-negative T cells are massively expanded in the MRL-*lpr* lupus strain under the influence of the recessive lymphoproliferation gene lpr (72). However, the surprising observation is that such double-negative T cells are found in lupus strains lacking the *lpr* gene (39,41). The origins and function of the double-negative T cells in MRL-*lpr* mice are not yet clear. Purified double-negative cells of MRL-*lpr* mice have no helper activity (73), although they do express α/β TCR in low levels (74). Indeed, the helper activity that was attributed previously to the double-negative cells of MRL-*lpr* mice (75) was most probably due to the presence of $CD4^+$, autoreactive T cells that are also expanded in these mice (64,66). By contrast, the purified double-negative Th cells and Th lines of non*lpr* lupus mice do indeed have the ability to augment the production of pathogenic anti-DNA autoantibodies (39,41). Recent studies have shown that most of these $CD4^-/CD8^-$ double-negative Th cells of SNF_1 mice express "forbidden" TCR Vβ genes (70). Products of certain TCR Vβ genes are known to respond strongly against certain autoantigens. For example, T cells expressing Vβ5, 11, or 17a encoded receptors strongly react with I-E (MHC class II) molecules; Vβ6, 8.1,

SWR

Phenotype: H-2^q, I-E^-, *Mls*^{a}, *Mls*^{c}

Genotype: Lacks V_β 5, 8, 9, 11, 12 & 13 genes

Mature T cells: Not Deleted

anti- I-E = V_β 17^+cells

anti-*Mls* = V_β 3^+ & V_β 6^+ cells

NZB

H-2^d, I-E^+, *Mls*^{a}, *Mls*^{c}

Full Complement of TCR V_β genes (V_β 17 nonfunctional)

Deleted or markedly reduced

anti- I-E = V_β 5^+ & V_β 11^+cells

anti-*Mls* = $V_\beta 3^+$, $V_\beta 6^+$, $V_\beta 8.1^+$ & $V_\beta 9^+$cells

(SWR X NZB) F_1

Complementation of TCR V_β & I-E genes from the NZB parent

I-E^+:- $V_\beta 5^+$, V_β 11^+ & V_β $17a^+$ mature T cells *should* be deleted

Mls^a, *Mls*^{c}, I-E^+ & H-$2^{d/q}$:- $V_\beta 3^+$, $V_\beta 6^+$, $V_\beta 8.1^+$ & $V_\beta 9^+$mature T cells *should* be deleted

FIGURE 2 The complementation of T-cell receptor Vβ and MHC class II genes in the (SWR × NZB) F_1 or SNF_1 progeny and the *expected* phenotype of mature peripheral T cells in these lupus-prone mice.

and 9 encoded TCRs respond to *Mls*^{a} products; and Vβ3 encoded TCRs are reactive to *Mls*^{c} products (58–60,76–81). Thymocytes expressing such strongly autoreactive TCRs are deleted early in thymic ontogeny, probably at the immature $CD4^+/CD8^+$ stage (82,83). Consequently, very few mature T cells expressing these "forbidden" receptors are found in the periphery of normal mouse strains that can express the corresponding autoantigens (58–60,76–81). The lupus-prone SNF_1 mouse is a useful model to analyze a role for the "forbidden" receptor-bearing T cells in systemic autoimmune disease (84) (Fig. 2). The SWR parents of SNF_1 mice do not express I-E molecules, therefore, $V\beta17a^+$ T cells are present in the peripheral lymphoid organs of SWR mice (58,70). As mentioned above, gene encoding the other I-E reactive TCRs, namely, Vβ5 and 11, are lacking in this strain. On the other hand, the NZB parents of SNF_1 mice express I-E molecules, and, therefore, mature T cells expressing the I-E reactive TCRs are markedly reduced in NZB mice (70). Similarly, the *Mls* products are nonstimulatory in the SWR strain, because they are $I\text{-}E^-$ and they have the $H\text{-}2^q$ haplotype. Therefore, T cells expressing the *Mls*-reactive Vβ6 and Vβ3 receptors are present in the periphery of SWR mice (59,70,78,81). The other genes encoding anti-*Mls* TCRs (Vβ8.1 and 9) are lacking in the SWR strain (69). By contrast, B cells of the NZB parents of SNF_1 mice can present *Mls* antigens, since they are $I\text{-}E^+$ and $H\text{-}2^d$ in haplotype. Therefore, mature T cells expressing the anti-*Mls* TCRs are markedly reduced in the NZB strain (70). Due to codominant inheritance of the relevant genes, the SNF_1 progeny is $I\text{-}E^+$, and it can present *Mls* antigens in stimulatory form. Furthermore, the SNF_1 mice have a full complement of TCR Vβ genes (57). Therefore, the SNF_1 mice are expected to delete mature T cells expressing the forbidden autoreactive TCRs (Fig. 2). However, the pathogenic autoantibody-inducing, double-negative Th cells that are found in the periphery of SNF_1 mice express forbidden autoreactive TCRs, such as Vβ6, Vβ8.1, and Vβ11 (70). In this regard, the double-negative Th cells of the non*lpr* SNF_1 mice are clearly distinct from those found in the MRL-lpr strain or in the thymuses of normal mice, since the latter are functionally inert and express Vβ8 TCRs predominantly but none of the autoreactive TCRs (85–87). The expression of “forbidden” TCRs by the double-negative Th cells of SNF_1 mice indicates an abnormality in the thymic deletion/selection process in this lupus strain, which probably results from the premature thymic atrophy known to occur in lupus mice (2,88). The strongly autoreactive thymocyte precursors of the mature double-negative Th cells could have escaped thymic deletion by their failure to express CD4 (and or CD8) antigens as suggested by other studies (82,83). Alternatively, the double-negative pathogenic autoantibody-inducing Th cells could arise from downregulation of CD4 antigens in autoreactive T cells in vivo, an endogeneous mechanism to diminish the intensity of autoreactivity. Double-negative cells that can differentiate into $CD4^+$ autoreactive T cells have been detected in normal mice (89), however, the double-negative Th-cell lines of SNF_1 mice are functionally competent by themselves, and they have maintained a stable double-negative phenotype over a year in culture (41,70). Similar types of double-negative T cells expressing an autoreactive TCR transgene are found in mice that have incorporated the autoreactive TCR gene in their germline, but those double-negative cells appear to be functionally inert (82,90). Thus, the functionally competent double-negative Th cells of non-*lpr* lupus mice (39) probably play an important role in the development of lupus nephritis.

C. Susceptible B Cells

The $CD4^+$ and $CD4^-/CD8^-$ Th cells can induce the production of pathogenic anti-DNA autoantibodies only when they are co-cultured with B cells from older prenephritic SNF_1 mice (39,41). However, these Th cells cannot induce the production of pathogenic autoantibodies when cultured with B cells from younger preautoimmune SNF_1 mice or with B cells from the NZB and SWR parents, even though the $CD4^+$ autoreactive Th cells can proliferate in the presence of such B cells (39,41). Therefore, the younger SNF_1 mice and the parental strains may be deficient in the select B-cell population that are committed to produce the pathogenic anti-DNA autoantibodies. Alternatively, this pathogenic autoantibody-producing B cell population may be in a more inducible state in the older SNF_1 mice due to an intrinsic defect.

V. HUMAN SLE: OLIGOCLONAL EXPANSION OF PATHOGENIC AUTOANTIBODY-PRODUCING B CELLS AND UNUSUAL T-HELPER CELLS

Human lupus is considered to be a heterogeneous disease with multiple underlying mechanisms, since numerous immunologic abnormalities have been documented in the human disease (91). However, many of these nonspecific defects could arise secondarily as a consequence of the disease. When we investigated lupus patients for the cellular mechanisms that specifically regulate the production of the pathogenic variety of anti-DNA autoantibodies, we obtained results that were analogous to the SNF_1 model (92). Lymphocytes from patients with active lupus nephritis uniformly produce highly cationic, IgG-class anti-DNA antibodies but not the lymphocytes of inactive patients. Th cells in the patients with active lupus play a central role in the production of these pathogenic variety of autoantibodies, and those Th cells consist of a $CD4^+$ subset as well as an unusual $CD4^-/CD8^-$, α/β TCR^+ double-negative subset (92) (Fig. 3). A small number ($\approx 0.3\%$) of these unusual α/β TCR^+, double-negative cells are also present in the peripheral blood of normal subjects, but in patients with active lupus the double-negative population expands more than 10-fold (92) (Fig. 4). These double-negative Th cells of human lupus may also express forbidden autoreactive TCRs like those in the SNF_1 mice, although such $V\beta$ TCRs have not yet been identified in humans. Double-negative T cells expressing α/β TCRs were subsequently detected in normal subjects by other investigators, but their function has not been determined (93–95). The striking feature of the Th cells in patients with active lupus is that they selectively increase the production of the pathogenic anti-DNA autoantibodies, but not total polyclonal IgG (92) (Fig. 3). Moreover, the cationic anti-DNA autoantibodies induced by the Th cells are markedly restricted in spectrotype, indicating again that the Th cells help a select

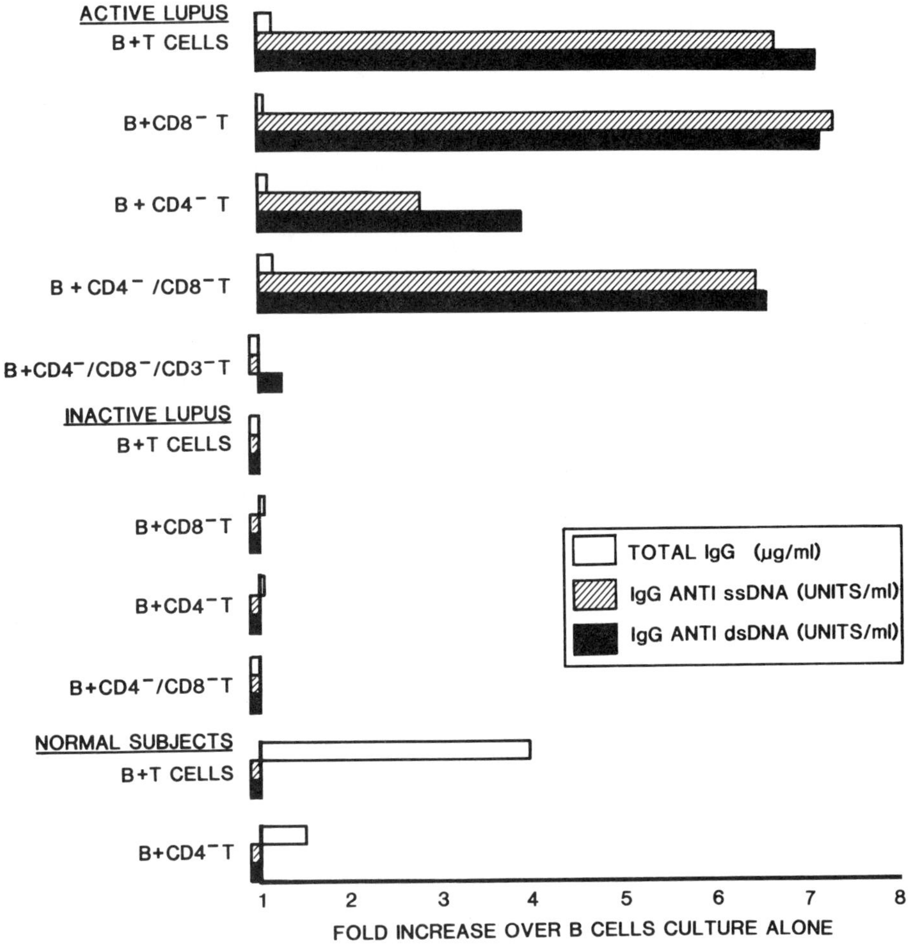

FIGURE 3 $CD4^+$ and double-negative ($CD4^-/CD8^-$) T cells from patients with active lupus nephritis preferentially augment the production of IgG class anti-DNA autoantibodies by autologous B cells. When cultured by themselves, B cells from the lupus patients produced 20- to 30-fold more total polyclonal IgG than those of normal subjects (92). However, unlike the increase in anti-DNA autoantibodies, no further increase in total IgG production occurred when the lupus B cells were co-cultured with autologous T cells. (Modified from Ref. 92.)

and oligoclonal population of B cells that are committed to produce these pathogenic autoantibodies in patients with active lupus nephritis (92). Recent studies with other lupus autoantibodies have also demonstrated the selective

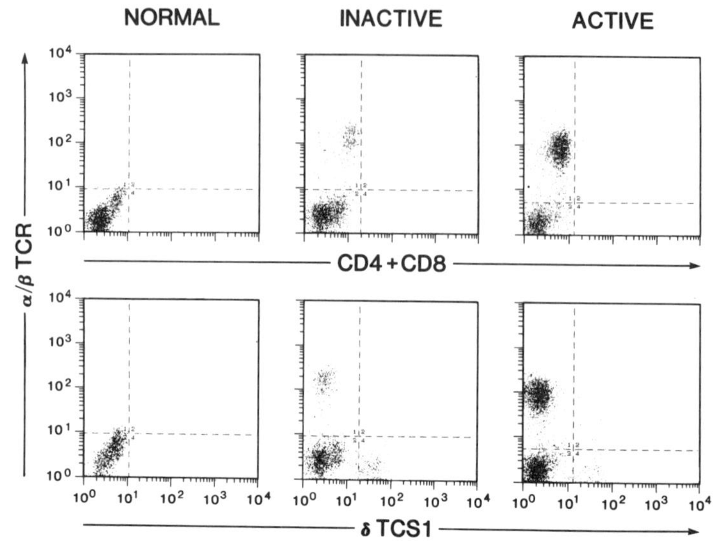

FIGURE 4 A marked expansion of α/β TCR$^+$, double-negative cells in patients with active lupus nephritis. Two-color immunofluorescence analysis (FACS dot plot) of purified double-negative (CD4$^-$/CD8$^-$) T cells obtained from peripheral blood T cells of normal subjects and patients with inactive and active SLE. The α/β TCR fluorescence is on Y axis and the X axis shows fluorescence for each of the other antigens as designated. Based on background staining with control antibodies, the dot plots were divided into four quandrants to identify unstained cells (lower left), cells that stained with both fluorochromes (upper right), and cells that stained with only one of the two fluorochromes (upper left and lower right). Top row: The cells were stained with anti-α/β TCR and anti-CD4 + anti-CD8 MAbs. Bottom row: The cells were stained with the anti-α/β TCR and the anti-γ/δ TCR MAbs. The latter stains a subset of γ/δ T cells. (Reproduced with permission from Ref. 92.)

nature of B cell response in human SLE (96,97). As in the SNF_1 mice, pathogenic autoantibody-inducing Th cell lines with either CD4$^+$ or double-negative phenotypes can be derived from patients with active lupus nephritis (92,98). Only 10–15% of T-cell lines derived from different patients with active lupus have the capability to induce pathogenic autoantibodies (98), suggesting again that a select population of Th cells mediate this particular type of help.

These studies in the lupus-prone SNF_1 mice and in human SLE indicate that there are distinct populations of T and B cells involved in the production of pathogenic anti-DNA autoantibodies. Further characterization of the structure and specificities of the receptors expressed by these particular lymphocyte subsets will help us to understand the underlying mechanisms for SLE.

ACKNOWLEDGMENTS

This work was supported by National Institutes of Health grants RO1 CA31789 and AR 39157. Sumati Rajagopalan's previous (maiden) name was Shivakumar.

REFERENCES

1. Koffler, D., Carr, R. I., Agnello, V., Thoburn, R., and Kunkel, H. G. 1971. Antibodies to polynucleotides in human sera: Antigenic specificity and relation to disease. *J. Exp. Med., 134*: 294–312.
2. Theofilopoulos, A. N., and Dixon, F. J. 1985. Murine models of systemic lupus erythematosus. *Adv. Immunol., 37*: 269–390.
3. Ternynck, T., and Avrameas, S. 1986. Murine natural monoclonal autoantibodies: A study of their polyspecificities and their affinities. *Immunol. Rev., 94*: 99–112.
4. Datta, S. K., Stollar, B. D., and Schwartz, R. S. 1983. Normal mice express idiotypes related to autoantibody idiotypes of lupus mice. *Proc. Natl. Acad. Sci. USA, 80*: 2723–2727.
5. Souroujon, M., White-Scharff, M. E., Andre-Schwartz, J., Gefter, M. L., and Schwartz, R. S. 1988. Preferential autoantibody reactivity of the preimmune B cell repertoire of normal mice. *J. Immunol., 140*: 4173–4179.
6. Manohor, V., Brown, E., Lieserson, W. M., and Chused, T. M. 1982. Expression of Lyt-1 by a subset of B lymphocytes. *J. Immunol., 129*: 532–538.
7. Hayakawa, K., Hardy, R. R., Honda, M., Herzenberg, L. A., Steinberg, A. D., and Herzenberg, L. A. 1984. Ly-1 B cells: Functionally distinct lymphocytes that secrete IgM autoantibodies. *Proc. Natl. Acad. Sci. USA., 81*: 2494–2498.
8. Casali, P., Burastero, S. E., Nakamura, M., Inghirami, G., and Notkins, A. L. 1987. Human lymphocytes making rheumatoid factor and antibody to ssDNA belong to Leu-1^+ B cell subset. *Science, 236*: 77–81.
9. Homberg, D. 1987. High connectivity natural autoantibodies preferentially use 7183 and QUPC 52 V_H families. *Eur. J. Immunol., 17*: 399–403.
10. Ghosh, S., and Campbell, A. M. 1986. Multispecific monoclonal antibodies. *Immunol. Today, 7*: 217–222.
11. Datta, S. K. 1984. Anti-DNA antibody idiotypes in normal and lupus mice. In *Regulation of the Immune System* (Sercarz, E., Cantor, H., and Chess, L., eds.), UCLA symposium on molecular and cellular biology, Vol. 18. Alan R. Liss, New York, pp. 877–886.
12. Datta, S. K., Naparstek, Y., and Schwartz, R. S. 1986. In vitro production of an anti-DNA idiotype by lymphocytes of normal subjects and patients with systemic lupus erythematosus. *Clin. Immunol. Immunopathol., 38*: 302–318.
13. Kearney, J. F., and Vakil, M. 1986. Idiotype-directed interactions during ontogeny play a major role in the establishment of adult B cell repertoire. *Immunol. Rev., 94*: 39–50.

14. Marion, T. N., Dzierzak, E. A., Lee, H. S., Adams, R. L., and Janeway, C. A. 1984. Non-dinitrophenyl-binding immunoglobulin that bears a dominant idiotype (Id 460) associated with anti-dinitrophenyl antibody is specific for an antigen on *Pasteurella pneumotropica*. *J. Exp. Med.*, *159*: 221–232.
15. Paul, W. E., and Bona, C. 1982. Regulatory idiotypes and immune networks: A hypothesis. *Immunol. Today*, *3*: 230–234.
16. Davidson, A., Shefner, R., Livneh, A., and Diamond, B. 1987. The role of somatic mutation of immunoglobulin genes in autoimmunity. *Ann. Rev. Immunol.*, *5*: 85–108.
17. Kabat, E. A., Nickerson, K. G., Liao, J., Grossbard, L., Osserman, E. F., Glickman, E., Chess, L., Robbins, J. R., Schneerson, R., and Yang, Y. 1986. A human monoclonal macroglobulin with specificity for α(2-8)-linked poly-N-acetyl neuraminic acid, the capsular polysaccharide of group B meningococci and *Escherichia coli* K1, which cross-reacts with polynucleotides and with denatured DNA. *J. Exp. Med.*, *164*: 642–654.
18. Koffler, R., Noonan, D. J., Levy, D. E., Wilson, M. C., Moller, N. P. H., Dixon, F. J., and Theofilopoulos, A. N. 1985. Genetic elements used for a murine lupus anti-DNA autoantibody are closely related to those for antibodies to exogenous antigens. *J. Exp. Med.*, *161*: 805–815.
19. Trepicchio, W., Maruya, A., and Barrett, K. J. 1987. The heavy chain genes of a lupus anti-DNA autoantibody are encoded in the germline of a nonautoimmune strain of mouse and conserved in strains of mice polymorphic for this gene locus. *J. Immunol.*, *139*: 3139–3145.
20. Dersimonian, H., Schwartz, R. S., Barrett, K. J., and Stollar, B. D. 1987. Relationship between human variable region heavy chain germ-line genes and genes encoding anti-DNA autoantibodies. *J. Immunol.*, *139*: 2496–2501.
21. Naparstek, Y., Duggan, D., Schattner, A., Madaio, M. P., Goni, F., Frangione, B., Stollar, B. D., Kabat, E. A., and Schwartz, R. S. 1985. Immunochemical similarities between monoclonal Waldenstrom's macroglobulins and monoclonal anti-DNA lupus autoantibodies. *J. Exp. Med.*, *161*: 1525–1538.
22. Monestier, M., Bonin, B., Migliorini, P., Dang, H., Datta, S., Kuppers, R., Rose, N., Maurer, P., Talal, N., and Bona, C. 1987. Autoantibodies of various specificities encoded by genes from the V_H J558 family bind to foreign antigens and share idiotopes of antibodies specific for self and foreign antigens. *J. Exp. Med.*, *166*: 1109–1124.
23. Shoenfeld, Y., Ben-Yehuda, O., Naparstek, Y., Wilner, Y., Frolichman, R., Schattner, A., Lavie, G., Joshua, H., Pinkhas, J., Kennedy, R. C., Schwartz, R. S., and Pick, A. I. 1986. The detection of a common idiotype of anti-DNA antibodies in the sera of patients with monoclonal gammopathies. *J. Clin. Immunol.*, *6*: 194–204.
24. Madaio, M. P., Carlson, J., Cataldo, J., Ucci, A., Migliorini, P., and Pankewycz, O. 1987. Murine monoclonal anti-DNA antibodies bind directly to glomerular antigens and form immune deposits. *J. Immunol.*, *138*: 2883–2889.
25. Isenberg, D. A., and Collins, C. 1985. Detection of cross-reactive anti-DNA antibody idiotypes on renal tissue-bound immunoglobulins from lupus patients. *J. Clin. Invest.*, *76*: 287–294.
26. DeHeer, D. H., and Edgington, T. S. 1976. Cellular events associated with

immunogenesis of anti-erythrocyte autoantibody responses of NZB mice. *Transplant Rev.*, *31*: 116–155.
27. Pennell, C. A., Arnold, L. W., Haughton, G., and Clarke, S. H. 1988. Restricted Ig variable region gene expression among Ly-1$^+$ B cell lymphomas. *J. Immunol.*, *141*: 2788–2796.
28. Moore, J. S., and Calkins, C. E. 1985. In vitro regulation of the pathogenic autoantibody response of New Zealand Black mice. I. Loss with age of suppressive activity in T cell populations. *J. Immunol.*, *134*: 3838–3844.
29. Reininger, L., Ollier, P., Poncet, P., Kaushik, A., and Jaton, J. C. 1987. Novel V genes encode vritually identical variable regions of six murine monoclonal anti-bromelain-treated red blood cell autoantibodies. *J. Immunol.*, *138*: 316–323.
30. Caulfield, M. J. Stanko, D., Schulze, D. H., and Calkins, C. E. 1989. Characterization of a pathogenic monoclonal antibody that dominates the spontaneous autoimmune response to self erythrocytes. *FASEB J. 3*: A495 (Abstract No. 1563).
31. Datta, S. K., Owen, F. L., Womack, J. E., and Riblet, R. J. 1982. Analysis of recombinant inbred lines derived from autoimmune (NZB) and high leukemia (C58) strains: Independent multigenic systems control B cell hyperactivity, retrovirus expression and autoimmunity. *J. Immunol.*, *129*: 1539–1544.
32. Raveche, E. S., Novotny, E. A., Hansen, C. T., Tjio, J. H., and Steinberg, A. D. 1981. Genetic studies in NZB mice. V. Recombinant inbred lines demonstrate that separate genes control autoimmune phenotype. *J. Exp. Med.*, *153*: 1187–1197.
33. Eastcott, J. W., Schwartz, R. S., and Datta, S. K. 1983. Genetic analysis of the inheritance of B cell hyperactivity in relation to the development of autoantibodies and glomerulonephritis in NZB × SWR crosses. *J. Immunol.*, *131*: 2232–2239.
34. Howie, J. B., and Helyer, B. J. 1968. The immunology and pathology of NZB mice. *Adv. Immunol.*, *9*: 215–268.
35. Datta, S. K., Manny, N., Andrzejewski, C., Andre-Schwartz, J., and Schwartz, R. S. 1978. Genetic studies of autoimmunity and retrovirus expression in crosses of New Zealand Black mice. I. Xenotropic virus. *J. Exp. Med.*, *147*: 854–871.
36. Gavalchin, J., Nicklas, J., Eastcott, J. W., Madaio, M. P., Stollar, B. D., Schwartz, R. S., and Datta, S. K. 1985. Lupus prone (SWR × NZB)F_1 mice produce potentially nephritogenic autoantibodies inherited from the normal SWR parent. *J. Immunol.*, *134*: 885–894.
37. Gavalchin, J., Seder, R. A., and Datta, S. K. 1987. The NZB × SWR model of lupus nephritis. I. Cross-reactive idiotypes of monoclonal anti-DNA antibodies in relation to antigenic specificity, charge and allotype. Identification of interconnected idiotype families inherited from the normal SWR and the autoimmune NZB parents. *J. Immunol.*, *138*: 128–137.
38. Gavalchin, J., and Datta, S. K. 1987. The NZB × SWR model of lupus nephritis. II. Autoantibodies deposited in renal lesions show a restricted idiotypic diversity. *J. Immunol.*, *138*: 138–148.
39. Datta, S. K., Patel, H., and Berry, D. 1987. Induction of a cationic shift in IgG anti-DNA autoantibodies. Role of T helper cells with classical and novel phenotypes in three murine models of lupus nephritis. *J. Exp. Med.*, *165*: 1252–1268.
40. Ebling, F., and Hahn, B. H. 1980. Restricted subpopulations of DNA antibodies in

kidneys of mice with systemic lupus: comparison of antibodies in serum and renal eluates. *Arthritis Rheum.*, *23*: 392–403.
41. Sainis, K., and Datta, S. K. 1988. $CD4^+$ T cell lines with selective patterns of autoreactivity as well as $CD4^-$ $CD8^-$ T helper cell lines augment the production of idiotypes shared by pathogenic anti-DNA autoantibodies in the NZB × SWR model of lupus nephritis. *J. Immunol.*, *140*: 2215–2224.
42. Dang, H., and Harbeck, R. J. 1984. The in vivo and in vitro glomerular deposition of isolated anti-double-stranded-DNA antibodies in NZB/W mice. *Clin. Immunol. Immunopathol.*, *30*: 265–278.
43. Mannik, M., Gauthier, V. J., Stapleton, S. A., and Agodoa, L. Y. C. 1987. Immune complexes with cationic antibodies deposit in glomeruli more effectively than cationic antibodies alone. *J. Immunol.*, *138*: 4209–4217.
44. Gauthier, V. J., and Mannik, M. 1990. Noncationized antibodies in immune complexes are deposited in glomeruli by the presence of a small fraction of cationized antibodies. *J. Immunol.* *145*: 3348–3352.
45. Rennke, H. G, Cotran, R. S., and Venkatachalam, M. A. 1975. Role of molecular charge in glomerular permeability. Tracer studies with cationized ferritin. *J. Cell Biol.*, *67*: 638–646.
46. Kanwar, Y. S., and Farquhar, M. G. 1976. Anionic sites in glomerular basement membrane. In vivo and in vitro localization to the laminae rarae by cationic probes. *J. Cell. Biol.*, *81*: 137–153.
47. Ghatak, S., O'Keefe, T., Imanishi-Kari, T., and Datta, S. K. 1990 Selective strain distribution pattern of a germline V_H gene for a pathogenic anti-DNA autoantibody family. *International Immunol.* *2*: 1004–1012.
48. O'Keefe, T. L., Bandyopadhyay, S., Datta, S. K., and Imanishi-Kari, T. 1990. Variable region sequences of an idiotypically connected family of pathogenic anti-DNA autoantibodies. *J. Immunol.* *144*: 4275–4283.
49. Hahn, B. H., and Ebling, F. M. 1987. Idiotype restriction in murine lupus; high frequency of three public idiotypes on serum IgG in nephritic NZB/NZW F_1 mice. *J. Immunol.*, *138*: 2110–2118.
50. Shlomchik, M. J., Marshak-Rothstein, A. M., Wolfowicz, C. B., Rothstein, T. L., and Weigert, M. G. 1987. The role of clonal selection and somatic mutation in autoimmunity. *Nature*, *328*: 805–811.
51. Schlomchik, M. J., Aucoin, A. H., Pisetsky, D. S., and Weigert, M. G. Structure and function of anti-DNA autoantibodies derived from a single autoimmune mouse. *Proc. Natl. Acad. Sci. USA*, *84*: 9150–9154.
52. Duchosal, M. A., Kofler, R., Balderas, R. S., Aguado, M. T., Dixon, F. J., and Theofilopoulos, A. N. 1989. Genetic diversity of murine rheumatoid factors. *J. Immunol.*, *142*: 1737–1742.
53. Panosian-Sahakian, N. ,Klotz, J. L., Ebling, F., Kronenberg, M., and Hahn, B. 1989. Diversity of Ig V gene segments found in anti-DNA autoantibodies from a single (NZB × NZW)F_1 mouse. *J. Immunol.*, *142*: 4500–4506.
54. Madaio, M. P., Hodder, S., Schwartz, R. S., and Stollar, B. D. 1984. Responsiveness of autoimmune and normal mice to nucleic acid antigens. *J. Immunol.*, *132*: 872–876.
55. Datta, S. K., and Schwartz, R. S. 1976. Autoimmunization in the graft-versus-host reaction. *Transplant Rev.*, *31*: 44–78.

56. Vanderveen, F., Rolnik, A. G., and Gleichmann, E. 1981. Diseases caused by reactions of T lymphocytes to incompatible structures of the major histocompatibility complex. IV. Autoantibodies to nuclear antigens. *Clin. Exp. Immunol.*, *46*: 589–595.
57. Ghatak, S., Sainis, K., Owne, F. L., and Datta, S. K. 1987. T cell receptor β and I-Aβ chain genes of normal SWR mice are linked with the development of lupus nephritis in NZB × SWR crosses. *Proc. Natl. Acad. Sci. USA*, *84*: 6850–6853.
58. Kappler, J. W., Roehm, N., and Marrack, P. 1987. T cell tolerance by clonal elimination in the thymus. *Cell*, *49*: 273–280.
59. MacDonald, R. H., Schneider, R., Lees, R. K., Howe, R. C., Acha-Orbea, H., Festenstein, H., Zinkernagel, R. M., and Hengartner, H. 1988. T cell receptor Vβ use predicts reactivity and tolerance to *Mls*^{a}-encoded antigens. *Nature*, *332*: 40–45.
60. Pullen, A. M., Marrack, P., and Kappler, J. W. 1988. The T cell repertoire is heavily influenced by tolerance to polymorphic self-antigens. *Nature*, *335*: 796–801.
61. Knight, J. G., and Adams, D. D. 1978. Three genes for lupus nephritis in NZB × NZW mice. *J. Exp. Med.*, *147*: 1653–1660.
62. Hiroshe, S., Nagasawa, R., Sekikawa, I., Hamaoki, M., Ishida, Y., Sato, H., and Shirari, T. 1983. Enhancing effects of H-2 linked NZW genes on the autoimmune traits of (NZB × NZW)F_1 mice. *J. Exp. Med.*, *158*: 228–233.
63. Cohen, P. L., Rapoport, R., and Eisenberg, R. A. 1986. Characterization of functional T cell lines derived from MRL mice. *Clin. Immunol. Immunopathol.*, *40*: 485–496.
64. Weston, K. M., Ju, S. T., Lu, C. Y., and Sy, M. S. 1988. Autoreactive T cells in MRL/MP-*lpr*/*lpr* mice. Characterization of lymphokines produced and analysis of antigen presenting cells required. *J. Immunol.*, *141*: 1941–1948.
65. Ando, D. G., Sercarz, E. E., and Hahn, B. H. 1987. Mechanisms of T and B cell collaboration in the in vitro production of anti-DNA antibodies in the NZB/NZW F_1 murine SLE model. *J. Immunol.*, *138*: 3185–3190.
66. Santoro, T. J., Portanova, J. P., and Kotzin, B. L. 1988. The contribution of L3T4+ T cells to lymphoproliferation and autoantibody production in MRL-*lpr*/*lpr* mice. *J. Exp. Med.*, *167*: 1713–1718.
67. Rosenberg, Y. J., Goldsmith, P. K., Ohara, J., Steinberg, A. D., and Ohriner, W. 1986. Ia antigen expression and autoimmunity in MRL-*lpr*/*lpr* mice. *Ann. NY Acad. Sci.*, *475*: 251–266.
68. Wofsy, D, and Seaman, W. E. 1985. Successful treatment of autoimmunity in NZB/NZW F_1 mice with monoclonal antibody to L2T4. *J. Exp. Med.*, *161*: 378–391.
69. Behlke, M., Chou, H., Huppi, K., and Loh, D. Y. 1986. Murine T-cell receptor mutants with deletions of β-chain variable region genes. *Proc. Natl. Acad. Sci. USA*, *83*: 767–771.
70. Adams, S., Zordan, T., Sainis, K., and Datta, S. K. 1990. T cell receptor Vβ genes expressed by IgG anti-DNA autoantibody inducing T cells in lupus nephritis: Forbidden receptors and double negative T cells. *Eur. J. Immunol.* *20*: 1435–1443.
71. Yanagi, Y., Hirose, S., Nagasawa, R., Shirai, T., Mak, T. W., and Tada, T. 1986. Does the deletion within T cell receptor β-chain gene of NZW mice contribute to autoimmunity in (NZB × NZW)F_1 mice? *Eur. J. Immunol.*, *16*: 1179–1182.

72. Davidson, W. F., Dumont, F. J., Bedigian, H. G., Fowlkes, B. J., and Morse, H. C. Phenotypic, functional and molecular genetic comparisons of the abnormal lymphoid cells of C3H-*lpr*/*lpr* and C3H-*gld*/*gld* mice. *J. Immunol., 136*: 4075–4084.
73. Budd, R., Cerottini, J. C., and MacDonald, H. R. 1986. Cultured Lyt-2$^-$L3T4$^-$ T lymphocytes from normal thymus or *lrp* mice express a broad spectrum of cytolytic activity. *J. Immunol., 137*: 3734–3741.
74. Nemazee, D. A., Studer, S., Steinmetz, M., Dembic, Z., and Kiefer, M. 1985. The lymphoproliferating cells of MRL-*lpr*/*lpr* mice are a polyclonal population that bear the T lymphocyte receptor for antigen. *Eur. J. Immunol., 15*: 760–764.
75. Prud'homme, G. J., Park, C. L., Fieser, T. M., Kofler, R., Dixon, F. J., and Theofilopoulos, A. N. 1983. Identification of a B cell differentiation factor(s) spontaneously produced by proliferating T cells in the murine lupus strain of the *lpr*/*lpr* genotype. *J. Exp. Med., 157*: 730–742.
76. Kappler, J. W., Staerz, U., White, J., and Marrack, P. C. 1988. Self-tolerance eliminates T cells specific for Mls-modified products of the major histocompatibility complex. *Nature, 332*: 35–40.
77. Bill, J. Kanagawa, O., Woodland, D. L., and Palmer, E. 1989. The MHC I-E molecule is necessary but not sufficient for the clonal deletion of Vβ11-bearing T cells. *J. Exp. Med., 169*: 1405–1419.
78. Vacchio, M. S., and Hodes, R. J. 1989. Selective decreases in T cell receptor Vβ expression. Decreased expression of specific Vβ families is associated with expression of multiple MHC and non-MHC gene products. *J. Exp. Med., 170*: 1335–1346.
79. Happ, M. P., Woodland, D. L., and Palmer, E. A. 1989. A third T cell receptor β chain variable region gene encodes reactivity to Mls-1^a gene products. *Proc. Natl. Acad. Sci. USA, 86*: 6293–6296.
80. Fry, M. A., Cotterman, M. M., and Matis, L. A. 1989. The influence of self MHC and non-MHC antigens on the selection of an antigen-specific T cell receptor repertoire. *J. Immunol., 143*: 2723–2729.
81. Anderson, G. D., Bannerjee, S., David, C. A. 1989. MHC class II A_α and E_α molecules determine the clonal deletion of Vβ6$^+$ T cells. Studies with recombinant and transgenic mice. *J. Immunol., 143*: 3757–3761.
82. Kisielow, P., Bluthman, H., Staerz, U. D., Steinmetz, M., and von Boehmer, H. 1988. Tolerance in T cell receptor transgenic mice involves deletion of nonmature CD4$^+$8$^+$ thymocytes. *Nature, 333*: 742–746.
83. Fowlkes, B. J., Schwartz, R. H., and Pardoll, D. M. Deletion of self reactive thymocytes occur at a CD4$^+$8$^+$ precursor stage. *Nature, 334*: 620–623.
84. Datta, S. K. 1989. A search for the underlying mechanisms of systemic autoimmune disease in the NZB × SWR model. *Clin. Immunol. Immunopathol., 51*: 141–156.
85. Singer, P. A., McEvilly, R. J., Noonan, D. J., Dixon, F. J., and Theofilopoulos, A. N. 1986. Clonal diversity and T cell receptor β chain variable region expression in enlarged lymph nodes of MRL-*lpr*/*lpr* ice. *Proc. Natl. Acad. Sci. USA, 83*: 7018–7022.
86. Kotzin, B. L., Babcock, S. K., and Herron, L. R. 1988. Deletion of potentially self-reactive T cell receptor specificities in L3T4$^-$, Lyt-2$^-$ T cells of *lpr* mice. *J. Exp. Med., 168*: 2221–2229.

87. Singer, P. A., Balderas, R. S., McEvilly, R. J., Bobardt, M., and Theofilopoulos, A. N. 1989. *J. Exp. Med., 170*: 1869–1877.
88. Gershwin, M. E., Ikeda, R. M., Kruse, W. L., Wilson, F., Shifrine, M., and Spangler, W. 1978. Age dependent loss in New Zealand mice of morphological and functional characteristics of thymic epithelial cells. *J. Immunol., 120*: 971–976.
89. Morisset, J., Trannoy, E., deTalance, A., Spinella, S., Debre, P., Godet, P., and Seman, M. Genetics and strain distribution of concanavalin A-reactive Lyt-2^-, L3T4^- peripheral precursors of autoreactive T cells. *Eur. J. Immunol., 18*: 387–395.
90. Sha, W. C., Nelson, C. A., Newberry, R. D., Kranz, D. M., Russell, J. H., and Loh, D. Y. 1988. Positive and negative selection of an antigen receptor on T cells in transgenic mice. *Nature, 336*: 73–76.
91. Tsokos, G. C., and Balow, J. E. 1984. Cellular immune responses in systemic lupus erythematosus. *Prog. Allergy, 35*: 93–161.
92. Shivakumar, S., Tsokos, G. C., and Datta, S. K. 1989. T cell receptor α/β expressing double negative (CD4^-/CD8^-) and CD4^+ T helper cells in humans augment the production of pathogenic anti-DNA autoantibodies associated with lupus nephritis. *J. Immunol., 143*: 103–112.
93. Porcelli, S., Brenner, M. B., Greenstein, J. L., Balk, S. P., Terhorst, C., and Bleicher, P. A. 1989. Recognition of cluster of differentiation 1 antigens by human CD4^-CD8^- cytolytic T lymphocytes. *Nature, 341*: 447–450.
94. Londei, M., Verhoff, A., De Berardinis, P., Kissonerghis, M., Grubeck-Loebenstein, B., and Feldman, M. 1989. Definition of a population of CD4^-8^- T cells that express the $\alpha\beta$ T-cell receptor and respond to interleukins 2, 3 and 4. *Proc. Natl. Acad. Sci. USA, 86*: 8502–8506.
95. Groh, V., Fabbi, M., Hochstenbach, F., Maziarz, R. T., and Strominger, J. L. 1989. Double negative (CD4^-CD8^-) lymphocytes bearing T-cell receptor α and β chains in normal human skin. *Proc. Natl. Acad. Sci. USA, 86*: 5059–5063.
96. Gharavi, A. E., Chu, J. L., and Elkon, K. B. 1988. Autoantibodies to intracellular proteins in human systemic lupus erythematosus are not due to random polyclonal B cell activation. *Arthritis Rheum., 31*: 1337–1345.
97. Kalunian, K. C., Panosian-Sahakian, N., Ebling, F. M., Cohen, A. H., Louis, J. S., Kaine, J., Hahn, B. H. 1989. Idiotypic characteristics of immunoglobulins associated with systemic lupus erythematosus. Studies of antibodies deposited in the glomeruli of humans. *Arthritis Rheum., 32*: 513–522.
98. Rajagopalan, S., Zordan, T., Tsokos, G. C., and Datta, S. K. 1990. Pathogenic anti-DNA autoantibody inducing T helper cell lines from patients with active lupus nephritis: Isolation of CD4 /CD8 T helper cell lines that express the γ/δ T-cell receptor. *Proc. Natl. Acad. Sci. USA, 87*: 7020-7024.

9

The Autoimmune T-Cell Receptor in Experimental Disease

Ellen Heber-Katz
The Wistar Institute, Philadelphia, Pennsylvania

I. INTRODUCTION

In 1875, Louis Pasteur made the serendipitous finding that his rabies vaccine induced an autoimmune disease. He multiply injected vaccine into patients and found that they eventually came down with a syndrome known as postvaccine encephalitis (PVE). The "obvious" explanation was that the rabies virus was causing this. However, the vaccine was produced in rabbit brain, and it became clear that some component of the brain itself was responsible for PVE (1,2). It is now known that at least several myelin-associated proteins, myelin basic protein (MBP), a structural molecule found in the myelin sheath of the central nervous system (CNS), and proteolipid protein (PLP), do indeed cause encephalitis, neurological damage, and paralysis (3,4, reviewed in Refs. 5,6). These proteins are responsible for the induction of antigen-specific T cells, which find their way to the brain and spinal cords and cause inflammation and demyelination resulting in a disease known as experimental allergic encephalomyelitis, or EAE, and represents the first model of an experimentally induced T-cell–mediated autoimmune disease.

Since that time, many such experimental diseases have been described. What makes these diseases particularly important is the parallel in symptomatology with spontaneously occurring human disease. In a more theoretical vein, it is clear from these diseases that autoimmune-reactive T cells in general are *not* necessarily eliminated during ontogeny as previously suggested (7,8), but are present in significant numbers and are very real in their ability to cause disease. The fact that autoimmune disease is not the common state of affairs begs for an explanation for the regulation of such T cells as well. In fact, regulatory cells are readily found after recovery from such diseases and have also been easy to induce (9–12).

This chapter shall cover these experimental diseases and shall also discuss an unusual finding that seems to relate many of these autoimmune diseases, their T cells, and their antigen receptors making them look as if they share a common pathway. First, however, it is important to review some basic aspects of T-cell immunology.

A. T Cells and Their Recognition of Antigen

In general, T cells recognize antigen on the surface of a major histocompatibility complex (MHC) identical antigen-presenting cell, a cell type which includes dendritic cells, macrophages, and B cells. This phenomenon is known as MHC-restricted antigen recognition and has been explained by the fact that antigen is presented in association with the MHC molecules, class I or class II, found at high concentrations on the surface of such antigen-presenting cells (reviewed in Ref. 13). Furthermore, antigen most likely exists in its presented form as processed protein or a small peptide (14). It is now believed that, in fact, antigen binds to the Ia molecule in a specific manner and controls the antigen specificity of T cells of given haplotypes (15–19). It follows, then, that animals of different haplotypes will respond to different antigenic peptide determinants. Though this is not always true, such as in viral infections (20–22), it certainly is true in cases in which the antigen is limiting. One might also expect that in experimental autoimmune diseases, one would find that antigenic determinants that cause disease vary from strain to strain and also between species. This is in fact true.

B. Restricted Usage of T-Cell Receptor Genes

T cells recognize antigen in association with MHC through a specific receptor. Diversity in this receptor is generated by the use of genetically defined component parts which can recombine; other mechanisms resulting in diversity are used as well. The receptor is a disulfide-linked heterodimer made up of two chains, the alpha and beta chains, which function together as an antigen receptor (23–27). There are four different gene segments—the variable (V), diversity (D), joining (J), and constant (C) regions—which come together in random fashion and are expressed as a single protein molecule (28,29). For the mouse, the alpha (α) chain has at least 100 V genes and up to 100 J gene segments to choose from, but does not have a D region. The beta (β) chain has 30 defined V genes, 15 J, and 2 D gene segments. Besides the use of many different gene segments, diversity also is generated at the point at which these genes join. This is known as junctional diversity and occurs with (1) the irregular joining of the V-D-J segments, (2) the deletion of germline nucleotides, and (3) the random addition of nucleotides. Thus, it is this region that seems to be important in the antigenic differences seen by given TcRs. There have been several systems studied in which restricted usage of T-cell receptor genes have been reported (30–33). The most complete study employed the T-cell response to the C-terminal peptide of cytochrome c. In a given strain of mouse, the B10.A, it was found that the majority of clones use one particular V_α region, V_α 11, and also a particular J region, Jα 84. The V region of the beta chain is also of highly restricted heterogeneity, though it varies according to the MHC restriction fine specificity of the T cells (30,33,34), with the junctional region of this chain conserved.

II. EXPERIMENTAL ALLERGIC ENCEPHALOMYELITIS

Experimental allergic encephalomyelitis is a disease in which inflammatory cells migrate into the central nervous system through the blood-brain barrier and classically result in perivascular cuffing by lymphocytes and demyelination. The most well-studied causative antigen, P_1 protein or myelin basic protein (MBP), a molecule of molecular weight 18,000, is a major component of the myelin sheath surrounding nerve fibers and is synthesized and maintained by the oligodendrocyte in the CNS and by the Schwann cell in the peripheral nervous system (PNS). P_1 is found not only in CNS myelin but also in PNS myelin. Thus, it is interesting that P_1 or MBP induces disease and encephalitogenic T cells, which are found mainly in the CNS and not in the PNS. Encephalitogenic T-cell determinants have been mapped throughout the length of the MBP molecule with given determinants assigned to different strains and species with little overlap. Furthermore, synthetic peptides of the appropriate sequence can induce MBP-specific T cells and disease (3,4,6).

Though the first experiments done that suggested limited heterogeneity and autoregulation in a T-cell population involved the allograft response (35–37), an experiment done in 1981 by Cohen and collaborators (38) gave the first indication that T cells involved in EAE were also of limited clonality and could be autoregulated. The experiment involved T cells from Lewis rats specific for the MBP antigen, which could be adoptively injected into normal animals and cause severe paralysis within a few days. These cells were kept as a long-term line and thus were thought to have been selected for a single or only a few clones. These cells, when attenuated by X-irradiation or mitomycin treatment, could be injected into rats without causing any disease symptoms or histology; however, the animals that received these cells were now resistant to further disease. This resistance was shown to be EAE specific. To explain such resistance, one must rely on a regulatory response directed to an antigenic determinant unique to these cells, and the most likely candidate would be a determinant present on the T-cell receptor. Further, this result implied that self-antigenic determinants were shared between the injected cells and the cells causing disease. Finally, these results indicated that the T-cell response to EAE was mono- or pauci-idiotypic or possibly that the response itself was mono- or pauciclonal, i.e., derived from only a few cells. This was an important finding, which if true would offer the possibility of treating autoimmune diseases such as EAE in an anti-idiotypic fashion.

A. Monoclonal Anti-T-Cell Receptor Antibodies

One experiment to examine the possibility of monoidiotypy in EAE was the generation of a monoclonal antibody against a T cell which responded to the encephalitogenic determinant of MBP. In the case of the Lewis rat, which has the Rt-1^1 MHC haplotype, the major encephalitogenic determinant is located in residues 68–88 of guinea pig or rat MBP. The monoclonal antibody, 10.18, was made in a BALB/c mouse against a Lewis rat 68–88-specific T-cell hybridoma, could block antigen-specific T-cell responses, could immunoprecipitate the T-cell receptor, and most importantly, could block disease induction at low concentrations. This antibody could bind to most, if not all, T cells specific for the encephalitogenic determinant of MBP, 68–88, but not T cells specific for an irrelevant antigen (39). This antibody has the unusual property, however, of only binding to activated T cells and could be specific for a conformational change in the receptor. Whether this antibody is specific for the TcR alpha or beta chain is not known, and one possibility is that it is recognizing the α β dimer. These findings do indeed demonstrate that the EAE T-cell response in the rat is monoidiotypic and subject to anti-idiotypic control.

Similar studies were done in the mouse with previously defined antibodies specific for the V region of the TcR beta chain. These antibodies demonstrated that the majority of encephalitogenic T cells from PL/J and B10.PL mice [animals of the H-2^u MHC haplotype that recognizes residues 1–9 of MBP as the major encephalitogenic determinant (40–42)] used the TcR Vβ8 (43–45). Those same antibodies, F23.1 (46) and KJ-16 (47), could also block disease induction or ongoing disease. In another strain of mouse, the SJL (of the H-2^s MHC haplotype which recognizes residues 81–114 of MBP as the major encephalitogenic determinant), in which Vβ8 has been deleted from the genome, it was shown that Vβ 17 was the majority Vβ used (44,45). Antibody to this V region, however, could block disease, and it appears that in this case Vβ gene usage is more heterogeneous than in the PL/J mouse.

B. T-Cell Receptor Gene Usage in EAE

A second type of analysis of the EAE autoimmune T-cell response involved the examination of TcR gene elements used by these T cells. In the case of the Lewis rat, a cDNA library was made from the same T cell used to generate the 10.18 antibody and examined for TcR positive clones (50,51). Since these were the first rat TcR genes sequences, the analysis was done in terms of homology to the mouse sequences. The beta chain used had a V region which was most homologous to the mouse Vβ8.2 (79% at the amino acid level), a J region homologous to the Jβ1.1 (94% a.a. homology), and Dβ1 identical with the mouse. The alpha chain used a V region homologous to the Vα2.1 (77% a.a. homology) and the Jα TA39 (70% homologous). Using these V regions as probes to examine the shared receptor usage in the other EAE-specific T cells, every T cell that was specific for the encephalitogenic determinant of MBP was found to use some member of the Vβ8 family. In the mouse this is a three-member family, and the V region probe does not distinguish these members from one another. As for the alpha V region, approximately 70% of the T cells examined used Vα2 (this is thought to be a six-member family). The cells examined were both T-cell hybridomas and T-cell clones; the latter were shown to be encephalitogenic upon transfer. As far as a correlation between antigen specificity and usage of these V regions, it was also shown that T cells specific for another antigen such as ovalbumin or for antigen determinants of MBP which were not encephalitogenic did not use these V regions. Furthermore, it was found that these V regions were not highly represented in a normal T-cell population found in the spleen or in a mitogen (ConA)-stimulated T-cell population. Thus, it did appear that these V regions were idiosyncratic of T-cell populations specific for a given antigenic determinant of MBP, specifically the encephalitogenic determinant. As discussed above, this is not unique to an autoimmune population since it had already been shown that the T-cell response to cytochrome c displayed similarly restricted heterogeneity in response to a given peptide determinant of cytochrome.

These results along with the anti-idiotypic antibody data confirmed Cohen's predictions that this response was indeed monoidiotypic and that it was possible to have a regulatory response which could be directed to the Vβ8 determinants on disease-causing T cells. However, examination of the clones tested above indicated that the T-cell response itself was not monoclonal since an MBP-specific T-cell population which was 100% 10.18 positive had TcR rearrangement patterns (using a constant region probe on Southern blot analysis), which showed that all T cells examined were actually different from one another and did not derive from a single parent cell (52). One important aspect of the above analysis was that the fine specificity of the Vα2, Vβ8-positive T-cell clones were not the same, with three different 68–88 specific fine specificities identified (50). Without sequence data, however, it is impossible to know which part of the receptor is responsible for these differences.

A second study in the Lewis rat also using MBP 68–88-specific encephalitogenic T cells showed similar results; i.e., Vβ8.2 again was being used with either Jβ1.1 or Jβ1.3 and a conserved D region. Vα2 was again used (53).

In a study to analyze T-cell receptor gene usage in the mouse, encephalitogenic T cells from PL/J and (PL/J × SJL) F_1 mice were examined. These cells were specific for residues 1 through 9 of MBP. Again, limited heterogeneity in TcR usage was seen. Sequencing of the receptors from these clones showed 80% usage of Vβ8.2 with Jβ2.7, 2.3, and 2.5 in descending frequency. Each beta chain VJ group used a specific junctional region sequence even though this junctional region is generally found to be highly variable. All of the clones used the same member of the Vα4 family, VαPJR-25 (45).

In a second study, B10.PL mice were examined (44). This mouse strain, which also is $H\text{-}2^u$, recognizes the MBP encephalitogenic determinant, residues 1–9. It was found that 80% of the clones used Vβ8.2; however, unlike PL/J, all of the clones used only Jβ2.7. Vα usage was more heterogeneous than in the PL/J with 58% Vα2 and 42% Vα4. All alpha chains used the same Jα39 sequence. Again, from both studies it is clear that there is a molecular basis for shared idiotypy.

C. Conservation of a TcR V Gene Combination in Autoimmune Disease–Inducing T Cells

From what has been presented so far, we are confronted with the unusual fact that TcR molecules (1) involved in the recognition of different antigenic determinants of MBP, residues 68–88 and 1–9, (2) recognizing different MHC molecules, $Rt\text{-}1^l$ and $H\text{-}2^u$, and (3) derived from two different species, mouse and rat, use similar gene elements. Perhaps the "easiest" explanation is that this common usage is mere coincidence. However, the more satisfying explanation is that these clones share something besides their TcR V regions. One feature of these cells is that they recognize antigen + MHC and the two together could be antigenically cross-reactive. When comparing the 1–9 and 72–84 minimal encephalitogenic determinants of the PL/J mouse and the Lewis rat, five residues are shared. To determine the importance of these similarities, functional studies were done by cross-presenting each of the two determinants with the two different antigen-presenting cells (APC). Thus whole MBP or either peptide was added to culture with Lewis T cells and PL/J APC or to cultures of PL/J T cells and Lewis APC. No antigen presentation was seen (54). Thus, it does not appear that antigenic cross-reactivity can easily explain the shared usage of Vα2 and Vβ8.

To determine the generality of this usage of paired V gene combination, examination of three other EAE-susceptible strains of rat whose MBP-specific T cells could cause EAE upon transfer into syngeneic hosts was carried out (54,55). Such T cells recognized antigenic determinants of MBP other than 68–88 and different from one another and recognized Ia molecules of different haplotypes. They again showed usage of this TcR Vα2Vβ8 combination. Lack of positive results in antigen cross-presentation experiments as described above supported the notion that this shared Vα2Vβ8 usage was not due to recognition of the same antigen–Ia complex. Also, the 10.18 antibody which recognized a shared idiotype bound to T cells of two out of three of the rat strains, a finding which suggests that the antibody is not recognizing Vβ8.

The Vα2Vβ8 combination was seen in another T-cell population in the Lewis rat (56). In this case the Ia isotype recognized was different (I-E instead of I-A) and the antigenic determinant was also different, residues 87–99 of MBP. This determinant was seen as the dominant encephalitogenic determinant upon a second challenge of MBP.

Two strains of rats resistant to EAE, LeR (57), and BN (55) were also examined. Here, MBP-specific T cells could be induced and transfer disease to normal X-irradiated hosts. These T cells were found to use Vα2Vβ8 in the case of BN and Vα4Vβ8 in the case of LeR.

Finally, preliminary data in yet a third species, the guinea pig, has indicated that an MBP-specific T-cell population again hybridizes with the Vβ8 and Vα2 probes (S. Goldman and E. Heber-Katz, unpublished data).

Given the fact that the EAE TcR V gene combination Vα2Vβ8 appeared to be so frequently used, we proposed a relationship between neurologic pathogenesis and the use of this receptor combination, which we have called the V-region disease hypothesis (54). Essentially, the TcR would have two separate functions. One would be to recognize antigen plus MHC and could be localized to the junctional regions of the α and β chains. The second function is linked to pathogenesis, and we proposed a neurologically relevant ligand independent of "antigen" which would be recognized by a site on the TcR receptor made up of the Vα2Vβ8 combination. We thus examined two other autoimmune diseases which were inducible by other antigens of the nervous system, inducing inflammation at different sites in the body, EAN and EAU, to see if the T cells involved also used this same V-region combination.

III. OTHER DISEASES IN WHICH A "UNIQUE" Vα2Vβ8 TcR COMBINATION IS USED

A. Experimental Allergic Neuritis

Experimental allergic neuritis (EAN) is an autoimmune disease which is adoptively transferred by T cells specific for the peripheral nerve myelin protein, P_2 (58). This protein is a major structural protein of molecular weight 15,000 and differs from P_1 in its amino acid sequence. It is found mainly in the peripheral myelin sheath made by Schwann cells, but small quantities exist in the CNS (as identified in rabbits). Injection of this protein in CFA causes demyelination and paralysis and is similar in symptomatology and thus considered to be a model for Guillain-Barre syndrome in humans. In the Lewis rat, a synthetic peptide of residues 53–78 of the bovine P_2 protein has been shown to be neuritic (59,60). Analysis of the TcR gene usage in long-term T-cell lines specific for this peptide and known, upon adoptive transfer, to cause severe disease has shown that again both $V\alpha2$ and $V\beta8$ are strongly represented, whereas in a normal T-cell population these V regions are not predominant. Furthermore, use of the anti-idiotype has indicated that these EAN-inducing T cells are positive for the 10.18 anti-idiotype (61). Examination of clonal populations which cause disease has not been carried out, but these results support the idea of a common neurologically associated ligand.

B. Experimental Allergic Uveoretinitis

Experimental allergic uveoretinitis (EAU) is an autoimmune response to the neural autoantigen, retinal S-antigen, a retinal rod photoreceptor cell protein, and the interphotoreceptor retinoid-binding protein (IRBP) and is considered to be an animal model for human uveitis (62,63). This experimental disease is also a T-cell–mediated disease induced by injection of the autoantigens emulsified in CFA. An analysis has been made of TcR gene usage in T-cell lines that can respond to the whole S-antigen but are specific for either pathogenic or nonpathogenic antigenic determinants (64). A perfect correlation has been found with T cells that are pathogenic and use TcR $V\beta8$ genes and with T cells that are nonpathogenic and do not use $V\beta8$. Furthermore, three out of four T-cell lines which are pathogenic used $V\alpha2$ (65). These percentages are the same when T-cell clones and hybridomas that cause EAE were examined. This provides a third case of experimentally induced neurologic disease in which this V gene combination exists and is associated with disease.

C. Adjuvant Arthritis

Adjuvant or autoimmune arthritis (AA) is an experimental disease induced by the injection of complete Freund's adjuvant (CFA) containing *Mycobacterium tuberculosis* into animals and has some characteristics similar to rheumatoid arthritis in humans including severe inflammation of the joints. Disease-inducing T-cell lines and clones from such immunized rats respond to PPD and to collagen, and it has recently been shown that a heat shock protein (HSP) derived from *M. tuberculosis* is the specific antigen (66–68). Analysis of these clones has revealed usage of $V\beta8.2$ (Van Eden and Cohen, unpublished data). Also, a PPD-specific T-cell line which can transfer disease has revealed usage of both Vβ8 and Vα2 (Clark and Heber-Katz, unpublished data). Such data again support the V-region disease hypothesis, but AA is not a neurologic disease. On the other hand, it is a sequestered antigen which may require a shared ligand to allow recirculation into that region. One aspect of the diseases described above is that they are all induced by high concentrations of self-antigen in CFA. It would be of interest to examine spontaneously occurring autoimmune diseases.

IV. DISEASES IN WHICH THE Vα2Vβ8 TcR COMBINATION IS NOT USED

A. Diabetes

Insulin-dependent diabetes mellitus (IDDM) is a disease in which T cells are found to infiltrate the pancreas and have a destructive effect on the insulin-producing beta cells. Two spontaneous disease models exist, one in the nonobese diabetic (NOD) mouse and one in the BioBreeding (BB) rat. In the NOD mouse, interesting results from Janeway et al. (69) have demonstrated that the T-cell clones of both the CD4 and CD8 phenotype which are reactive to pancreatic islet cell antigens (the exact antigenic determinants are not known) are necessary for transfer of severe insulitis. Both cell types have been found to be TcR Vβ5 positive. At present no information is available on TcR gene usage in the BB rat.

It is interesting that in a spontaneous autoimmune disease there is again restricted heterogeneity, however, it is not Vα2Vβ8. NOD mice are lacking the Ia isotype, I-E. When NOD transgenics are made to express I-E, however, the animals become resistant to spontaneous diabetes (68). Concomitant with this resistance is the elimination of the $V\beta5^+$ T-cell population, presumably occurring during maturation in the thymus (70). One might conclude that only a T-cell population in I-E negative mice can cause this disease. However, the BB rat is I-E positive, yet still gets diabetes, a situation similar to that seen in the human, and this BB model will be important to study.

B. Spontaneous Autoimmune Disease Induced by Neonatal Thymectomy

In 1971, it was shown that (B6 × A/J) F_1 mice thymectomized at an early age were subject to the autoimmune disease ovarian dysgenesis (71). Recent analysis of TcR V gene usage has revealed an interesting correlation (72). In normal adult F_1 mice, the Vβ11 subset is deleted in the peripheral T-cell population. However, in F_1 mice thymectomized at 1–4 days after birth, the Vβ11 subset is 10 times as high as that in normals. Whether this Vβ11 subset is actually involved in disease remains to be determined, but would again support the notion that a restricted set of TcR positive T cells is involved in organ-specific spontaneous autoimmune disease.

V. CONCLUSION

The study of T-cell receptor gene usage in experimental autoimmune diseases has revealed several things. First, it is clear that responses to given self-antigenic determinants result in populations of T cells which share T-cell receptor genes and provide the possibility of anti-idiotypic immune intervention in specific disease. This finding appears to be true in spontaneously induced disease as well, in which the antigens have not been identified.

Second, we have found unusual degrees of similarities in V regions used by T cells, not only in a particular disease, but even when the antigens are different. Furthermore, there is even sharing in different and seemingly unrelated diseases. What this means is at present unknown, however, we have proposed the V-region disease hypothesis, which states that the disease is in part defined by the V regions of the T-cell receptor and not the antigen. This T-cell receptor with a given V gene combination (Vα2Vβ8) would recognize a second ligand, other than antigen+ MHC, which could allow pathogenic cells to migrate to sites of disease. Since this receptor or V gene combination is seen with many diseases, this ligand would not be disease-site specific. Disease specificity would then be conferred by the antigen-specific part of the T-cell receptor. Theoretical issues aside, if this finding is also true in human disease, than shared idiotypy may exist for many different antigens and different diseases as well, and one could imagine the possibilities for broad-based immune regulation.

REFERENCES

1. Bassoe, P., and Grinker, R. R. 1930. Human rabies and rabies vaccine encephalitis. A clinicopathological study. *Arch. Neurol. Psychiatr.*, *23*: 1138–1145.
2. Rivers, T. M., and Schwentker, F. F. 1935. Encephalomyelitis accompanied by myelin destruction experimentally produced in monkeys. *J. Exp. Med.*, *61*: 689–695.
3. Shapira, R. McKneally, S. S., Chou, F., and Kibler, R. F. 1971. Encephalitogenic fragment of myelin basic protein. Amino acid sequence of bovine, rabbit, guinea pig, monkey, and human fragments. *J. Biol. Chem.*, *246*: 4630–4639.
4. Dunkley, P. R., and Carnegie, P. R. 1974. Amino acid sequences of the smaller basic protein from rat brain myelin. *Biochem. J.*, *141*: 243–257.
5. Bergstrand, H. 1977. Immunochemistry of encephalitogenic protein. In *Immunochemistry of Proteins*, Vol. 1. (Atassi, ed.). Plenum Press, New York, p. 315.
6. Hashim, G. A. 1978. Myelin basic protein: Structure, function, and antigenic determinants. *Immunol. Rev.*, *39*: 60–95.
7. Burnet, F. M. 1959. *The Clonal Selection Theory of Acquired Immunity*. Cambridge University Press, New York.
8. Nossal, G. J. V. 1983. Cellular mechanisms of immunological tolerance. *Ann. Rev. Immunol.*, *1*: 33–62.
9. Lider, O., Reshef, T., Beraud, E., Ben-Nun, A., and Cohen, I. R. 1988. Anti-idiotypic

network induced by T cell vaccination against experimental autoimmune encephalomyelitis. *Science, 239*: 181–183.
10. Ellerman, K. E., Powers, J. M., and Brostoff, S. W. 1988. A suppressor T lymphocyte cell line for autoimmune encephalomyelitis. *Nature, 331*: 265–267.
11. Sun, D., Qin, Y., Chluba, J., Epplen, J. T., and Wekerle, H. 1988. Suppression of experimentally induced autoimmune encephalomyelitis by cytolytic T-T cell interactions. *Nature, 332*: 843–845.
12. Howell, M. D., Winters, S. T., Olse, T. Powell, H. C., Carlo, D. J., and Brostoff, S. W. 1989. Vaccination against experimental allergic encephalomyelitis with synthetic T cell receptor peptides. *Science, 246*: 668–670.
13. Schwartz, R. H. 1985. T lymphocyte recognition of antigen in association with gene products of the major histocompatibility complex. *Ann. Rev. Immunol., 3*: 239–261.
14. Allen, P. 1987. Antigen processing at the molecular level. *Immunol. Today, 8*: 270–273.
15. Rosenthal, 1978. Determinant selection and macrophage function in genetic control of the immune response. *Immunol. Rev., 40*: 136.
16. Benacerraf, B. 1978. A hypothesis to relate the specificity of T lymphocytes and the activity of I region-specific Ir genes in macrophages and B lymphocytes. *J. Immunol., 120*: 1809.
17. Heber-Katz, E., Hansburg, D., and Schwartz, R. S. 1983. The Ia molecule of the antigen-presenting cell plays a critical role in immune response gene regulation of T cell activation. *J. Mol. Cell. Immunol., 1*: 3.
18. Babbit, B. P., Allen, P. M., Matsueda, G., and Unanue, E. R. 1985. Binding of immunogenic peptides to Ia histocompatibility molecules. *Nature, 317*: 359.
19. Buus, S., Sette, A., Colon, A., Miles, C., and Grey, H. M. 1987. The relation between MHC restriction and the capacity of Ia to bind immunogenic peptides. *Science, 235*: 1353.
20. Yamashita, K., and Heber-Katz, E. 1989. Lack of immunodominance in the T cell response to herpes simplex virus glycoprotein D after administration of infectious virus. *J. Exp. Med., 170*: 997.
21. Mills, K. H., Skehel, J. J., and Thomas, D. B. 1986. Extensive diversity in the recognition of influenza virus hemagglutinin by murine helper clones. *J. Exp. Med., 163*: 1477.
22. Atassi, M. A., and Kurisaki, J. 1984. A novel approach for localization of the continuous protein antigenic sites by comprehensive synthetic surface scanning antibody and T cell activity to several influenza hemagglutinin synthetic sites. *Immunol. Commun., 13*: 539.
23. Allison, J. P., and Lanier, L. L. 1987. Structure, function, and serology of the T cell antigen receptor complex. *Ann. Rev. Immunol., 5*: 503–540.
24. Hedrick, S. M., Cohen, D. I., Nielson, E. A., and Davis, M. M. 1984. Isolation of cDNA clones encoding T-cell specific membrane associated proteins. *Nature, 308*: 149.
25. Dembic, Z., von Boehmer, H., and Steinmetz, M. 1986. The role of T cell receptor α and β genes in MHC restricted antigen recognition. *Immunol. Today, 7*: 308.
26. Saito, T., and Germaine, R. N. 1987. Predictable acquisition of a new HMC

recognition specificity following expression of a transfected T cell receptor β chain gene. *Nature, 329*: 256.
27. Davis, M., and Bjorkman, P. J. 1988. T cell antigen receptor genes and T cell recognition. *Nature, 334*: 395.
28. Kronenberg, M., Siu, G., Hood, L. E., and Shastri, N. 1986. The molecular genetics of the T cell antigen receptor and T cell antigen recognition. *Ann. Rev. Immunol., 4*: 529–591.
29. Wilson, R. K., Lai, E., Concannon, P., Barth, K., and Hood, L. 1988. Structure, organization, and polymorphism of murine and human T cell receptor α and β chain gene families. *Immunol. Rev., 101*: 149–172.
30. Fink, P. J., Matis, L., McElliott, D. L., Bookman, M., and Hedrick, S. 1986. Correlations between T cell specificity and the structure of the antigen receptor. *Nature, 312*: 219.
31. Hochheschwender, U., Simon, H. G., Weltsien, H. U., Bartles, F., Becker, A., and Epplen, J. T. 1987. Dominance of one T cell receptor in the H-2K^b/TNP response. *Nature, 326*: 307.
32. Tan, K-N, Datlot, B. M., Gilmore, J. A., Kronman, A. C., Lee, J. H., Maxam, M. M., and Rao, A. 1988. The T cell receptor Vα3 gene segment is associated with reactivity to azobenene-arsonate. *Cell, 54*: 247.
33. Winoto, A., Urban, J. L., Lan, N. C., Governman, J., Hood, L., and Hansburg, D. 1986. Predominant use of a Vα gene segment in mouse T cell receptors for cytochrome c. *Nature, 324*: 679.
34. Sorger, S. B., Hedrick, S. M., Fink, P. J., Bookman, M. A., and Matis, L. A. 1987. Generation of diversity in T cell receptor repertoire specific for pigeon cytochrome c. *J. Exp. Med., 165*: 279–301.
35. Ramseier, H., and Lindenmann, J. 1969. F_1 hybrid animals: Reactivity against recognition structures of parental strain cells. *Pathol. Microbiol., 34*: 379.
36. Rose, N. 1975. Modification of hybrid responsiveness in local graft versus host reactions by injection of parental lymphocytes. *Transplantation, 20*: 248–254.
37. Woodland, R. T., and Wilson, D. B. 1977. The induction of specific resistance in F_1 hybrid rats to local graft-vs-host reaction: nature of the eliciting cell. *Eur. J. Immunol., 7*: 136–142.
38. Ben-Nun, A., Wekerle, H., and Cohen, I. R. 1981. Vaccination against autoimmune encephalomyelitis using attenuated cells of a T lymphocyte line reactive against myelin basic protein. *Nature, 292*: 60–62,
39. Owhashi, M., and Heber-Katz, E. 1988. Protection from EAE conferred by a monoclonal antibody against a shared idiotype on rat TcRs specific for MBP. *J. Exp. Med., 168*: 2153.
40. Pettinelli, C. B., Fritz, R. B., Chou, CH-J, and McFarlin, D. E. 1982. Encephalitogenic activity of guinea pig myelin basic protein in the SJL mouse. *J. Immunol., 129*: 1209.
41. Fritz, R. B., Jen Chou, C. H., and McFarlin, D. E. 1983. Induction of experimental allergic encephalomyelitis in PL/J and (SJL $\times$ PL/J)F_1 mice by myelin basic protein and its peptides: Localization of a second encephalitogenic determinant. *J. Immunol., 130*: 191.

42. Zamvil, S. S., Mitchell, D. J., Lee, N. E., Moore, A. C., Kitamura, K., Steinman, L., and Rothbard, J. B. 1986. T cell epitope of the autoantigen myelin basic protein that induce encephalomyelitis. *Nature, 324*: 258.
43. Zamvil, S.S., Mitchell, D. J., Lee, N. E., Moore, A. C., Waldorf, M. K., Saki, K., Rothbard, J. B., McDevitt, H. O., Steinman, L., and Acha-Orbea, H. 1988. Predominant expression of a T cell receptor Vβ gene subfamily in autoimmune encephalomyelitis. *J. Exp. Med., 167*: 263.
44. Urban, J., Kumar, V., Kono, D., Gomez, C., Horvath, S. J., Clayton, J., Ando, D. G., Sercarz, E.E., and Hood, L. 1988. Restricted used of TcR V genes in murine autoimmune encephalomyelitis raises possibilities for antibody therapy. *Cell, 54*: 577.
45. Acha-Orbea, H. Mitchell, D. J., Timmerman, L., Wraith, D. C., Taich, G. S., Waldor, M. K., Zamvil, S., McDevitt, H., and Steinman, L. 1988. Limited heterogeneity of TcRs from lymphocytes mediating autoimmune encephalomyelitis allows specific immune intervention. *Cell, 54*: 263.
46. Staerz, U. D., Rammensee, H. G., Benedetto, J. D., and Bevan, M. J. 1985. Characterization of a murine monoclonal antibody specific for an allotype determinant of T cell antigen receptor. *J. Immunol., 134*: 3994–4000.
47. Haskins, K., Hannum, C., White, J. Roehm, N., Kubo, R., Kappler J., and Marrack, P. 1984. The antigen specific MHC restricted receptor on T cells. VI. An antibody to a receptor allotype. *J. Exp. Med., 160*: 452–471.
48. Kono, D. H., Urban, J. L., Horvath, S. J., Ando, D. G., Saavedra, R. A., and Hood, L. 1988. Two minor determinants of myelin basic protein induce experimental allergic encephalomyelitis in SJL/J mice. *J. Exp. Med., 168*: 213.
49. Sakai, K., Sinha, A. A., Mitchell, D. J., Zamvil, S. S., Rothbard, J. B., McDevitt, H. O., and Steinman, L. 1988. Involvement of distinct T cell receptors in the autoimmune encephalitogenic response to nested epitopes of myelin basic protein. *P.N.A.S., 85*: 8608.
50. Happ, M. P., and Heber-Katz, E. 1988. Differences in the repertoire of the Lewis rat T cell response to self and non-self MBPs. *J. Exp. Med., 167*: 502.
51. Burns, F., Li, X., Shen, N., Offner, H., Chou, Y. K., Vandenbark, A. A., and Heber-Katz, E. 1989. Both rat and mouse TcRs specific for the encephalitogenic determinant of MBP use similar Vα and Vβ chain genes even though the MHC and encephalitogenic determinants being recognized are different. *J. Exp. Med., 169*: 27.
52. Happ, M. P., Kiraly, A. S., Offner, H., Vandenbark, A., and Heber-Katz, E. 1988. The autoreactive T cell population in experimental allergic encephalomyelitis: T cell receptor β chain rearrangements. *J. Neuroimmunol., 19*: 191.
53. Chluba, J., Steeg, C., Becker, A., Wekerle, H., and Epplen, T. J. 1989. TcR β chain usage in MBP specific rat T lymphocytes. *Eur. J. Immunol., 19*: 279.
54. Heber-Katz, E., and Acha-Orbea, H., 1989. The V-region hypothesis: Evidence from autoimmune encephalomyelitis. *Immunol. Today, 10*: 164.
55. Li, X., Owhashi, M., Jones, R., Offner, H., Vandenbark, A. A., and Heber-Katz, E. 1990. Evolutionarily conserved V regions in autoimmune encephalitis. (In preparation.)
56. Offner, H., Hashim, G. A., Celnick, B., Galang, A., Li, X., Burns, F. R., Shen, N., Heber-Katz, E., and Vandenbark, A. A. 1989. T cell determinants of myelin

basic protein include a unique encephalitogenic I-E restricted epitope for Lewis rats. *J. Exp. Med., 170*: 355.

57. Blankenhorn, E., and Hickey, W. 1991. TcR gene usage in Lewis resistant (LeR) rats. (Submitted.)
58. Waksman, B. H., and Adams, R. D. 1955. Allergic neuritis: An experimental disease of rabbits induced by the injection of peripheral nervous tissue and adjuvants. *J. Exp. Med., 102*: 213–236.
59. Rostami, A., Burns, J. B., Brown, M. J., Rosen, J., Zweiman, B., Lisak, R. P., and Pleasure, D. E. 1983. Transfer of experimental allergic neuritis with P2 reactive T cells. *Ann. Neurol., 14*: 108.
60. Rostami, A. M., Ventura, E., Kimura, H., Brown, M. J., and Pleasure, D. E. 1988. Induction of severe experimental allergic neuritis (EAN) with a synthetic peptide corresponding to the 53-78 amino acid sequence of the myelin P2 protein. *Neurology, 38*: 375.
61. Clark, L., Heber-Katz, E., and Rostami, A. M. 1991. Shared T cell receptor gene usage in experimental allergic neuritis and encephalomyelitis. (Submitted.)
62. Wacker, W. B., Donoso, L. A., Kalsow, C. M., Yankelov, J. A., and Organisciak, D. T. 1977. Experimental allergic uevitis. Isolation, characterization, and localization of soluble uveitopathogenic antigen from bovine retina. *J. Immunol., 119*: 1949–1956.
63. Hirose, S., Kubawara, T., Nussenblatt, R. B., Wiggert, B., Redmond, T. M., and Gery, I. 1986. Uveitis induced in primates by IRBP. *Arch. Ophthalmol., 104*: 1698–1702.
64. Gregorson, D. S., Obritsch, W. F., Fling, S. P., and Cameron, J. D. 1986. S-antigen specific rat T cell lines recognize peptide fragments of S-antigen and mediate experimental autoimmune uveoretinitis and pinealitis. *J. Immunol., 136*: 2875–2882.
65. Gregorson, D. S., Li, X., Fling, S. P., Merryman, C. F., and Heber-Katz, E. 1989. Pathogenic Lew rat T cell lines specific for distinct sites on retinal S-antigen use similar TcR Vβ8 genes, nonpathogenic lines do not. *J. Cell Biochem., 13D*: 71.
66. Van Eden, W., Holoshitz, J., Nevo, Z., Frenkel, A., Klajman, A., and Cohen, I. R. 1985. Arthritis induced by a T lymphocyte clone that responds to *Mycobacterium tuberculosis* and to cartilage proteoglycans. *Proc. Natl. Acad. Sci. USA, 82*: 5117–5120.
67. Van Eden, W., Thole, J. E. R., van der Zee, R., Noordzij, A., van Embden, J. D. A., Hansen, E. J., and Cohen, I. R. 1988. Cloning of the mycobacterial epitope recognized by T lymphocytes in adjuvant arthritis. *Nature, 331*: 171–173.
68. Holoshitz, J., Klajman, A., Drucker, I., Lapidot, Z., Yaretzsky, A., Frenkel, A., Van Eden, W., and Cohen, I. R. 1986. T lymphocytes of rheumatoid arthritis patients show augmented reactivity to a fraction of mycobacteria cross-reactive with cartilage. *Lancet, 2*: 305–309.
69. Reich, E., Sherwin, R. S., Kanagawa, O., and Janeway, Jr., C. A. 1989. An explanation for the protective effect of the MHC class II I-E molecule in murine diabetes. *Nature, 341*: 326–328.

70. Nishimoto, H., Kikutani, H., Yamamura, K. I., and Kishimoto, T. 1987. Prevention of autoimmune insulitis by expression of I-E molecule in NOD mice. *Nature, 328*: 432–434.
71. Nishizuka, Y., and Sakakura, T. 1971. Ovarian dysgenesis induced by neonatal thymectomy in the mouse. *Endocrinology, 89*: 886.
72. Smith, H., Chen, I. M., Kubo, R., and Tung, K. S. 1989. Neonatal thymectomy results in a repertoire enriched in T cells deleted in adult thymus. *Science, 245*: 749–752.

10

TCR V Gene Usage in Autoimmunity

David N. Posnett
Cornell University Medical College, New York, New York
Kevin J. Horgan and Steven M. Friedman
The Hospital for Special Surgery, New York, New York

I. INTRODUCTION

A number of considerations implicate T cells as the primary contributors to the pathogenesis of many autoimmune diseases. First, a prototypical autoimmune disease in man, rheumatoid arthritis, is characterized by infiltration of synovial membranes by activated T cells. In the synovium, T cells, once activated, produce lymphokines that result in the activation of synoviocytes, which in turn produce prostaglandin E_2 and collagenase (1), which are thought to contribute to the inflammatory process resulting in joint destruction. Synovial T cells specific for *M. tuberculosis* antigens are found in the human disease and in the experimental model, rat adjuvant arthritis. The latter can be induced by a single injection of *M. tuberculosis* in Freund's adjuvant and can be transferred to irradiated rats with T cells specific for *M. tuberculosis* antigens (2). Recent studies have identified the pathogenic *M. tuberculosis* antigen as a heat shock protein: hsp 60 (3,4). Because of the high degree of evolutionary sequence conservation among heat shock proteins and the finding that they are very immunogenic, it has been postulated that pathogen-derived heat shock proteins may induce autoimmunity by molecular mimicry (5). Interestingly, synovial T cells from patients with rheumatoid arthritis can respond to mycobacterial hsp 60 and hsp 70, to *E. coli* hsp 60 and hsp 70, and to human hsp 70 (6). However, similar T cells may also be found in individuals without autoimmune disease (6,7), indicating that more needs to be learned about these T cells.

A hallmark of all autoimmune diseases in human is the striking association of susceptibility to a given disease with specific MHC-encoded allelic antigens. Thus, susceptibility to rheumatoid arthritis is related to the presence of a DR4 class II antigen. The third hypervariable region of the DRβI chain may contain residues responsible for RA susceptibility (8). These residues are putative contact residues of the antigen-binding pocket of the DR class II molecule and may influence antigen binding or interact with the T-cell receptor. Similarly, individual amino acid residues situated around the antigen-binding pocket of MHC molecules have been implicated in conferring susceptibility versus resistance to two other autoimmune diseases: insulin-dependent diabetes mellitus (9) and pemphigus vulgaris (10). These considerations imply that clinical autoimmunity is a consequence of the activation of normally quiescent clones of MHC-restricted autoantigen-reactive T cells.

A number of animal models for human autoimmune diseases have demonstrated that injection of a single clone of autoantigen-reactive MHC-restricted T cells may be sufficient to induce an autoimmune disease in an X-irradiated recipient animal (11,12). These animal models include adjuvant arthritis, mentioned above, and experimental allergic encephalomyelitis (EAE), a disease which serves as a model for multiple sclerosis and which is induced in susceptible mouse and rat strains by immunization with myelin basic protein (MBP). T-cell clones recognizing defined peptides of MBP can transfer the disease to X-irradiated recipient animals (12). The disease can be prevented by blocking interaction of the relevant TCR with Ag/MHC using either anti-TCR V region-specific monoclonal antibodies (MAbs) (13,14), or anti-Ia MAbs (18,19), or modified MBP peptide, which can bind to the MHC but no longer activates the relevant T-cell clone (20,21).

An important finding in these studies on EAE was that the disease-producing T-cell clones used a restricted number of V gene elements for their TCR. Murine Vβ8.2 gene products were used by these clones in >80% of cases (13,14), and MAbs specific for $V\beta 8.2^+$ TCRs could prevent disease produced by such clones. In multiple sclerosis (the human disease equivalent of EAE), T-cell clones derived from cerebrospinal fluid have also shown limited heterogeneity, suggesting oligoclonality (22). Most recently, several groups have successfully immunized animals with synthetic peptides corresponding to TCR sequences based on knowledge of which TCR V gene elements are used by T-cell clones producing EAE (15–17). These animals are protected against EAE. While it is still unclear how this protection is generated, these findings suggest that therapies for autoimmune diseases will be forthcoming and that knowledge of the composition of TCRs used by antoantigen reactive T-cell clones will be essential.

We have therefore initiated a screening approach to determine TCR V gene usage in a variety of human autoimmune diseases. There are currently two methods to determine TCR V gene usage: (1) monoclonal antibodies specific for subsets of TCR V gene products, and (2) polymerase chain reaction (PCR) amplification of TCR V gene cDNA. These methods will be discussed in detail below. It is worth considering the source of the T cells being examined. Clonal excess of autoreactive T cells may be found only at discrete locations relevant to the autoimmune process, for instance, the endocrine pancreas in IDDM. These locations are often inaccessible for study in humans. It is also important to consider the stage of the disease at which cells are obtained, since it is possible that the T cells responsible for initiating the autoimmune responses may represent a minor component of the inflammatory response during the chronic phase of the disease.

The present chapter summarizes primarily work performed in the authors' laboratories dealing exclusively with human systems. These studies include the demonstration of TCR V-region allotypes. Regarding TCR V gene usage, T cells bearing human Vβ8 gene products are expanded in a subset of patients with Crohn's disease and sarcoidosis. Similarly, studies with certain microbial superantigens have shown that these substances cause expansion of T-cell subsets that share TCR V gene products. Some of these T cells provide help to B cells in a cognate T-B interaction mediated by a superantigen bridge leading to potent polyclonal B-cell activation. Therefore, it is possible that superantigens play a role in initiating an autoimmune response.

II. ANTIBODIES TO HUMAN TCR V GENE PRODUCTS

Three types of monoclonal antibodies to human TCR α/β and gamma/delta molecules have been produced. Antibodies to gamma/delta TCR molecules are summarized elsewhere (23) and will not be further discussed, but also fall into the general categories outlined below. By far the most prevalent type of MAb is the clonotypic antibody, which recognizes only the TCR molecule of the immunizing T-cell clone or leukemia. The uses for such antibodies are therefore limited. Because of the similarity with immunoglobulin idiotypes, these MAbs have been termed "anti-idiotypic" or "Ti" antibodies. Although the specific determinants recognized by such MAbs have not been mapped in the majority of cases, it is likely that amino acids encoded by N-segment codons, produced by VDJ or VJ rearrangement, are involved. Such residues are thought to be the most diverse, to interact with antigen rather than MHC and to be located in the third hypervariable loop of the putative three-dimensional structure of the α/β TCR molecule (24,25). It is also possible that anticlonotypic MAbs recognize conformational epitopes such as epitopes defined by both α and β chains. The second category of MAb to TCR molecules encompasses anticonstant region MAbs, which will not be discussed here.

A third category of MAb to TCR molecules is also frequently observed. These MAbs react with small populations of T cells, usually between 1 and 10% (26,27). In most instances, they have been characterized as V gene–specific MAbs (Table 1). The TCR recognized by such a MAb all share the same or very similar V gene products. For instance, mRNA from S511$^+$ T cell lines has been reverse transcribed and amplified by PCR using primers specific for different Vβ gene subfamilies. Only Vβ12-specific primers amplified the TCR β chain from S511$^+$ T-cell lines (28). While these studies clearly identified S511 as an anti-Vβ12 MAb, it is not yet known whether all or only a subset of the 4 Vβ12 V genes are recognized or whether other related V genes can be recognized under different circumstances. Similarly, the MAb OT145 detects primarily Vβ6.7 gene products (29) but may also detect some other Vβ6 gene products of this large Vβ gene subfamily with an estimated 6–9 genes by counting cross-hybridizing bands on Southern blots.

Anti-V gene MAbs are possibly similar to certain MAbs directed to immunoglobulin V gene subsets, such as the anti-VkIIIa and anti-VkIIIb specificities of certain kappa chains (30). However, these MAbs seem to occur much more frequently when immunizing with TCRs compared to immunoglobulins. This could be due to the fact that TCR V genes do not undergo somatic hypermutation as do immunoglobulin V genes. Thus, V gene-specified epitopes of TCR are likely to be preserved, and MAbs recognizing these epitopes can accurately detect V gene usage by individual T cells. It is of interest that in the few instances of similar V gene–specific MAbs to immunoglobulin V genes such as the VkIIIb genes, these V genes are often used as germline sequences without much somatic mutation (30).

Finally, this subset of anti-TCR MAbs is obviously very useful for rapid assessment of V gene usage at the level of the mature membrane expressed TCR molecule. As discussed below, these MAbs have also been central to the definition of superantigens, which, like the MAbs themselves, also have specificity for subsets of V gene products (28,31,32).

MAbs specific for V gene products have been used extensively in murine and human studies. Yet little is known about the distribution of T-cell subpopulations that share usage of a particular TCR V gene and are identified by such MAbs. In the past, we have found that populations identified by anti-V gene-specific MAbs are composed of CD4$^+$ and CD8$^+$ T cells (33,34). Two-color fluorescence is best suited to detect a bias toward either CD4$^+$ or CD8$^+$ T cells in these small populations. In general, one finds that Vβ gene usage as identified by the MAbs listed in Table 1 is similar in the CD4$^+$ and CD8$^+$ subsets. Occasionally, a normal individual will have a skewed V gene usage, as presented in Table 2, where Vβ8 gene usage was five times more frequent among CD8$^+$ than among CD4$^+$ T cells.

TABLE 1 Monoclonal Antibodies with Specificity for Human V Gene Products

MAb	Immunogen	Specificity	Size of V gene family[a]	Ref.
S511	Sezary T-cell leukemia	Vβ12	4	26
C37	HPBALL	Vβ5.3	5	33
OT145	T-cell CLL	Vβ6.7	≈9	27
16G8	Jurkat	Vβ8	5	TCS[b]
Ti3a	Jurkat	Vβ8	5	89
F1	T-cell CLL	Vα2.3		TCS
LC4	T-cell CLL	Vβ5.1		90, TCS

[a]Vβ8.3, Vβ8.4, and Vβ8.5 are pseudogenes based on sequence analysis of these genes isolated from a single individual (48). For the other V gene famiies, it is not known how many genes are functional.
[b]T Cell Sciences, Inc., Cambridge, MA.

Another question regards V gene usage among different subsets of CD4$^+$ T cells: naive and memory T cells (35). These subsets can be distinguished by two-color analysis with an anti-CD45RA MAb (Leu-18), which reacts specifically with the higher molecular weight isoform of CD45 expressed by naive T cells (35). The data presented in Table 3 shows that, in two normal individuals, there were no differences in V gene usage between these two subsets. However, it may not be possible to generalize from these data, since it is quite possible that changes in V gene expression occur over time in an individual and that this is dependent on exposure to different antigenic stimuli (36). These considerations are important

TABLE 2 V Gene Expression in CD4 and CD8 Subsets from Normal Peripheral Blood T Cells

Population	CD3$^+$	CD4$^+$ CD8$^-$	CD8$^+$ CD4$^-$
CD3	100%	100%	100%
CD4	82.3	100	—
CD8	9.7	—	100
Vβ5 (C37)	2.6	2.7	2.2
Vβ6 (OT145)	4.4	4.4	6.8
Vβ8 (Ti3a)	2.8	3.2	15.9

Two-color fluorescence analysis with phycoerthin-labeled anti-CD3, CD4$^-$, and CD8$^-$ MAbs.

TABLE 3 Naive and Memory Cells Have Similar Expression of Particular Vβ Chains

Population		Donor 1210		Donor 1308	
		Naive	Memory	Naive	Memory
S511	(Vβ12)	1.8	1.7	1.9	1.4
OT145	(Vβ6.7)	5.4	5.5	3.5	3.1
C37	(Vβ5.3)	1.9	2.5	0.4	0.4
Ti3A	(Vβ8.1/8.2)	5.1	4.5	4.3	3.6
Total		14.2	14.2	10.1	8.5

Two-color fluorescence analysis (35).

in order to interpret analyses of Vβ gene usage in autoimmune disease where shifts in subpopulations of T cells are frequently observed.

The distribution of T cells sharing V gene usage among different tissues has also been investigated. Carrel et al. (37) have shown that Vβ8 and Vβ5 expression is similar in thymic cortex versus medulla, both in a fetal thymus and a pediatric thymus. We have similar results in a number of pediatric thymuses using, in addition, MAbs to Vβ6 and Vβ12 gene products (Table 4). Moreover, we have found that expression of Vβ12, Vβ5, Vβ6, and Vβ8 in a variety of tissues is quite similar to the levels found in peripheral blood (Table 4).

TABLE 4 V Gene Expression in Different Tissues

	Vβ12 (S511)	Vβ5 (C37)	Vβ6 (OT145)	Vβ8 (Ti3a or 16G8)	Ref.
Peripheral blood	1.7 ± 0.6[a]	3.2 ± 1.3	3.0 ± 1.8	4.5 ± 0.8	27,50,52
Mesenteric lymph nodes[b]	2.6 ± 0.3	2.6 ± 0.7	5.1 ± 0.5	4.3 ± 0.9	52
Synovial fluid[c]	1.5 ± 0.4	3.4 ± 1.1	2.9 ± 1.4		50
Thyroid tissue[a]	2.7 ± 1.0	3.8 ± 1.6	4.3 ± 1.4		51
Thymic cortex	1–3	2–4	<4	2–4	37
Thymic medulla	1–3	2–4	<4	2–4	37
Skin[e]	0.5–2	0.5–2	0–3		50
Colonic mucosa[f]	<3	<3	<3	<3	52

[a]Mean percentage of $CD3^+$ T cells that express Vβ (±SD).
[b]From patients with ulcerative colitis, diverticulitis, or colon carcinoma.
[c]From patients with rheumatoid arthritis.
[d]From patients with Graves' disease or thyroiditis.
[e]From patients with psoriasis.
[f]Uninvolved bowel mucosa from patients with ulcerative colitis, Crohn's disease, diverticulitis, or bowel cancer.

III. POLYMERASE CHAIN REACTION (PCR) TO DETERMINE TCR V GENE USAGE

The major current limitation of the use of MAbs to determine V gene expression is the absence of a complete panel of MAbs covering all possible V genes. For example, if the seven MAbs listed in Table 1 are pooled, 12–20% of $CD3^+$ T cells are stained. Since cDNA sequences of the majority of $V\beta$ and $V\alpha$ genes are known (38–40), several methods have been proposed to assay V gene usage at the level of mRNA. Variations of the PCR may be used to indirectly quantify V gene usage among a polyclonal population of T cells or to determine V gene usage by a clonal population. The latter case is straightforward. Only one functional message is usually found, and the nonfunctional allele, if present, is represented by a lesser amount of mRNA. In the former case, however, PCR systems should be quantitative and accurately represent the percentage of T cells expressing different V genes. This depends on the relative abundance of different messages between different cells, on the enzymatic efficiency of reverse transcriptase using different mRNA substrates (from different T cells), and on the efficiency of Taq polymerase using different cDNA substrates, different primers, and often different lengths of substrate for amplification. Surprisingly, PCR has nevertheless been used successfully to determine V gene usage in polyclonal T-cell populations (41). This was done with a panel of V gene primers corresponding to specific sequences of the 20 known $V\beta$ gene subfamilies. Each of these primers is then used in combination with a $C\beta$ primer to amplify cDNA (obtained by reverse transcription of mRNA). The amplified product can be visualized directly by staining with ethidium bromide, analyzed by Southern blotting with a $C\beta$ probe, or be labeled by inclusion of labeled primer in the PCR. The relative intensities of the various bands obtained with different V gene primers apparently correspond to V gene usage as measured at the cell surface (41).

An alternative PCR method ("anchored PCR") may also be useful (42). Here the V gene-specific primers are not necessary, and only a $C\beta$ or $C\alpha$ primer is used. Any potential bias introduced by the V gene primers is therefore avoided. The method involves cDNA synthesis from mRNA by reverse transcriptase, Tdt-tailing with dGTP nucleotides, for instance, and then amplification with a C-region–specific primer and a poly C–containing primer (42). The amplified product will contain a mixture of rearranged TCR β or α chains depending on which C-region primer is used. This mixture can be analyzed by hybridization with different probes specific for different V genes (Fig. 1) or cloned and sequenced. It is unclear whether this approach accurately reflects TCR V gene usage. In addition, it is not easy to quantify the PCR-amplified material, since this is often represented by a smear corresponding to many different lengths of amplified cDNAs (Fig. 1).

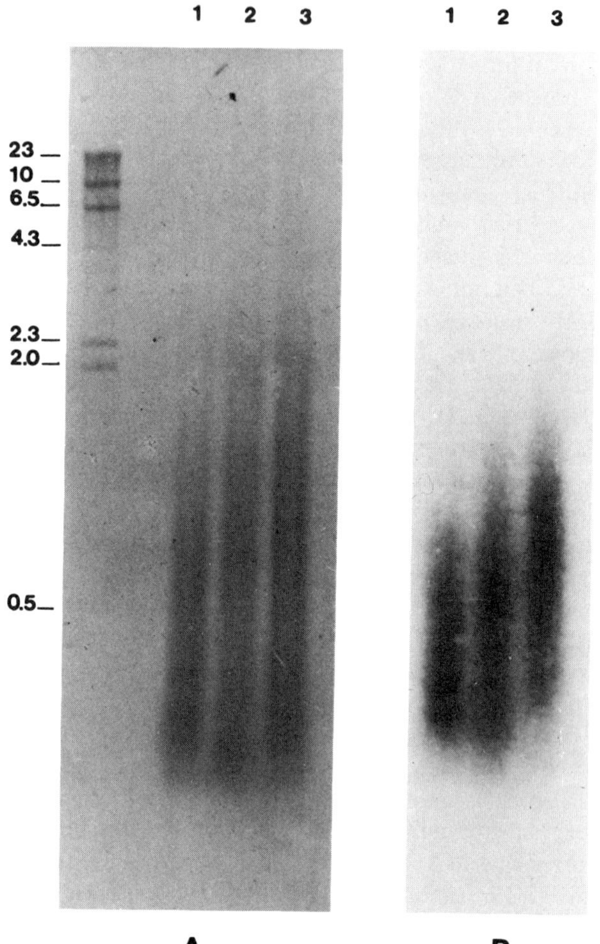

FIGURE 1 Anchored PCR with a TCR Cβ primer using the method of Loh et al. (42). The substrate was mRNA from the Jurkat T-cell line, which was reverse transcribed to cDNA. (A) Ethidium bromide staining of amplified DNA after 25 cycles of amplification. (B) Southern blot of the gel shown to the left, using a Vβ8 probe homologous to the Vβ region expressed by Jurkat. Lanes 1, 2, and 3 correspond to amplification conditions using 1.5 mM, 2.0 mM, or 2.5 mM MgCl, respectively.

IV. ALLELIC V GENE POLYMORPHISMS

When analyzing V gene expression in disease, it is important to consider germline-encoded differences from one individual to the other. That such differences exist was suggested by the finding that the epitope recognized the MAb OT145 (Vβ6) was not expressed in a significant proportion ($\approx$20%) of normal individuals (27). A second group of normal individuals had a high percentage of OT145$^+$ T cells in the peripheral blood (mean 4.5%), and a third group had an intermediary percentage of OT145$^+$ T cells (mean 2.1%). These groups were designated −/−, +/+, and +/−, respectively. In family studies, the three different phenotypes appeared to be inherited in an autosomal codominant mode. Moreover, the phenotypes were strongly linked to the ethnic background of the individuals examined (27). The −/− phenotype was frequent in American blacks, Hispanics, Filipinos, and Japanese, but rare in Caucasians and Chinese. The reverse was found for the +/+ phenotype. The basis for the polymorphic expression of the OT145-defined epitope has recently been discovered (29). The MAb OT145 recognized primarily Vβ6.7 gene products, and there are two functional alleles of Vβ6.7, termed Vβ6.7a and Vβ6.7b. The former corresponds to the "+" allele recognized by OT145, while the latter represents the "−" allele not recognized by the MAb. The two alleles differ only by two amino acids in the mature expressed protein. In the Vβ6.7b allele, a single nucleotide mutation results in a substitution from a serine to an arginine at position 38, and another single base mutation results in a substitution from a glycine to a glutamic acid at position 72. These are nonconservative changes from neutral to charged amino acids. In addition, position 72 is thought to be located close to the antigen/MHC binding site (25) and may therefore influence antigen/MHC reactivity or reactivity with superantigens.

The single base mutation responsible for the change at position 72 is located within a BamHI restriction site which is present in the Vβ6.7a allele and absent in the Vβ6.7 allele (29). Thus, individuals can now be readily genotyped with a BamHI RFLP. Comparison between genotypes and MAb OT145–defined phenotypes revealed a surprisingly accurate correlation: The OT145–defined phenotypes failed to match the BamHI RFLP in only 2 of 42 individuals (29). Thus, data obtained by phenotyping with the OT145 MAb can be used for studies on this polymorphic V gene.

An unanswered question is whether Vβ6.7 alleles are associated with susceptibility to a disease. To address this question, the distribution of OT145-phenotypes was examined in 14 different disease groups (Table 5). The distribution is similar in all groups. Small variations from one group to another are probably due to the small numbers of individuals in some of the groups and to the fact that the groups were heterogeneous in regard to ethnic composition. For instance, the UC group was primarily composed of Caucasians, while the leprosy group

TABLE 5

Group	n	OT145-defined phenotypes[a]		
		+/+	+/−	−/−
Normals (A)[b]	33	67%	21%	12%
Normals (B)	186	40	40	20
RA[c]	21	48	42	10
JRA	5	60	20	20
Graves' disease	27	55	30	15
ITP	39	46	39	15
Psoriasis	17	64	18	18
SLE	14	43	43	14
IDDM	8	50	25	25
Hemophilia	8	25	75	0
Leprosy	25	36	40	24
Allergy	13	62	32	15
UC	26	42	50	8
Crohn's disease	71	56	31	13
Sarcoidosis	15	46	39	15
Other	21	43	47	10

[a]Phenotypes are determined by the percentage of $OT145^+$ T cells in the peripheral blood (27): >3% (+/+); 0.5–3.0% (+/−); <0.5% (−/−).
[b]The two groups of normals were used as controls in two different studies: A, (52); B, (50).
[c]The disease groups are: RA, rheumatoid arthritis; JRA, juvenile rheumatoid arthritis; GD, Graves' disease; ITP, idiopathic thrombocytopenia; PSOR, psoriasis; SLE, systemic lupus erythematosus; IDDM, insulin-dependent diabetes mellitus; HPH, hemophilia; LEP, leprosy; ALL, allergy; UC, ulcerative colitis; CD, Crohn's disease; SARC, sarcoidosis; Other, mixed infectious and neoplastic diseases.

contained many non-Caucasians. Future studies will need carefully selected control groups, matched with disease groups in regard to ethnic background, just like studies on disease associations with HLA types.

Preliminary results (29,43,44) suggest that allelic polymorphism of TCR V genes is not a rare occurrence. Using PCR, we have found different alleles of the Vβ6.3 gene, and two alleles of the Vβ1 gene have also been described (43). It is not yet clear whether the number of allelic products at a given locus will be much higher, as with MHC genes. However, the apparent lack of large numbers of allelic products may be offset by an increased recombination frequency within TCR loci as compared to MHC, as described by Robinson and Kindt (45). This results in large numbers of different TCR haplotypes (45) and therefore considerable heterogeneity in the TCR germline V gene repertoire within a species.

Apart from allelic polymorphism resulting in TCR V gene allotypes as described for Vβ6.7, other genetic mechanisms may also contribute to polymorphic expression of V genes in man. Thus, two insertion/deletion polymorphisms within the TCR Vβ locus have been described, one of 30 kb and the other of 15 kb (46). It is possible that these insertion/deletion fragments contain functional V genes, which would not be available to individuals homozygous for the deletion allele.

Nonfunctional alleles can also be produced by point mutations resulting in a stop codon within the V gene exon, as described for one of the alleles of the murine Vβ17 gene (47). Point mutations leading to stop codons have been reported in human TCR V genes, for example, Vβ8.4 and Vβ8.5 (48). It is possible that these genes represent nonfunctional alleles and that putative functional alleles have not yet been sequenced because, often, the available sequences are derived only from a single individual. As yet, there are no examples of such an allelic system among human TCR V genes.

Similar allelic systems to those described above could represent the basis for observed disease associations with TCR loci (Table 6) (44). Of these, the association of multiple sclerosis with the TCR β locus is the most convincing since it is based on family studies (49) rather than analysis of unrelated populations. Thus, TCR loci may confer susceptibility for individual autoimmune diseases.

V. V GENE USAGE IN AUTOIMMUNE DISEASES

We have examined V gene usage using MAbs specific for V gene products as listed in Table 1. Over 200 normal donors and a similar number of patients with a variety of disorders have been examined (27,50). In general, isolated T cells from peripheral blood were used, although in some instances tissue samples from involved sites of autoimmune disease could also be obtained. The results are summarized in Figures 2 through 5. From these results, it is apparent that in most autoimmune diseases, there is no detectable variation in V gene usage among peripheral blood T cells. In some individual cases, high levels of T cells staining

TABLE 6 Disease Associations with TCR Loci

Disease	Method	RR	Ref.
Insulin-dependent DM	Bgl II—Cβ RFLP	2.08	91
Graves' disease	Bgl II—Cβ RFLP	16.7	92
Membranous nephropathy	Bgl II—Cβ RFLP	4.10	93
Autoimmune hypothyroidism	Taq I—Vα RFLP	2.7	94
Multiple sclerosis	Family studies with haplotype assignment of TCR β locus		49,95

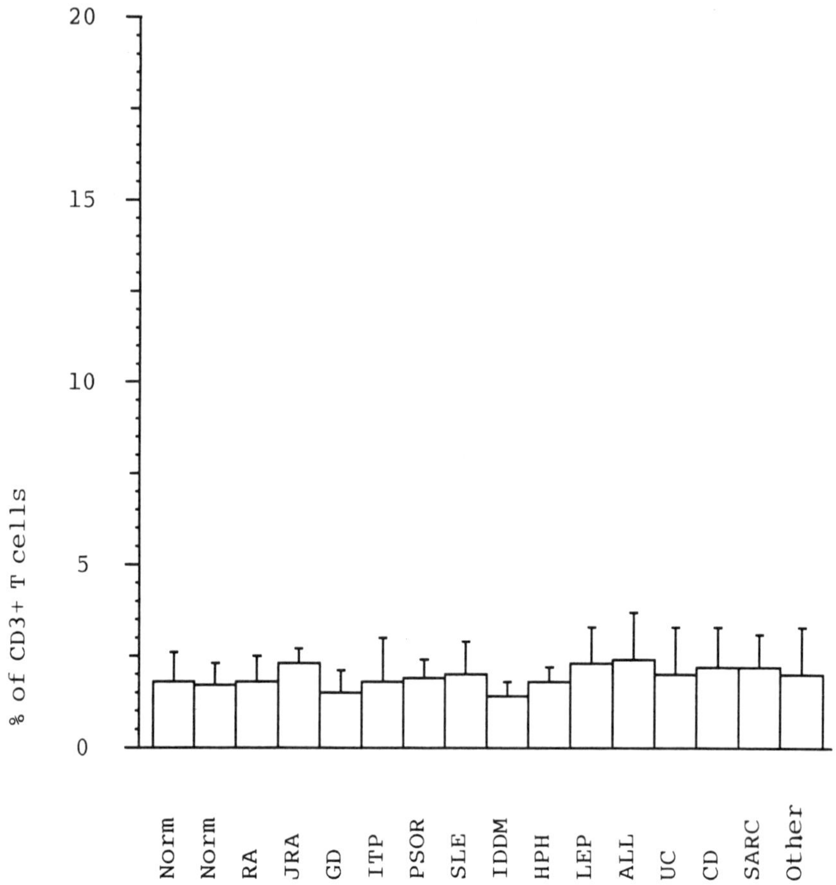

FIGURE 2 TCR Vβ12 gene usage. Abbreviations and the *n* values for the disease groups are given in Table 5. The bars represent mean values $\pm$ standard deviation.

with a given MAb were detected. Thus, a patient with SLE had 12% Vβ5.3$^+$ T cells, a patient with psoriasis had 19% Vβ6.7$^+$ T cells, and a patient with ITP had 24% Vβ6.7$^+$ cells in the peripheral blood (50). The latter patient was followed over a 2-year period, during which there were always 15–25% OT145$^+$ (Vβ6.7$^+$) T cells in the peripheral blood. This population of T cells was found to be exclusively CD8$^+$ CD4$^-$, and by Southern blotting with a Cβ probe it contained a rearranged band typical of a monoclonal population of T cells (50). In other cases, however, the increased expression of a Vβ gene is polyclonal and often appears to involve both CD4$^+$ and CD8$^+$ T cells (Table 7).

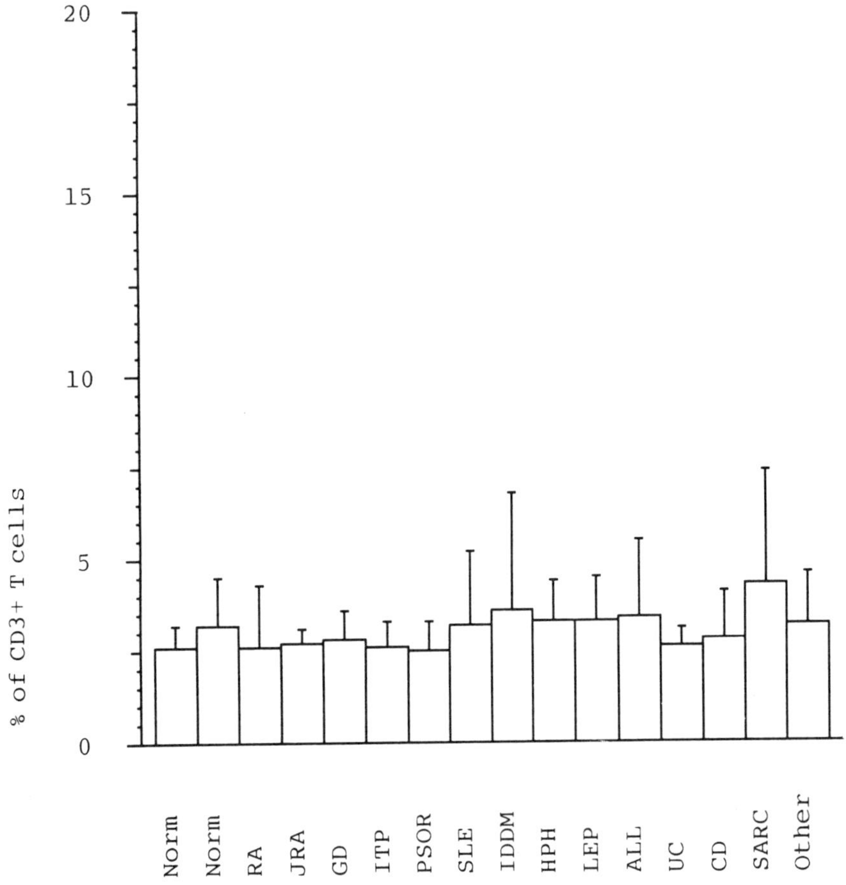

FIGURE 3 TCR Vβ5 gene usage. Abbreviations and the n values for the disease groups are given in Table 5. The bars represent mean values $\pm$ standard deviation.

In view of the largely negative findings in peripheral blood, we considered that disease-related T cells might be sequestered at relevant tissue sites. However, even T cells in tissue sites of autoimmunity such as the synovial fluid in RA (50), the involved skin in psoriasis (50), and the thyroid in Graves' disease (51) appear to use an evenly distributed repertoire of V genes (Table 4). There are of course several caveats. Only a minor portion of the repertoire was actually analyzed with the available MAbs, and Vα gene usage was not tested. In addition, it is possible that TCR V gene usage may vary over time and that findings

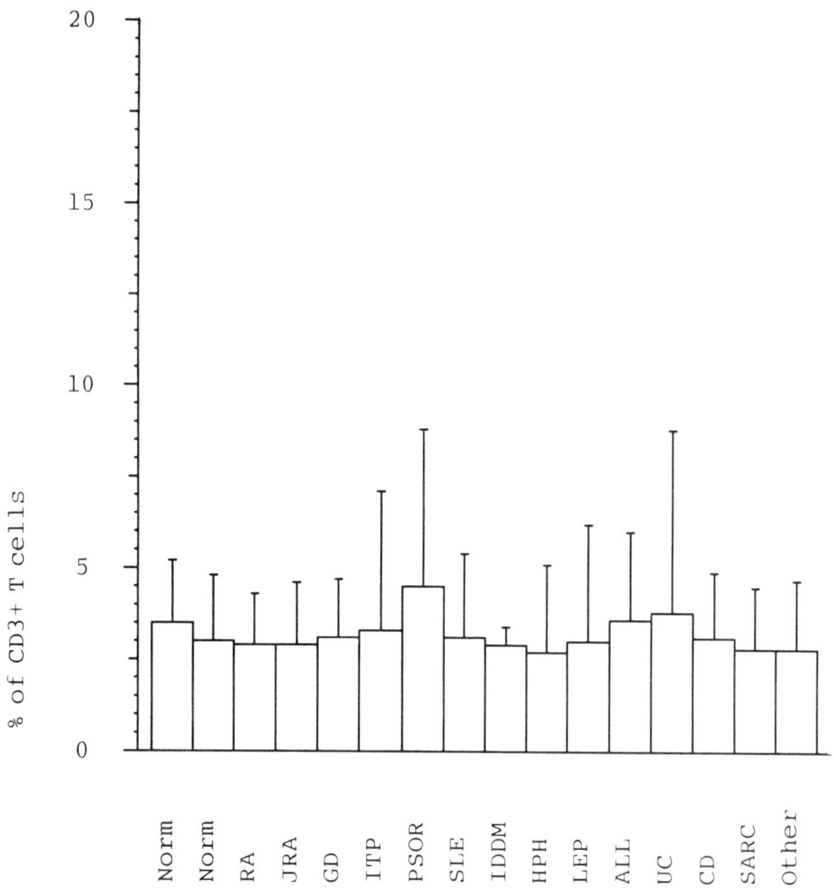

FIGURE 4 TCR Vβ6 gene usage. Abbreviations and the *n* values for the disease groups are given in Table 5. The bars represent mean values ± standard deviation.

obtained at later stages of the disease course may not reflect the T-cell clones initially involved in the pathogenesis of the disease.

VI. INCREASED Vβ8 GENE EXPRESSION IN CROHN'S DISEASE AND SARCOIDOSIS

Two striking examples of biased V gene expression were discovered as part of screening a variety of diseases. In Crohn's disease and in sarcoidosis, subsets of patients contained elevated numbers of V$\beta 8^+$ T cells in their peripheral blood

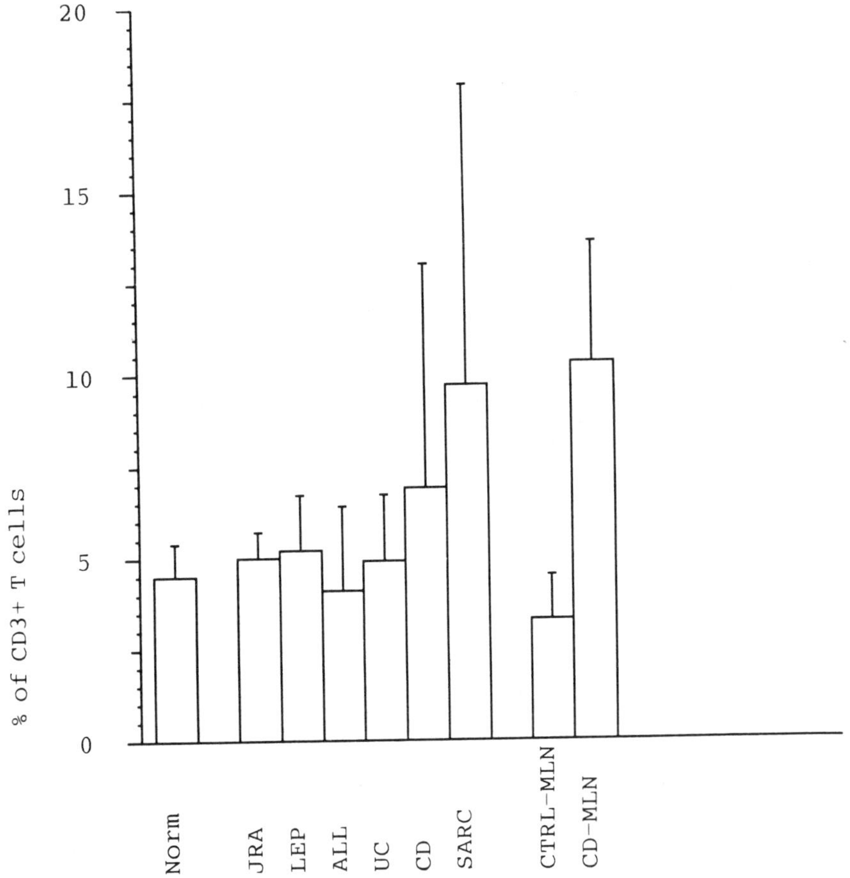

FIGURE 5 TCR Vβ8 gene usage. Abbreviations and the *n* values for the disease groups are given in Table 5. The bars represent mean values ± standard deviation.

(Fig. 5). These are two similar chronic granulomatous diseases, both of unknown etiology. In Crohn's disease, we found that 20% of patients had elevated V$\beta8^+$ T cells, using 7.2% Ti3a$^+$ T cells as a cutoff value representing the mean +2SD of the normal group (52). The patient with the highest value had 39% V$\beta8^+$ T cells. Moreover, it was clear that the V$\beta8^+$ T cells were concentrated in mesenteric lymph nodes (MLN) draining the diseased bowel (52). Over 60% (9/15) of MLN samples from patients with Crohn's disease had elevated V8$^+$ T cells as compared to 0% (0/9) of MLN samples from control patients with ulcerative

TABLE 7

A. V gene expression in CD4 and CD8 subsets in a patient with Crohn's disease (pbl)

Population	$CD3^+$	$CD4^+$ $CD8^-$	$CD8^+$ $CD4^-$
CD3	100%	100%	100%
CD4	66.2	97.8	>0.1
CD8	35.2	2.3	100
Vβ12 (S511)	2.2	2.5	2.3
Vβ5 (C37)	4.1	3.1	4.8
Vβ6 (OT145)	3.4	5.6	2.9
Vβ8 (Ti3a)	8.4	8.3	5.6
Tac	—	6.0	3.9

B. V gene expression in CD4 and CD8 subsets in Crohn's disease mesenteric LN

Population	$CD3^+$	$CD4^+$ $CD8^-$	$CD8^+$ $CD4^-$
CD3	100%	100%	100%
CD4	83.7	100	—
CD8	20.8	—	100
Vβ5 (C37)	4.5	3.6	4.7
Vβ6 (OT145)	4.4	4.5	3.6
Vβ8 (Ti3a)	5.2	5.2	5.1

C. V gene expression in CD4 and CD8 subsets in Crohn's disease mesenteric LN

Population	$CD3^+$	$CD4^+$ $CD8^-$	$CD8^+$ $CD4^-$
CD3	100%	100%	100%
CD4	77.8	100	—
CD8	23.0	—	100
Vβ5 (C37)	2.3	2.0	3.2
Vβ6 (OT145)	3.0	3.9	2.0
Vβ8 (Ti3a)	4.3	3.6	8.3

colitis, diverticulitis, or colon cancer (Fig. 5). This represents a significant increase in $V\beta8^+$ expression in a large number of patients with Crohn's disease (52). In further studies, it was shown that the $V\beta8^+$ T cells were polyclonal $CD4^+$ and $CD8^+$ T cells. In Table 7, data are shown on a patient with elevated Vβ8 expression in the peripheral blood (8.4% $Ti3a^+$ T cells). The CD4 and CD8 T-cells subsets were isolated indirectly by depleting the reciprocal population with MAb and complement. Both CD4 and CD8 populations contain $Ti3a^+$ T cells, although there is a slight enrichment of Vβ8 expression in the CD4 population.

In two MLN samples where normal Vβ8 expression was observed, two-color immunofluorescence showed equal distribution of $V\beta8^+$ cells between CD4 and CD8 populations or a slight bias for Vβ8 expression in the CD8 population (Table 7). These slight variations in V gene expression between $CD4^+$ and $CD8^+$ T cells are similar to those occasionally observed among normal donors (Table 2). Crohn's disease and ulcerative colitis are two related diseases together considered as inflammatory bowel disease (IBD). Ten percent of patients with Crohn's disease have close relatives with IBD. Eight two-generation families with several members affected with IBD were examined for Vβ8 expression (52). Relatives of probands with high Vβ8 expression had normal levels of $V\beta8^+$ T cells whether or not they were also affected with IBD. A set of identical twins, both with Crohn's disease, were also discordant for Vβ8 expression. These studies failed to show genetic regulation of Vβ8 gene expression, but did not exclude this possibility.

In summary, the elevated levels of $V\beta8^+$ T cells appeared to be due to a gut-associated immune response. These cells are found in the mesenteric lymph nodes but not in the lamina propria of the affected mucosa. They are, therefore, probably related to the afferent, but not the efferent, limb of a gut-associated immune response. The identity of the putative antigen is not yet known. Recently, a superantigen (see below) specifically reacting with $V\beta8^+$ T cells has been described, staphylococcal enterotoxin E (SEE) (28). This superantigen or a similar bacterial product could gain access through inflamed gut tissues and cause a proliferative response of $V\beta8^+$ T cells. An alternative hypothesis was suggested by the finding that several Vβ8-reactive MAbs cross-react with an epithelial cell antigen present on epithelial cells of different tissue origins but prominently on epithelial cells of colonic mucosa (52). It was suggested that a human autoantibody might have the same cross-reactivity pattern as these MAbs (52). Such a putative autoantibody would be expected to be mitogenic for $V\beta8^+$ T cells. Some preliminary evidence in favor of the presence of such autoantibodies was obtained using two sera from patients with Crohn's disease (53).

In sarcoidosis, similar results have been obtained by Moller et al. (54), and we have confirmed their findings (Fig. 5). In our studies, 40% of patients (5/13) have elevated blood levels of $V\beta8^+$ T cells. Here also it appears that the $V\beta8^+$ T cells are concentrated at the site of the disease (in the bronchial lavage fluid). The $V\beta8^+$ cells are polyclonal and comprise both $CD4^+$ and $CD8^+$ T cells. PCR amplification and sequencing of the VDJ junctional areas of the TCR β chains from these $V\beta8^+$ T cells has suggested that they are oligoclonal, i.e., reactive with a specific antigen (55).

It is of interest that Crohn's disease and sarcoidosis are both similar chronic granulomatous diseases. Granuloma formation involves the interaction of antigen-presenting cells and T lymphocytes. It is therefore particularly intriguing that the same Vβ8 genes are selectively overexpressed in these two diseases.

VII. STUDIES WITH MYCOPLASMA ARTHRITIDIS SUPERANTIGEN (MAM)

Monoclonal antibodies recognizing TCR V gene products have helped to define a unique group of potent T-cell activators, which have been termed superantigens (28,31). Recognized superantigens include murine self antigens,both Mls loci gene products (56,57) and a B-cell–specific antigen (58), as well as a group of microbial products, the staphylococcal enterotoxins (SE) (28,31), the pyrogenic enterotoxin A of group A streptococci (59), and a soluble glycoprotein produced by mycoplasma arthritidis (60,61).* Superantigens share a number of intriguing characteristics which distinguish them from conventional antigens. Superantigens bind selectively and with high affinity to relatively nonpolymorphic regions of MHC class II molecules (62–64). The precise regions of MHC class II molecules to which a particular superantigen binds are currently being defined; however, there is evidence that some microbial superantigens display MHC class II isotype binding preference (see below). Another relatively unique finding is that T-cell recognition of superantigens does not require antigen processing. Thus, in the absence of antigen processing and in an MHC nonrestricted manner, superantigen–MHC class II complexes on the antigen-presenting cell surface trigger the proliferation of superantigen-reactive T cells (62–65). Perhaps most intriguing, superantigen recognition is, in large measure, dictated by TCR Vβ gene usage (28,31,41). Thus, a particular superantigen is recognized by virtually all T cells that utilize a selected subfamily or a restricted group of TCR Vβ genes. Superantigen recognition is little influenced by other polymorphic TCR gene elements or by cell surface expression of the CD4 or CD8 antigens (66). Thus, superantigen bound to MHC class II is recognized equally well by CD4$^+$ and CD8$^+$ cells, although the functional consequences of this recognition differ (see below). Finally, the microbial products that function as superantigens are among the most potent mitogens known, inducing T-cell proliferation at concentrations of 10^{-9}–10^{-11} M (61,67).

A. MAM Recognition and Response in Man

From the standpoint of this review, it is important to consider that, in vivo, microbial superantigens could activate and markedly expand a given T-cell population defined by its TCR V gene expression. These activated T cells may include normally quiescent autoreactive cells, which then mediate autoaggression (see below). With the pathogenic potential of superantigens in mind, we have investigated the response of human T cells to the *Mycoplasma arthritidis*-derived superantigen (MAM). This choice was made in view of the chronic inflammatory arthritis which *Mycoplasma arthritidis* induces in selected strains of mice (60,68) and early reports of *Mycoplasma* cultured from the bone marrow of patients with SLE (69,70).

*The endogenous murine superantigens have now been shown to be endogenous retroviral gene products and some of the microbial superantigens are encoded by viral plasmids (97–100).

B. MHC Class II Isotype Restriction of MAM Presentation

Although superantigens bind to relatively nonpolymorphic regions, there is evidence for preferential interactions of selected superantigens with particular MHC class II isotypes (63,71). Perhaps the best characterized MHC class II binding preference of a microbial superantigen has been provided by Cole's studies of MAM (72). These studies demonstrate that expression of the chain of IE is required and sufficient for MAM presentation. This is of interest as the α chain is a relatively nonpolymorphic structure. The more polymorphic β chain, so crucial for conventional antigen presentation, plays little if any role in MAM binding and presentation.

We have performed analogous studies to demonstrate the nature of human MHC class II isoforms that can serve as MAM-presenting structures. Utilizing murine L-cell transfectants which express human DR or DQ antigens as superantigen-presenting cells, we analyzed the proliferative responses of human T-cell lines (TCL) reactive with either the SEs or MAM. The results show that SEB and SEE are presented by both MHC class II antigen transfectant cells but not by untransfected L cells. In contrast, MAM is selectively presented by transfectants which express DR, the human analog of the murine IE antigen.

C. Human TCR V Gene Usage in Response to MAM

In the mouse, MAM-reactive T cells and T-cell hybridomas have been characterized with respect to TCR Vβ gene usage. The majority of MAM-reactive murine T cells are Vβ8 or Vβ6 positive (72,73).

Studies of MAM reactivity in man have demonstrated clonal restriction, in that approximately 5% of alloreactive T-cell clones tested were responsive to MAM (66). In order to investigate TCR V gene usage among human MAM-reactive T cells, we activated PBL by coculture with MAM, SEE, or the polyclonal T-cell mitogen, PHA. After 4 days, activated T cells and resting populations were isolated by discontinuous Percoll gradient centrifugation. Efficient isolation of the relevant superantigen-reactive T-cell population was confirmed by functional assay. Thus, the activated T-cell "blast" populations respond with a vigorous and accelerated proliferative response to the sensitizing superantigen, while the resting T cells proliferative to control stimuli (PHA, anti-CD3 MAb, or an irrelevant superantigen) but are unresponsive to the sensitizing superantigen (74). The superantigen-reactive T-cell blast populations were analyzed for TCR V gene usage by indirect immunofluorescence (Table 8). The most striking and consistent finding is the uniform absence of Vβ5 (C37$^+$) or Vβ6 (OT145$^+$) expressing T cells in the MAM-reactive T-cell pool. In some studies Fl$^+$ T cells are enriched in the MAM-responsive T-cell blasts, increasing two- to threefold over the percentage of Fl$^+$ T cells in the resting pool. SEE-reactive T cells are also depleted in Vβ5 and Vβ6 positive T cells, but are enriched in Vβ8$^+$, rather than

TABLE 8 Vβ Gene Usage in Superantigen-Activated T Cells[a]

	PHA		MAM		SEE	
	Blasts	Resting	Blasts	Resting	Blasts	Resting
Vβ12 (S511)	4.0	1.7	2.3	1.7	4.2	1.7
Vβ5 (C37)	1.7	2.0	0.4	2.1	0.5	1.3
Vβ6 (OT145)	2.3	2.0	0.0	1.4	0.8	4.3
Vβ8 (16G8)	4.0	4.4	3.8	4.0	13.3	2.4
Vα2.3 (Fl)	2.5	3.7	7.0	2.7	4.1	3.2

[a]PBl were stimulated for 4 days with the indicated superantigen or PHA. IL-2 was added to 10% on the fourth day. Blasts were separated from small resting T cells by density centrifugation on a discontinuous Percoll gradient, cultured overnight, and then analyzed by immunofluorescence.

in Fl^+, T cells (Table 8), consistent with a prior report (28). T-cell lines repetitively triggered with X-irradiated autologous APCs and MAM and expanded in the presence of IL-2 retain an elevated percentage of Fl-expressing cells. However, the percentage of Fl^+ cells does not increase beyond 10–15%. This data suggests that while Fl^+ cells are likely to be MAM reactive, there is a significant population of MAM-reactive T cells which are not recognized by the currently available pool of TCR V gene–specific MAbs. More recent data with a new MAb called C1, specific for Vβ17 products, has shown that 50–60% of MAM-reactive T cells are routinely positive. Thus Vβ17 gene products represent the major V gene used by MAM-reactive T cells (unpublished data, Posnett DN, Friedman SM).

VIII. SUPERANTIGENS AND AUTOIMMUNITY

The dual affinity of superantigens for selected TCR Vβ gene products and MHC class II molecules, coupled with their recognition by T cells in the absence of processing, suggested to us that bacterial superantigens may perturb the immune system in a manner analogous to that seen in experimentally induced graft versus host disease (GVHD). The sequelae of GVHD have long represented a provocative model of non–organ specific autoimmune disease (75–78). For example, GVHD may be characterized by hypergammaglobulinemia, autoantibody formation, and immune complex–mediated organ system damage which mimics systemic lupus erythematosus (SLE) (77). These autoimmune phenomena are mediated by abnormal T-helper (T_h)–B-cell cooperation, across MHC disparities, in which donor-derived allospecific T_h cells recognize and interact with MHC class II antigens on the surface of recipient B cells (76,77). While GVHD is an attractive model of human SLE, it has been difficult to understand how the abnormal T_h–B-cell interaction central to this model could arise spontaneously. We would

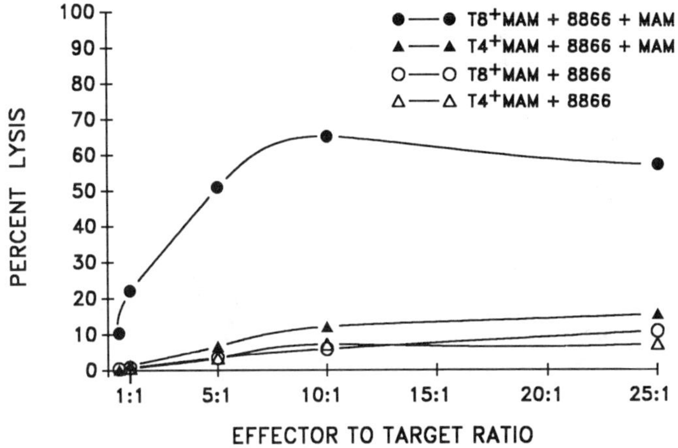

FIGURE 6 $CD4^+$ or $CD8^+$ MAM-reactive TCL cells were cocultured for 4 hours with ^{51}Cr-labeled human lymphoblastoid B-cell line cells (8866) in the presence or absence of MAM. Percent cytotoxicity was calculated.

suggest that microbial superantigens could provide an answer. For example, any B cell, regardless of its specificity for antigen, may bind a superantigen and be rendered a target of cognate T-cell help by superantigen-specific T_h cells (Fig. 8). To explore this question, MAM-reactive $CD4^+$ human T-cell blasts were cocultured with autologous B cells or B cells obtained from the peripheral blood of HLA-typed normal donors. After 10 days in culture, supernatants were harvested and assayed by ELISA for total IgM content as a measure of polyclonal B-cell activation. Little IgM was produced in B-cell cultures supplemented with MAM alone or MAM plus unselected autologous T cells. In marked contrast, a striking polyclonal IgM response was induced in cultures containing both MAM-reactive $CD4^+$ T-cell blasts and MAM (74). As expected, the polyclonal B-cell response triggered is MAM-dependent, but not MHC restricted (74).

Antibody production by resting B cells requires direct cognate cell–cell interaction with antigen-speific T_h cells as well as the action of lymphokines (79–83). Recent studies of GVHD in chimeric mice have demonstrated that autoantibody production in this model is also dependent on cognate T_h–B-cell interaction (84). In order to postulate a role for superantigens in the in vivo activation of normally quiescent (resting) autoreactive B cells, it is crucial to demonstrate that superantigens can promote a productive T_h–resting B-cell interaction. To address this question, purified (>98% sIg^+) high density, resting tonsillar B cells were isolated by Percoll gradient density centrifugation. MAM-pulsed resting B cells proved to be excellent activators of and targets for MAM-reactive $CD4^+$ T-cell help in the absence of exogenous MAM (74). These data demonstrate that a microbial superantigen, bound to the surface of resting human B cells, is an effective means of activating superantigen reactive T_h cells, which, in turn, trigger polyclonal immunoglobulin production by the superantigen-bearing B-cell population. We would point out that similar results have recently been reported with the staphylococcal toxic shock syndrome toxin (85). It remains to be determined if the superantigen bridge between T_h-cell TCR and B-cell MHC class II molecules serves only to ensure the release of lymphokines in close proximity to the surface of the superantigen-bearing B cell or also provides those B-cell activation signals which occur via TCR engagement of B-cell MHC class II during a normal immune response (86–88).

While $CD4^+$ MAM-reactive T cells mediate MAM-dependent help for B-cell activation, we noted that MAM-reactive TCL, comprised of both CD4 and CD8 cells, often provide little help for B-cell activation. This suggested restriction of helper activity to the $CD4^+$ MAM-reactive T-cell subset. While both $CD4^+$ and $CD8^+$ MAM-reactive T-cell blasts proliferate in response to MAM, only $CD4^+$ cells provide MAM-dependent help for B-cell activation as assessed by immunoglobulin production (Table 9) (74).

The function of $CD8^+$ MAM-reactive T cells was explored by measuring cytotoxicity against ^{51}Cr-labeled targets. The results demonstrate that only MHC class II positive target cells, incubated with MAM, are lysed by superantigen reactive $CD8^+$ TCL (Fig. 6). These studies demonstrate that $CD4^+$ and $CD8^+$ superantigen reactive T cells differ markedly in their superantigen-dependent functions. $CD4^+$ T cells provide help for superantigen-bearing B cells, and $CD8^+$ T cells lyse superantigen-bearing cells. It will be important to determine if, in any individual, particular TCR V gene families are utilized preferentially by the $CD4^+$ or $CD8^+$ subset. As noted above (Table 2), some individuals show marked subset skewing of TCR gene usage. Utilizing the Fl MAbs, we analyzed MAM-reactive TCL derived from two normal donors. These preliminary studies

TABLE 9 $CD4^+$ Superantigen-Reactive T Cells Provide Help for B-Cell Differentiation in the Presence of Superantigen

Culture conditions			IgM secretion (ng/ml)
Responder cells	Th cell	Stimulus	
B	—	media	30
B	—	MAM	30
B	$CD4^+$ MAM_{xr}	media	60
B	$CD8^+$ MAM_{xr}	media	30
B	$CD4^+$ MAM_{xr}	MAM	7350
B	$CD4^+$ MAM_{xr}	MAM	40

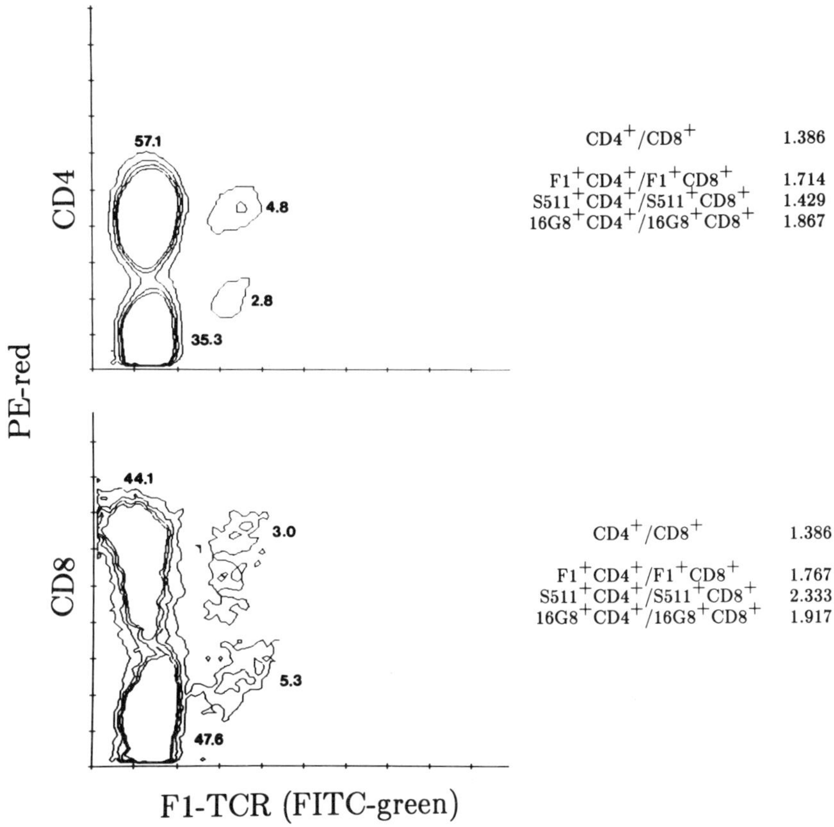

FIGURE 7 T-cell subset distribution of Fl^+ T cells in MAM-reactive T-cell lines. Double staining was performed with CD4 and CD8 in red, but Fl or other TCR MAbs (S511, 16G8) in green. Only the FACS data with Fl are shown. The percentages of cells in each cell population are indicated in the graph. Ratios were always calculated based on both the double staining with CD4 and the double staining with CD8, allowing an estimate of the experimental error by comparison of the data. There appears to be no difference between the CD4/CD8 distribution of Fl^+ cells as compared to $S511^+$ or $16G8^+$ cells.

(Fig. 7) revealed equal distribution of Fl^+ cells in the two T-cell subsets. Similar results have also been obtained with the MAb C1 (Vβ17).

We would postulate that, in the susceptible host, exposure to a microbial superantigen could be an initiating factor in systemic autoimmune disease (Fig. 8). Microbial superantigens can be thought of as providing a superantigen bridge between T_h cell TCR and MHC class II antigens on the surface of all B cells. Those B cells (B_1 in Fig. 8) that receive a second signal via antigen mediated

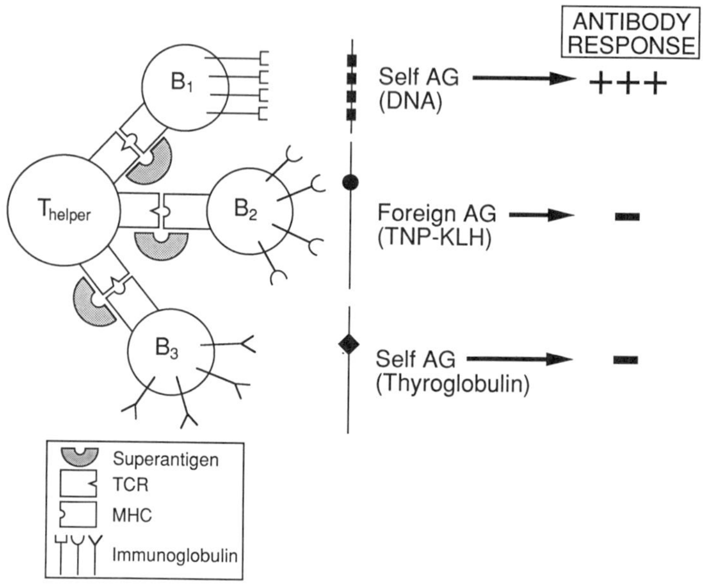

FIGURE 8 Superantigen mediated autoimmunity. Superantigens provide T-helper-cell–B-cell bridges for cognate help, thus explaining the GVHD model for non–tissue specific (systemic) autoimmunity.

cross-linking of membrane Ig molecules will proceed to maximal maturation and differentiation. The continuous presence of self antigens may lead to the preferential production of autoantibodies. As in the GVHD model, certain multivalent antigens will provide an effective second signal, while monovalent epitopes on globular proteins cannot (B_2 and B_3 in Fig. 8).

IX. SUMMARY

New fundamental insights into the structure of MHC Ag-presenting molecules and TCR molecules have resulted in rapid progress in our understanding of autoimmunity and in particular of the disease model EAE. It is apparent that one needs to study three components of an immune response: (1) the peptide antigen; (2) the autoantigen-presenting MHC molecule; and (3) the TCR molecule used by the autoimmune T cell. A number of different effective therapeutic approaches can be derived from structural information on these three components (13–21). In human autoimmune disease, very little is known about these components. We have summarized some initial efforts to identify TCR molecules that may participate in autoimmune responses. The methods available to determine TCR V gene usage in polyclonal T cells are being perfected. Knowledge of the peptide antigen involved (i.e., HSP peptide in rheumatoid arthritis?) and the MHC molecules involved (DR4, DR1, in rheumatoid arthritis) will allow in vitro studies with T-cell clones that are autoantigen specific and appropriately restricted by MHC molecules that impart disease susceptibility. Such studies have the potential to identify TCR V gene involved in the autoimmune response. This structural information may be used to synthesize peptide vaccines consisting of pathogenic TCR-V sequences for individual autoimmune diseases (15,16,18).

It is also important to understand TCR disease susceptibility genes. Evidence for disease susceptibility genes and evidence for TCR V gene allelic products was discussed in Sec. III. The exact structures of the alleles imparting disease susceptibility should provide valuable data for future vaccine development. In addition, germline genetic information on the presence or absence of susceptibility alleles allows screening of individuals who may be at high risk for a given disease. In this way, for example, one could identify candidates for vaccine therapy and avoid large-scale vaccination of populations that are not at risk.

Finally, we presented data in Secs. VII and VIII that microbial superantigens such as MAM may be involved in the pathogenesis of certain autoimmune diseases (74). There are major differences between tissue-specific autoimmune diseases and generalized autoimmunity, as in the prototypical human disease SLE. The pathogenetic mechanisms leading to different disease expressions require much further work. We have proposed a mechanism by which superantigens such as MAM may result in a GVHD-like immune response and could result in production of autoantibodies to a variety of multivalent antigens, such as DNA and cell surface antigens typically seen in SLE (96).

ACKNOWLEDGMENTS

This work was supported in part by the National Institutes of Health (CA42046, CA49283, AI18263), the Irvington Institute for Medical Research and the National Foundation for Ileitis and Colitis. DNP is an Investigator of the Cancer Research Institute. The Flow Cytometry Core Facility was supported in part by grant P60-AR38520 awarded by the National Institutes of Health.

REFERENCES

1. Dayer, J. M., Graham, R., Russell, G., and Krane, S. 1977. Collagenase production by rheumatoid synovial cells: stimulation by a human lymphocyte factor. *Science, 195*: 181–183.
2. Holoshitz, J., Naparstek, Y., Ben-Nun, A., and Cohen, I. R. 1983. Lines of T lymphocytes induce or vaccinate against autoimmune arthritis. *Science, 219*: 56–58.
3. van Elden, W., Thole, J. E. R., van der Zee, R., Noordzij, A., van Embden, J. D. A., Hensen, E. J., and Cohen, I. R. 1988. Cloning of the mycobacterial epitope recognized by T lymphocytes in adjuvant arthritis. *Nature, 331*: 171–173.

4. Young, D., Lathigra, R., Hendrix, R., Sweetser, D., and Young, R. A. 1988. Stress proteins are immune targets in leprosy and tuberculosis. *Proc. Natl. Acad. Sci. USA, 85*: 4267–4270.
5. Young, R. A., and Elliot, T. J. 1989. Stress proteins, infection, and immune surveillance. *Cell, 59*: 5–8.
6. Lamb, J. R., Bal, V., Mendez-Samperio, P., Mehlert, A., So, A., Rothbard, J., Jindal, S., Young, R. A., and Young, D. B. 1989. *Int. Immunol., 1*: 191–196.
7. Munk, M. E., Schoel, B., Modrow, S., Karr, R. W., Young, R. A., and Kaufmann, S. H. E. 1989. Thymocytes from healthy individuals with specificity to self epitopes shared by the mycobacterial and human 65-kilodalton heat shock protein. *J. Immunol., 143*: 2844–2849.
8. Gregersen, P., K., Silver, J., and Winchester, R. J. 1987. The shared epitope hypothesis: An approach to understanding the molecular genetics of susceptibility to rheumatoid arthritis. *Arthr. & Rheum., 30*: 1205–1213.
9. Todd, J. A., Bell, J. I., and McDevitt, H. O. 1987. HLA-DQβ gene contributes to susceptibility and resistance to insulin-dependent diabetes mellitus. *Nature, 329*: 599.
10. Sinha, A. A., Brautbar, C., Szafer, F., Friedmann, A., Tzfoni, E., Todd, J. A., Steinman, L., and McDevitt, H. O. 1988. A newly characterized HLA DQβ allele associated with pemphigus vulgaris. *Science, 239*: 1026–1028.
11. Holoshitz, J., Matitian, A., and Cohen, I. R. 1984. Arthritis induced in rats by cloned T lymphocytes responsive to mycobacteria but not to collagen type II. *J. Clin. Invest., 73*: 211–215.
12. Zamvil, S., Nelson, P., Trotter, J., Mitchell, D., Knobler, R., Fritz, R., and Steinman, L. 1985. T cell clones specific for myelin basic protein induce chronic relapsing paralysis and demyelination. *Nature, 317*: 355–358.
13. Acha-Orbea, H., Mitchell, D. J., Timmerman, L., Wraith, D. C., Tausch, G. S., Waldor, M. K., Zamvil, S. S., McDevitt, H. O., and Steinman, L. 1980. Limited heterogeneity of T cell receptors from lymphocytes mediating autoimmune encephalomylitis allows specific immune intervention. *Cell, 54*: 263–273.
14. Urban, J. L., Kumar, V., Kono, D. H., Gomez, C., Horvath, S. J., Clayton, J., Ando, D. G., Sercarz, E. E., and Hood, L. 1988. Restricted use of T cell receptor V genes in murine autoimmune encephalomyelitis raises possibilities for antibody therapy. *Cell, 54*: 577–592.
15. Vandenback, A. A., Hashim, G., and Offner, H. 1989. Immunization with a synthetic T cell receptor V-region peptide protects against experimental autoimmune encephalomyelitis. *Nature, 341*: 541–544.
16. Howell, M. D., Winters, S. T., Olee, T., Powell, H. C., Carlo, D. J., and Brostoff, S. W. 1989. Vaccination against experimental allergic encephalomyelitis with T cell receptor peptides. *Science, 246*: 668–670.
17. Janeway, C. A. 1989. Immunotherapy by peptides? *Nature, 341*: 482–483.
18. Srinam, S., Topham, D. J., and Carroll, L. 1987. Haplotype specific suppression of experimental allergic encephalomyelitis with anti-IA antibodies. *J. Immunol., 139*: 1485–1489.
19. Steinman, L., Rosenbaum, J. T., Srinam, S, and McDevitt, H. O. 1981. In vivo effects

of antibodies to immune response gene products: prevention of experimental allergic encephalomyelitis. *Proc. Natl. Acad. Sci. USA, 78*: 7111–7114.

20. Wraith, D. C., Smilek, D. E., Mitchell, D. J., Steinman, L., and McDevitt, H. O. 1989. Antigen recognition in autoimmune encephelomyelitis and the potential for peptide-mediated immunotherapy. *Cell, 59*: 247–255.
21. Urban, J. L., Horvath, S. J., and Hood, L. 1989. Autoimmune T cells: Immune recognition of normal and variant peptide epitopes and peptide-based therapy. *Cell, 59*: 257–271.
22. Hafler, D. A., Duby, A. D., Lee, S. J., Benjamin, D., Seidman, J. G., and Weiner, H. L. 1988. Oligoclonal T lymphocytes in the cerebrospinal fluid of patients with multiple sclerosis. *J. Exp. Med., 167*: 1313–1322.
23. Triebel, F., and Hercend, T. 1989. Subpopultions of human peripheral T gamma delta lymphocytes. *Immunology Today, 10*: 186–188.
24. Davis, M. M., and Bjorkman, P. J. 1988. T-cell antigen receptor genes and T-cell recognition. *Nature, 334*: 395–402.
25. Chothia, C., Boswell, D. R., and Lesk, A. M. 1988. The outline structure of the T cell α/β receptor. *EMBO J., 7*: 3745–3755.
26. Bigler, R. D., Fisher, D., Wang, C. Y., Rinnooy-Kan, E., and Kunkel, H. G. 1983. Idiotype molecules on the cells of a human T cell leukemia. *J. Exp. Med., 158*: 1000.
27. Posnett, D. N., Wang, C. Y., and Friedman, S. M.1986. Inherited polymorphism of the human T cell antigen receptor detected by a monoclonal antibody. *Proc. Natl. Acad. Sci. USA, 83*: 7888–7892.
28. Kappler, J., Kotzin, B., Herron, L., Gelfand, E., Bigler, R. D., Boylston, A., Carrel, S., Posnett, D. N., Choi, Y. W., and Marrack, P. 1989. Vβ-specific stimulation of human T cells by staphylococcal toxins. *Science, 244*: 811–813.
29. Li, Y., Szabo, P., Robinson, M. A., Dong, B., and Posnett, D. N. 1990. Allelic variations in the human T cell receptor Vβ6.7 gene products. *J. Exp. Med., 171*: 221–230.
30. Posnett, D. N. 1989. Idiotypes of rheumatoid factors. In *Monographs in Allergy: Autoantibodies to Immunoglobulins*. (F. Shakib, ed.). S. Karger AG, Basel, pp. 61–73.
31. White, J., Herman, A., Pullen, A. M., Kubo, R., Kappler, J. W., and Marrack, P. 1989. The Vβ-specific superantigen staphylococcal enterotoxin B: stimulation of mature T cells and clonal deletion in neonatal mice. *Cell, 57*: 27–35.
32. Marrack, P., and Kappler, J. 1988. The T cell repertoire for antigen and MHC. *Immunology Today, 9*: 308–315.
33. Wang, C. Y., Bushkin, Y., Pica, R., Lane, C., McGrath, H., and Posnett, D. N. 1986. A monoclonal antibody detecting a shared determinant on the human T cell antigen receptor molecule. *Hybridoma, 5*: 179–190.
34. Bigler, R. D., Posnett, D. N., and Chiorazzi, N. 1985. Stimulation of a subset of normal resting T lymphocytes by a monoclonal antibody to a crossreactive determinant of the human T cell antigen receptor. *J. Exp. Med., 161*: 1450–1463.
35. Sanders, M. E., Makgoba, M. W., and Shaw, S. 1988. Human naive and memory T cells: Reinterpretation of helper-inducer and suppressor-inducer subsets. *Immunology Today, 9*: 195–199.

36. Burton, D. A., Shepherd, G. M., Siskind, G. W., and Posnett, D. N. 1990. T cell receptor variable gene expression: Analysis in ragweed sensitive patients during allergen exposure. *Intl. Arch. Allergy Appl. Immunol., 91*: 306–310.
37. Carrel, S., Isles, P., Schreyer, M., Vacca, A., Salvi, S., Giuffre, L., and Mach, J. P. 1986. Expression on human thymocytes of the idiotypic structures (Ti) from two leukemia T cells lines, Jurkat and HPBALL. *Eur. J. Immunol., 16*: 649–652.
38. Tillinghast, J. P. Behlke, M. A., and Loh, D. Y. 1986. Structure and diversity of the human T cell receptor β chain variable region genes. *Science, 233*: 879–883.
39. Toyonaga, B., and Mak, T. W. 1987. Genes of the T cell antigen receptor in normal and malignant T cells. *Ann. Rev. Immunol., 5*: 585–620.
40. Wilson, R. K., Lai, E., Concannon, P., Barth, R. K., and Hood, L. E. 1988. Structure, organization and polymorphism of murine and human T cell receptor alpha and beta chain gene families. *Immunol. Rev., 101*: 149–172.
41. Choi, Y., Kotzin, B., Herron, L., Callahan, J., Marrack, P., and Kappler, J. 1989. Interaction of *Stephylococcus aureus* toxin "superantigens" with human T cells. *Proc. Natl. Acad. Sci. USA, 86*: 8941–8945.
42. Loh, E. Y., Elliott, J. F., Cwirla, S., Lanier, L. L., and Davis, M. M. 1989. Polymerase chain reaction with single sided specificity: analysis of T cell receptor delta chain. *Science, 243*: 217–220.
43. Robinson, M. A. 1989. Allelic sequence variations in the hypervariable region of a TCR β chain: Correlation with restriction length polymorphism in human families and populations. *Proc. Natl. Acad. Sci. USA, 86*: 9422–9426.
44. Posnett, D. N. 1990. Allelic variations of human TCR V gene products. *11*: 368–373
45. Robinson, M. A., and Kindt, T. J. 1987. Genetic recombination within the human T cell receptor α chain gene complex. *Proc. Natl. Acad. Sci. USA, 84*: 9089–9093.
46. Seboun, E., Robinson, M. A., Kindt, T. J., and Hauser, S. C. 1989. Insertion/deletion-related polymorphisms in the human T cell receptor β gene complex. *J. Exp. Med., 170*: 1263–1270.
47. Wade, T., Bill, J., Marrack, P. C., Palmer, E., and Kappler, J. W. 1988. Molecular basis for the nonexpression of Vβ17 in some strains of mice. *J. Immunol., 141*: 2165–2167.
48. Siu, G., Strauss, E. C., Lai, E., and Hood, L. E. 1986. Analysis of a human Vβ gene subfamily. *J. Exp. Med., 164*: 1600–1614.
49. Seboun, E., Robinson, M. A., Doolittle, T. H., Ciulla, T. A., Kindt, T. J., and Hauser, S. L. 1989. A susceptibility locus for multiple sclerosis is linked to the T cell receptor β chain complex. *Cell, 57*: 1095–1100.
50. Posnett, D. N., Gottlieb, A., Bussel, J. B., Friedman, S. M., Chiorazzi, N., Li, Y., Szabo, P., Farid, N. R., and Robinson, M. A. 1988. T cell antigen receptors in autoimmunity. *J. Immunol., 141*: 1963–1969.
51. Teng, W. P., Cohen, S. B., Posnett, D. N., and Weetman, A. P. 1990 T cell receptor phenotypes in autoimmune thyroid disease. *J. Endocrinol. Invest., 13*: 339–342.
52. Posnett, D. N., Schmelkin, I., Burton, D. A., August, A., McGrath, H., and Mayer, L. F. 1990 T cell antigen receptor V gene usage: Increases in Vβ8$^+$ T cells in Crohn's disease. *J. Clin. Invest., 85*: 1770–1776.

53. Posnett, D. N., McGrath, H., and Mayer, L. 1989. Human auto-antibody to a T cell antigen receptor V region. *FASEB, 3*: A302 (Abstract).
54. Moller, D. R., Konishi, K., Kirby, M., Balbi, B., and Crystal, R. G. 1988. Bias toward use of a specific T cell receptor β-chain variable region in a subgroup of individuals with sarcoidosis. *J. Clin. Invest., 82*: 1183–1191.
55. Moller, D. R., Banks, T. C., and Crystal, R. G. 1989. Evidence that sarcoidosis is a specific antigen driven disorder causing clonal expression of selected T cells at sites of disease. *Clin. Rev., 37*: 558A.
56. Kappler, J., Staerz, U., White, J., and Marrack, P. 1988. Self-tolerance eliminates T cells specific for MLS-modified products of the major histocompatibility complex. *Nature, 332*: 35–40.
57. MacDonald, H. R. 1988. T cell receptor Vβ use predicts reactivity and tolerance to MIS^a-encoded antigens. *Nature, 332*: 40–45.
58. Kappler, J., Roehm, N., and Marrack, P. 1987. T cell tolerance by clonal elimination in the thymus. *Cell, 49*: 273–280.
59. Fleisher, B. 1989. Bacterial toxins as probes for the T cell antigen receptor. *Immunology Today, 10*: 262–264.
60. Cole, B. C., Daynes, R. A., and Ward, J. R. 1981. Stimulation of mouse lymphocytes by a mitogen derived from mycoplasma arthritidis. I. Transformation is associated with an H-2-linked gene that maps to the IE/IC subregion. *J. Immunol., 127*: 1931–1936.
61. Atkin, C. L., Cole, B. C., Sullivan, G. J., Washburn, L. R., and Wiley, B. B. 1986. Stimulation of mouse lymphocytes by a mitogen derived from *Mycoplasma arthritidis*. V. A small basic protein from culture supernatants is a potent T cell mitogen. *J. Immunol., 137*: 1581.
62. Fraser, J. D. 1989. High-affinity binding of staphylococcal enterotoxins A and B to HLA-DR. *Nature, 339*: 221–223.
63. Mollick, J. A., Cook, R. G., and Rich, R. R. 1989. Class II MHC molecules are specific receptors for staphylococcus enterotoxin A. *Science, 244*: 817–820.
64. Scholl, P., et al. 1989. Toxic shock syndrome toxin 1 binds to major histocompatibility complex II molecules. *Proc. Natl. Acad. Sci. USA, 86*: 4210–4214.
65. Carlson, R., Fischer, H., and Sjogren, H. O. 1988. Binding to staphylococcal enterotoxin A to accessory cells is a requirement for its ability to activate human T cells. *J. Immunol., 140*: 2484–2488.
66. Matthes, M., Schrezenmeier, H., Homfeld, J., Heisher, S., Malissen, B., Kirchner, H., and Fleisher, B. 1988. Clonal analysis of human T cell activation of the *Mycoplasma arthritides* mitogen (MAS). *Eur. J. Immunol., 18*: 1733–1737.
67. Fleischer, B., and Schrezenmeier, H. 1988. T cell stimulation by staphylococcal enterotoxins. Clonally variable response and requirement for major histocompatibility complex class II molecules on accessory or target cells. *J. Exp. Med., 167*: 1697–1707.
68. Cole, B. C., Washburn, L. R., and Taylor-Robinson, D. 1985. In *The Mycoplasmas*, Vol. IV (S. Razin and M. F. Barile, eds.). Academic Press, Inc., New York, p. 107.
69. Jansson, E., Vainio, U., and Tuuri, S. 1971. Cultivation of a mycoplasma from the bone marrow in systemic lupus erythematosus disseminatus. *Acta Rheumatol. Scand., 17*: 233.

70. von Bonsdorff, C-H., Jansson, E., Vainio, U., and Tuuri, S. 1973. Ultrastructure of a mycoplasma recovered from the bone marrow in systemic lupus erythematosis. *Ann. Rheum. Dis.*, *32*: 25.
71. Herrmann, T., Accolla, R. S., and MacDonald, H. R. 1989. Different staphylococcal enterotoxins bind preferentially to distinct major histocompatibility complex class II isotypes. *Eur. J. Immunol.*, *19*: 2171–2176.
72. Cole, B. C., Kartchnu, D. R., and Wells, D. J. 1989. Stimulation of mouse lymphocytes by a mitogen derived from Mycoplasma arthritides. VII. Responsiveness is associated with expression of a product(s) of the Vβ gene family present on the T cell receptor α/β for antigen. *J. Immunol.*, *142*: 4131.
73. Cole, B. C., Kartchner, D. R., and Wells, D. J. 1989. Stimulation of mouse lymphocytes by a mitogen derived from Mycoplasma arthritidis. VIII. Selective activation of T cells expressing distinct Vβ T cell receptors from various strains of mice by the "superantigen" MAM. *J. Immunol.*, *142*: 4131–4137.
74. Tumang, J. R., Posnett, D. N., Cole, B. C., Crow, M. K., and Friedman, S. M. 1990. Helper T cell dependent human B cell differentiation mediated by a microbial "superantigen" bridge. *J. Exp. Med.*, *171*: 2153–2158.
75. Allison, A. C., Denman, A. M., and Barnes, R. D. 1971. Cooperating and controlling functions of thymus-derived lymphocytes in relation to autoimmunity. *Lancet*, *i*: 135.
76. Rolink, A. O., Radaszkiewicz, T., Pals, S. T., Van der Meer, W. G. J., Gleichmann, E. 1982. Allosuppressor and allohelper T cells in acute and chronic graft versus host disease. I. Allosuppressor cells rather than killer T cells appear to be the decisive effector cell in lethal graft versus host disease. *J. Exp. Med.*, *155*: 150.
77. Gleichmann, E., van Elven, E. H., van der Veen, F. M. 1982. A systemic lupus erythematosus (SLE)-like disease in mice induced by abnormal T-B cell cooperation. Preferential formation of autoantibodies characteristic of SLE. *Eur. J. Immunol.*, *12*: 152.
78. van Elven, E. H., van der Veen, F. M., Rolink, A. G., Issa, P., Duin, T. M., and Gleichmann, E. 1981. Diseases caused by reactions of T lymphocytes to incompatible structures of the major histocompatibility complex. *J. Immunol.*, *127*: 2435–2538.
79. Anderson, J., Schreier, M. H., and Melchers, F. 1980. T cell dependent B cell stimulation is H-2 restricted and antigen dependent only at the resting B cell level. *Proc. Natl. Acad. Sci. USA*, *77*: 1612–1624.
80. Asano, S. Y., Singer, A., and Hodes, R. J. 1981. Role of the major histocompatibility complex in T cell activation of B cell subpopulations. *J. Exp. Med.*, *154*: 1100–1115.
81. Principato, M. A, Thompson, G. S., and Friedman, S. M. 1983. A cloned major histocompatibility complex-restricted trinitrophenyl-reactive human helper T cell line which activates via two distinct pathways. *J. Exp. Med.*, *158*: 1444–1454.
82. Hirohata, S., Jelinek, D. F., and Lipsky, P. E. 1988. T cell dependent activation of B cell proliferation and differentiation by immobilized monoclonal antibodies to CD3. *J. Immunol.*, *140*: 3736–3744.
83. Julius, M. H., von Boehmer, H., and Sidman, C. L. 1982. Dissociation of two signals required for activation of resting B cells. *Proc. Natl. Acad. Sci. USA*, *79*: 1989–1993.

84. Morris, S. C., Cheek, R. L., Cohen, P. L., and Eisenberg, R. A. 1990. Autoantibodies in chronic graft versus host result from cognate T-B interactions. *J. Exp. Med.*, *171*: 503–517.
85. Mourad, W., Scholl, P., Diaz, A., Geha, R., and Chatila, T. 1989. The staphylococcal toxic shock syndrome toxin 1 triggers B cell proliferation and differentiation via major histocompatibility complex-unrestricted cognate T/B cell interaction. *J. Exp. Med.*, *170*: 2011.
86. Palacios, R., Martinez-Mara, O., and Guy, K. 1983. Monoclonal antibodies against HLA-DR antigens replace T helper cells in activation of B lymphocytes. *Proc. Natl. Acad. Sci. USA, 80*: 3456–3460.
87. Cambier, J. C., Newell, M. K., Justement, L. B., McGuire, J. C., Leach, C. L., and Chen, Z. Z. 1987. Ia binding ligands and cAMP stimulate nuclear translocation of PKC in B lymphocytes. *Nature, 327*: 629.
88. Guy, R., and Hodes, R. J. 1989. Antigen-specific, MHC-restricted B cell activation by cell-free Th2 cell products. Synergy between antigen-specific helper factors and IL-4. *J. Immunol., 143*: 1433–1440.
89. Acuto, O., Campea, T. J., Royes, H. D., Hussey, R. E., Poole, C. B., and Reinherz, E. L. 1985. Molecular analysis of T cell receptor V gene expression. Evidence that a single Ti Vβ gene family can be used in formation of V domains on phenotypically and functionally diverse T cell populations. *J. Exp. Med., 161*: 1326–1343.
90. Maecker, H. T., Levy, R. 1989. Prevalence of antigen receptor variants in human T cell lines and tumors. *J. Immunol., 142*: 1395–1404.
91. Hoover, M. L., Black, R. E., Ball, E., Alford, M., Marks, J., Stastny, P., and Capra, J. D. 1989. Polymorphisms of the human T cell receptor alpha and beta chain genes and their relationship to insulin dependent diabetes mellitus. In *Immunobiology of HLA*, Vol. 2: *Immunogenetics and Histocompatibility*, Springer Verlag, New York, N.Y.
92. Demaine, A. G., Millward, B. A., Vaughan, R. W., and Welsh, K. I. 1987. T cell receptor β gene polymorphisms are associated with certain autoimmune diseases. *J. Cell. Biochem., 11D*: 225.
93. Demaine, A. G., Vaughan, R. W., Taube, D. H., and Welsh, K. I. 1988. Association of membranous nephropathy with T-cell receptor constant β chain and immunoglobulin heavy chain switch region polymorphisms. *Immunogenetics, 27*: 19–23.
94. Weetman, A. P., So, A. K., Roe, C., Walport, M. J., and Foroni, L. 1987. T cell receptor α chain V region polymorphism linked to primary autoimmune hypothyroidism but not Graves disease. *Human Immunol., 20*: 167–173.
95. Beall, S. S., Concannon, P., Charmley, P., McFarland, H. F., Gatti, R. A., Hood, L. E., McFarlin, D. E., and Biddison, W. E. 1989. The germline repertoire of T cell receptor β chain genes in patients with chronic progressive multiple sclerosis. *J. Neuroimmunol., 21*: 59–66.
96. Friedman, S. M., Posnett, D. N., Tumaug, J. R., Cole, B. C., Crow, M. K. 1991. A potential role for microbial superantigens in the pathogenesis of systemic autoimmune disease. *Arthritis Rheum.*, in press.
97. Marrack, P., Kushnir, E., and Kappler, J. 1991. A maternally inherited superantigen encoded by a mammary tumour virus. *Nature, 349*: 524–526.

98. Frankel, W. N., Rudy, C., Coffin, J. M., and Huber, B. T. 1991. Linkage of Mls genes to endogenous mammary tumour viruses of inbred mice. *Nature, 349*: 526–528.
99. Woodland, D. L., Happ, M. P., Gollob, K. J., and Palmer, E. 1991. An endogenous retrovirus mediating deletion of the $\alpha\beta$ T cells? *Nature, 349*: 529–530.
100. Dyson, P. J., Knight, A. M., Fairchild, S., Simpson, E., and Tomonari, K. 1991. Genes encoding ligands for deletion of Vβ11 T cells cosegregate with mammary tumour virus genomes. *Nature, 349*: 531–532.

11

MHC and Autoimmune Diseases: Susceptibility to Rheumatoid Arthritis Associated with a Hydrophobic Strip of α Helix Encoded by Several MHC Alleles

Robert Winchester and Edward Dwyer
Hospital for Joint Diseases and New York University Medical Center, New York, New York

I. INTRODUCTION

Rheumatoid arthritis is a chronic systemic autoimmune disease characterized by infiltration of activated T lymphocytes and mononuclear cells into numerous organs, notably the joints, in parallel with the presence of abundant amounts of B and plasma cells. Some of the latter secrete autoantibodies primarily directed to IgG molecules, forming immunoreactive complexes capable of activating effector systems such as that involving complement. Tissue inflammation and destruction result from both the humoral and cellular arms of the autoimmune response. There is a clear genetic basis for susceptibility to this immune response, and we have estimated that something on the order of two or three genes are involved in determining the genetic liability to develop the disease phenotype (1). At least one of these genes is located in the class II region of the MHC as first shown with MLC typing and subsequently serologic analysis (2–4). However, several distinct serologic specificities such as DR4, DR1, and DRw6 have been associated with susceptibility (3–12). This complicates the interpretation of the genetic basis of the disorder with the possibility of heterogeneity in the disease, raising the question of whether one or several entirely different immune recognition events underlie the untoward autoimmune response or responses. Related to the answer for this question are the central issues in the pathogenesis of RA: What is the antigen or equivalent phenomenon that drives the immune system, and does this occur at the level of T-cell recognition involving MHC class II structures?

In this chapter we approach these questions by briefly reviewing the relevant data. A "segregation analysis" approach is used tht exploits ethnic differences in haplotype organization and gene sequence to map susceptibility into a small region of the *DRβ* chain gene shared by each of the *DRβ* chain alleles that predispose toward inheritance of the disease. These alleles are seen to encode a single equivalent region of polymorphic residues in a hydrophobic strip of α helical conformation oriented towards the T-cell receptor. From this we make the inference that rheumatoid arthritis originates from what can be designated as a unitary immune recognition event initiated by particular class II MHC molecules interacting with T-cell receptors probably expressed on cells of the CD4 lineage. We point out that the distinctive conformation of the α helix has certain attributes associated with determinants recognized by T cells that suggest speculations on certain T-cell mechanisms that could be involved in the disease.

II. DISEASE ASSOCIATION OF RHEUMATOID ARTHRITIS WITH CLASSIC HLA SPECIFICITIES: A PROBLEM OF MULTIPLE SUSCEPTIBILITY MARKERS DIFFERING AMONG ETHNIC GROUPS

The starting point of this analysis is that the best characterized marker of genetic susceptibility to RA is associated with certain MHC class II serologic specificities. The HLA specificity DR4 was found to be increased in many studies of rheumatoid arthritis, but the increased risk for the disease was not of an equivalent intensity in all groups that were studied, as reflected by heterogeneity in the calculated relative risk value (3–10). Most notably, rheumatoid arthritis was not encountered at an elevated frequency among DR4 positive Jewish people and certain other groups, such as East Indians and southern Spaniards (8–10).

That these genetic differences could still be attributed to structural differences of class II gene products predominating in the DR4 haplotypes of those populations became evident with studies delineating the subtypes of DR4 recognized by MLC typing (13,14). Of the five principal subtypes of DR4 readily recognized by this system, Dw4, Dw14, and Dw15 were found to be most prevalent in ethnic groups that exhibited a strong association of the rheumatoid arthritis with DR4, while Dw10 and Dw13 were predominant in those populations that had weak or no associations of rheumatoid arthritis with DR4 (2,15–18). This suggested that the DR4 subtypes were differentially associated with susceptibility.

Further complicating this analysis was the observation that in three ethnic groups—East Indians, southern Spaniards and Jews—DR1 but not DR4 was identified as the predominant DR allele associated with susceptibility (8–10). In fact, among the populations with predominant DR4-associated susceptibility, DR1 could be shown to be associated if the effect of the preponderant association with DR4 was corrected.

III. STRUCTURE OF THE CLASS II MOLECULES

The description of the conformation of the MHC class I molecule by Bjorkman et al. (19) permitted the visualization of a presumptive class II molecule conformation (20,21) depicted in Figure 1, which illustrates the three diversity (hypervariable) regions of the DRβ chain. Two are located in the β-pleated sheet floor of the antigen-binding cleft, and the third is located in an α helix in the margin of the cleft. In the case of the DR molecule, these three regions contain virtually all of the significant polymorphisms of the heterodimer because the α chain is monomorphic.

IV. USE OF ETHNIC DIFFERENCES IN THE STRUCTURE OF THE MHC CLASS II ALLELES TO MAP THE LOCATION OF SUSCEPTIBILITY IN A SEGREGATION TYPE OF ANALYSIS

There are two possible explanations for the basis of disease susceptibility with an HLA specificity: either the trait of developing the disease is controlled by a polymorphic gene in linkage disequilibrium with the HLA marker allele, or the disease is due to the direct action of the allelic product itself. Mapping of susceptibility is difficult in conventional serologic studies. Serologic typing using polyclonal antisera does not permit precise assignment of alleles because of the highly linked series of genes comprising the *DR* and *DQ* subregions (Fig. 2). These act both as immunogens to yield complex typing sera and as linked antigens to render the typing more complex. Indeed, the absence of observed recombination in this region of the MHC is a significant obstacle that prevents conventional segregation analysis in families to be used as a tool in mapping susceptibility.

However, the fact that in different ethnic groups susceptibility to rheumatoid arthritis varies in relationship to the particular Dw subtypes of DR4 that are the characteristic of that ethnic group afforded an opportunity to approach the genetic basis of developing the disease. Accordingly, we set out to analyze DR4 haplotypes, initially at the level of molecularly defined epitopes recognizable by monoclonal antibodies (22–25) and, in parallel, undertook studies of the gene structure (26–28). With the anticipation that the structural differences responsible for the different subtypes of DR4 delineated by MLC typing (13) would illuminate the problem of rheumatoid arthritis susceptibility, an extensive effort was made to sequence the relevant *DQ* and *DR* subregion genes in the *DR4* haplotype (26). This was followed by an analysis of the structure of DR1 alleles in individuals with rheumatoid arthritis (29).

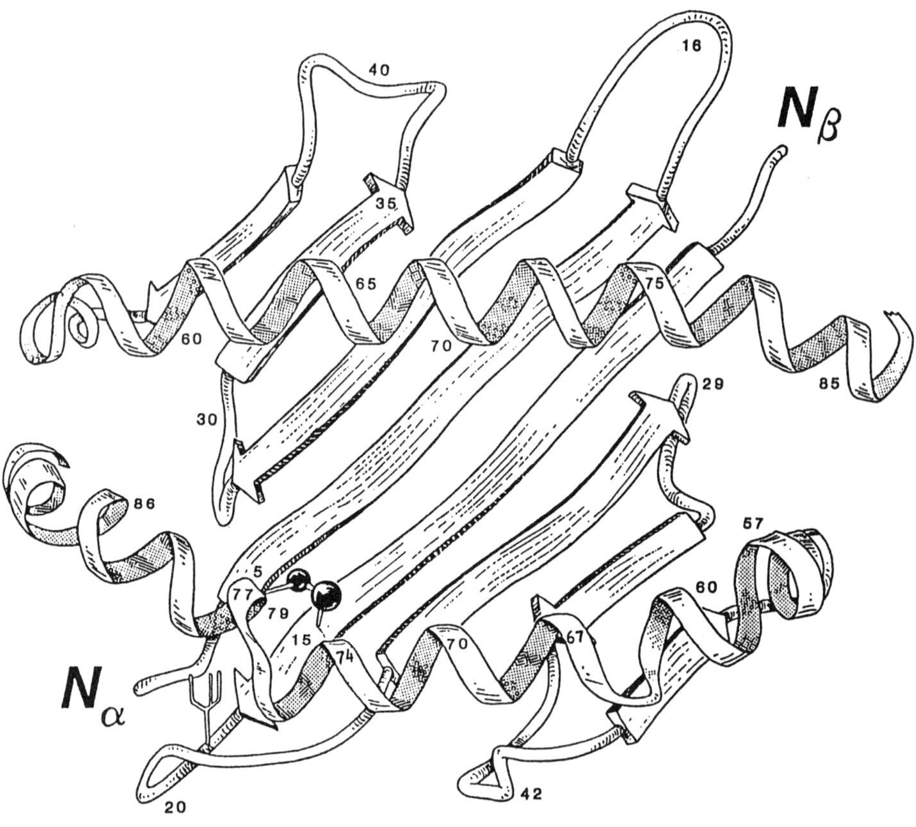

FIGURE 1 A hypothetical model of the class II antigen-binding domains based on the tertiary structure model of Bjorkman et al. (19) for the class I molecule and the approach to computer projections for secondary structure used by Norcross and Kanehisha (see Ref. 21). The N terminus of the α chain begins at the lower left and after providing the four left-hand strands of β-pleated sheet assumes an α helical structure and forms the upper margin of the antigen-binding cleft. The β-chain N terminus is at the upper right. This chain provides the β-pleated sheet on the right and the lower strand of α helix. A disulfide bond links residues 16 and 79. An oligosaccharide moiety lies just on the other side of the α helix in this region.

The results of the sequence determinations in the different DR4 haplotypes summarized schematically in Figure 3 can be used in a sort of segregation analysis to define the locus and its alleles that are most closely associated with susceptibility to rheumatoid arthritis (30). As an example, *DQβ* and *DQα* chain genes

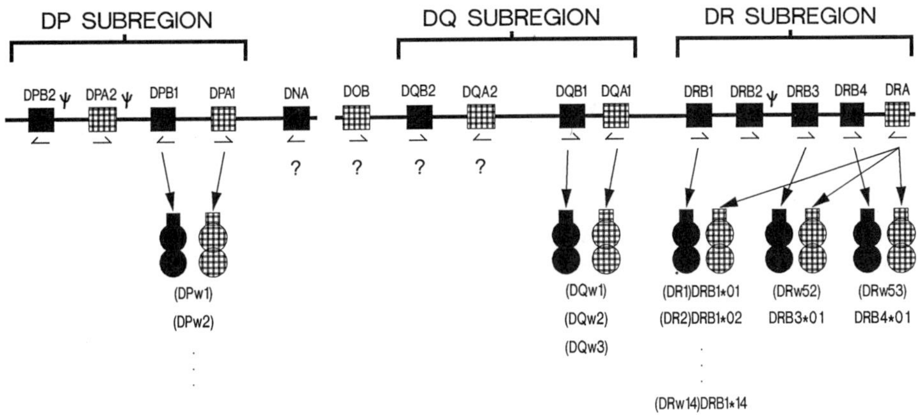

FIGURE 2 The organization of the class II genes and their products. Both the new and old terminologies are shown. The three subregions each contain an α-chain gene and one or more β-chain genes. The interaction of the chains encoded in each subregion forms the three principal MHC class II isotypes: DR, DQ, and DP molecules. Some allelic series are shown. While information on the specific analogs of haplotypes is still incomplete, it is proposed that the B3 gene is intact and expressed in the DRw52 haplotypes, while the B4 gene is intact and expressed in the DRw53 haplotypes, indicating that the β_2 chain encoding DRw52 or DRw53 specificities is pseudoallelic.

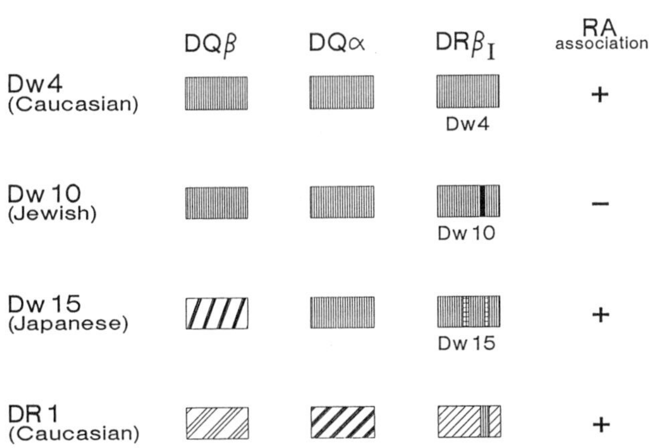

FIGURE 3 A "segregation"-type analysis of susceptibility to rheumatoid arthritis using the presence or absence of an association between disease and structurally distinct haplotypes in different ethnic groups to map sequences likely to be responsible for disease predisposition.

can be excluded as critical genetic factors because certain identical alleles at each locus are shared by the different Dw haplotypes that encode the DR4 specificity; for example, the Dw4 and Dw10 varieties of DR4 are disparate for association with rheumatoid arthritis, yet share identical DQβ and DQα chains. Similarly the *DR*β_2 (BIII, *DRB3*) and *DR*α (*DRA*) chain loci can be eliminated because of the invariant nature of *DRw53* and DRα gene products encoded by the *DRw53* haplotypes or in all DR types, respectively. The only locus with sufficient allelic heterogeneity to account for the pattern of its association or lack is the *DR*β_I (*DRB1*) (30,31).

Reciprocally, the identification of this β chain locus greatly diminished the likelihood that gene products of tightly linked genes other than the known class II MHC products are involved, rendering the oft-invoked hypothesis of a mysterious non-MHC class II–linked polymorphic gene as the responsible agent for susceptibility quite unlikely. Also of importance to the exclusion of this hypothesis were studies on the genomic organization of the MHC class II genes performed in multiple laboratories, in the case of DR4, most notably that of Strominger and colleagues (32). The central finding was that there was no evidence for an open reading frame encoding an additional HLA or non-HLA gene in this region. Moreover, identical RFLP analysis of Dw10 and Dw13 individuals with those having other varieties of DR4 argued against the existence of novel haplotype-specific genes or events in the haplotypes that were not formally sequenced at the genomic level (33).

V. MAPPING OF SUSCEPTIBILITY INTO A SEQUENCE OF RESIDUES OF THE THIRD DIVERSITY REGION OF THE DR4 DRβ CHAIN GENE

An analysis of the differences in the inferred amino acid sequence of *DR*β*1* genes present in the various DR4 subtypes allowed the intragenic region most likely responsible for susceptibility to be mapped. Table 1 illustrates the inferred amino acid sequences of the DR4 β chain variants. The primary finding is that the significant sequence variations in the Dw10 subtype of DR4 that is not associated with rheumatoid arthritis susceptibility was found to be in the third diversity region. This has two implications, the first of which is that the amino acid sequence of the first and second diversity regions for the DR4 alleles are not in themselves sufficient to confer susceptibility to rheumatoid arthritis. The second implication derives from the changes in the Dw10 DR4 third diversity region that involve the substitution of Ile at position 67 and Asp and Glu at positions 70 and 71, respectively.

This change from the sequence of the Dw4 prototype third diversity region was a critical finding in suggesting the importance of the third diversity region as a site of special relevance to rheumatoid arthritis. The consensus residues

TABLE 1 Locations of Significant Variability Among DR1 and DR4 β Chains

									10										20											30										40									
DR2w2	G	D	T	R	P	R	F	L	Q	Q	D	K	Y	E	C	H	F	F	N	G	T	E	R	V	R	F	L	H	R	D	I	Y	N	Q	E	E	D	L	R	F	D	S	D	V	G	E	Y	R	A
DR1									W		L		F													L		E		C		Y	N				S	V									Y		
DR1NA16									W		L		F													L		E		C		Y	N				S	V									Y		
DR4w14									E		V		H													F		D		Y		Y	H				Y	V									Y		
DR4w4									E		V		H													F		D		Y		Y	H				Y	V									Y		
DR413									E		V		H													F		D		Y		Y	H				Y	V									Y		
DR4w15									E		V		H													F		D		Y		Y	H				Y	V									Y		
DR4w10									E		V		H													F		D		Y		Y	H				Y	V									Y		

	50										60										70										80										90					
DR2w2	V	T	E	L	G	R	P	D	A	E	Y	W	N	S	Q	K	D	F	L	E	D	R	R	A	A	V	D	T	Y	C	R	H	N	Y	G	V	G	E	S	F	I	V	Q	R	R	V
DR1								D										L			Q	R			A											V	G									
DR1NA16								D										L			Q	R			A											G	V									
DR4w14								D										L			Q	R			A											V	V									
DR4w4								D										L			Q	K			A											V	G									
DR4w13								D										L			Q	R			E											V	G									
DR4w15								S										L			Q	R			A											V	G									
DR4w10								D										I			D	E			A											V	V									

permissive for the development of rheumatoid arthritis are, from position 67 and ending at position 74: *Leu*-Leu-Glu-*Gln-Arg or Lys*-Arg-Ala-*Ala*. The sequence of the Dw13 allele that also is not associated with susceptibility resembles the sequences of Dw4, Dw14, and Dw15 alleles with the important difference that, as with the Dw10 allele, there is a highly nonconservative amino acid substitution involving, again, a change to a negatively charged residue. However, the Glu is located at position 74, not at 71 as in the Dw10 β chain.

VI. RELATION OF THE THIRD DIVERSITY REGION OF DR1 AND DRw6AMALA TO CERTAIN DR4 ALLELES

Inasmuch as DR1 is serologically unrelated to DR4, yet both specificities are associated with rheumatoid arthritis, the structural analysis of the DR1 haplotype affords an important approach to determining whether the interpretation of the molecular basis of susceptibility is a valid notion. As predicted, the sequence analysis of DR1, including that of a distinctive DR1 β1 chain from a rheumatoid arthritis patient (DR1NASC), also revealed a third diversity region sequence that was essentially identical to the DR4 subtypes associated with disease susceptibility (Tables 1 and 2) (27,28,31,34). Lang et al. report an increase in Dw6 among German patients with rheumatoid arthritis (11). Similarly, Nepom et al. have recently identified a variety of DRw6, DRw6AMALA, which is associated with susceptibility to rheumatoid arthritis (12). Of great interest, the sequence of the third diversity region of this allele is also identical to the third diversity sequence shared by Dw14 and DR1 (Table 2). Accordingly, it should specify a conformationally equivalent structure. The sequence of the alleles encoding DR1 and DRw6 specificities both differ markedly from DR4 in the first two diversity regions, where the residues are found that are primarily responsible for the different serologic reactivity. With the exception of positions 28 and 32, there is no homology in these two diversity regions to suggest that susceptibility is encoded by these two regions of the DRβ chain. Moreover, the third diversity sequence is not found in other DR alleles that are not associated with susceptibility to rheumatoid arthritis (Table 2).

The interpretation that the diversity of the MHC associations could be accounted for by a single structure common to the products of otherwise distinct alleles was initially reported by Gregersen et al. as the "shared epitope theory," and was the first instance of an attempt to relate the molecular basis of disease susceptibility to a particular conformation (31). The term "epitope" referred analogously to structures detected by antibodies and did not refer to the term "epitope" in the terminology of the MHC molecule–T-cell receptor interaction. In view of the fact that the function of this shared structure is in interactions with a T-cell receptor or with an antigenic peptide, we also refer to the common structure as a shared conformation to reflect its conformational equivalence (30).

TABLE 2 Major Sites of Sequence Polymorphism Among DRβ Chain Alleles Illustrating Patchwork Pattern of Developing Variability from Recombination of a Smaller Number of Antecedent Genes

	Amino acid positions in DRβ chain diversity regions										
	First			Second				Third			
	9	11	13	26	28	30	37	67	70	71	74
DR1 βI	W	L	F	L	E	C	S	L	Q	R	A
DR1 Cetus	W	L	F	L	E	C	S	I	D	E	A
DR2 Dw2βI	Q	D	Y	F	H	D	D	F	D	R	A
DR2 Dw12βI	Q	D	Y	F	H	G	N	F	D	R	A
DR2 AZHβI	Q	D	Y	F	H	G	N	I	Q	R	A
DR3 βI	E	S	S	Y	D	Y	H	L	Q	K	R
DR3 DQWa	E	S	S	F	E	Y	H	L	Q	K	R
DR4 Dw4	E	V	H	F	D	Y	Y	L	Q	K	A
DR4 Dw14	E	V	H	F	D	Y	Y	L	Q	R	A
DR4 Dw15	E	V	H	F	D	Y	Y	L	Q	R	A
DR4 Dw10	E	V	H	F	D	Y	Y	I	D	E	A
DR5 Dw5βI	E	S	S	F	D	Y	Y	F	D	R	A
DR5 JVM	E	S	S	F	D	Y	Y	I	D	E	A
DRw6a βI	E	S	S	F	D	Y	N	I	D	E	A
DRw6b βI	E	S	S	F	D	Y	F	L	R	E	E
DR6 Amala	E	S	S	F	E	Y	N	L	Q	R	A
DR7 βI	W	G	Y	F	E	L	F	I	D	R	Q
DRw8 βI	E	S	G	F	D	Y	Y	F	D	R	L
DR9 βI	K	D	F	Y	H	G	N	F	R	R	E
DRw10 βI	E	V	F	L	E	R	Y	L	R	R	A
Dw2 βIII	W	P	R	F	D	Y	S	I	Q	A	A
AZH βIII	W	P	R	F	D	Y	S	F	D	R	A
DRw52aβIII	E	R	S	Y	D	H	F	L	Q	K	R
DRw52βIII	E	R	S	F	E	H	Y	L	Q	K	R
DRw52cβIII	E	R	S	F	E	Y	L	L	Q	K	R
DRw53βIII	E	A	C	N	I	Y	Y	L	R	R	E

VII. MAPPING SUSCEPTIBILITY INTO THE STRIP OF AN α HELIX PRESUMED TO BE FACING THE T-CELL RECEPTOR

Since the requirement for susceptibility appear to be a mosaic of nonpolar hydrophobic residues at the extreme positions 67 and 74, while the intervening positions of 70 and 71 require a neutral hydrophilic and a positively charged residue, respectively, it is of interest to consider the spatial distribution of the residues in this conformational analysis. Would the residue side chains primarily lie in the antigen-binding cleft, or would they point toward the T-cell receptor, or would they even be seemingly random in their distribution?

The Edmundson wheel diagram of the position of residues in an α helix, illustrated in Figure 4, gives some insight into the possible relationships of the amino acid polymorphisms relevant to susceptibility. The diagram illustrates a model of the predicted secondary structure of the DRβ1 α helix oriented from the right end of the antigen-binding cleft. By this model, residues 70 and 74 face upward toward the T-cell receptor and are thought of as having a major role in determining the T-cell receptor repertoire (35), whereas residue 71 faces into the antigen-binding cleft and is involved in binding antigenic peptides.

The polymorphic residues in this region of the third diversity region are grouped into permissive and nonpermissive residues according to their presence or absence in specific locations in alleles that are associated, or not, with susceptibility to rheumatoid arthritis (Table 3). If the permissive and nonpermissive amino acid substitutions are isolated according to the Edmundson wheel analysis into those comprising each of the three principal strips of the α helix, the critical variations that characterize individuals with rheumatoid arthritis are found in the strip of

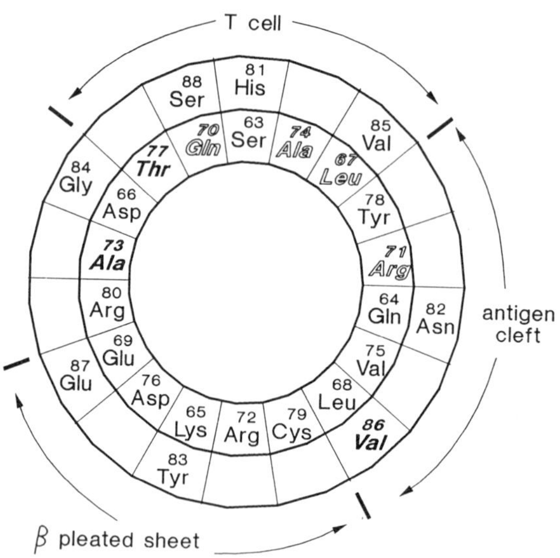

FIGURE 4 Edmundson wheel diagram showing the relation of axially contiguous residues in an α helix. The orientation of the α helix is likely determined by residue 79, which forms a disulfide link with the β-pleated sheet floor of the antigen cleft. Three principal strips of helix are shown: one facing the antigen binding cleft, one the β-pleated sheet infrastructure and outside of the helix, and one facing the T cell. Residues, 67, 70, and 74 appear vertically aligned, forming the strip of helix presumably oriented more upwards toward the T-cell receptor than into the antigen-binding cleft.

TABLE 3 Association of Hydrophobicity in T-Cell Strip of DRβ Chain Helix with Susceptibility to Rheumatoid Arthritis

	Amino acid position								
DR types	63	67	70	74	77	81	85	Mean hydrophobicity	RA associated?
DR1βI	S	L	Q	A	T	H	V	−.84	Yes
DR1NASC	S	L	Q	A	T	H	A	−.84	Yes
DR4w4	S	L	Q	A	T	H	V	−.84	Yes
DR4w14	S	L	Q	A	T	H	V	−.84	Yes
DR4w15	S	L	Q	A	T	H	V	−.84	Yes
DR6 Amala	S	L	Q	A	T	H	V	−.84	Yes
DR4w10	S	I	D	A	T	H	V	−.28	No
DR4w13	S	L	Q	E	T	H	V	−.14	No
DR5w5	S	F	D	A	T	H	V	−.42	No
DR2w2	S	F	D	A	T	H	V	−.42	No
DR3w3	S	F	D	R	N	H	V	+.40	No
DR6a	S	I	D	A	T	H	V	−.28	No
DR6b	S	F	R	A	T	H	V	−.42	No
DR7	S	I	D	Q	T	H	V	−.14	No
DR9	S	F	R	E	T	H	V	+.28	No
DRw10	S	L	R	A	T	H	V	−.28	Yes
BOT/OUT[a]	K	E	R	D	C	Y	E	+2.34	N/A
Cleft DR4[b]	T	L	R	V	Y	N	G	−.44	N/A

[a]BOT/OUT is the bottom-outside strip of helix which is invariant.
[b]Cleft DR4 is the strip of helix facing the antigen binding cleft in DR4w4.
N/A = Not applicable.

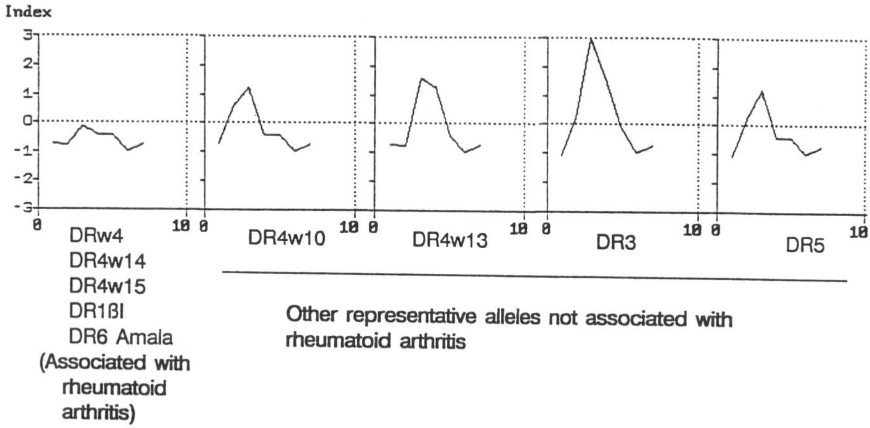

FIGURE 5 The hydrophobicity plots by the Hopp and Woods method of the strip of helix from residues 63 to 85 encompassing polymorphic residues 67, 70, and 74. According to the Edmundsom wheel algorithm, the sequence associated with rheumatoid arthritis susceptibility is the most hydrophobic of the various third diversity regions, as shown by the plot of the left-most graph. Positive values of the ordinate reflect the extent of calculated hydrophilicity.

helix facing the T-cell receptor. That is, substitution at positions 70 or 74 by a nonpermissive negatively charged residue removes susceptibility to rheumatoid arthritis that otherwise would be encoded by this conformation.

It is of special interest that the overall strip of helix determined by the polymorphisms associated with rheumatoid arthritis is the most hydrophobic of all third diversity regions, as shown by Hopp and Woods plots of this strip of helix. Figure 5 contrasts representative linear sequences of hydrophobicity of each third diversity region in Table 2 calculated by the Hopp and Woods algorithm, using a two-residue field for the strip of helix. The sequence of the strip of helix associated with susceptibility to RA is distinctive in its uniform moderately hydrophobic character. All of the other strip-of-helix sequences have a distinct hydrophilic maximum of varying magnitude at about position 71. It appears that the presence of nonpermissive side chains that have different chemical, spatial, and, perhaps most importantly, more hydrophilic and charge interaction properties appears to alter the functional character of the α helix and prevents the other DRβ chain alleles from operating as a susceptibility determinant for rheumatoid arthritis.*

*There is one exception to this generalization. The *DRw10* allele is also related to susceptibility (24,25,27,30), accounting for a small proportion of cases, and differs from the consensus sequence by substitution of Arg for Gln at position 70. This could imply an expanded concept of the shared epitope: Leu-Leu-Glu-Gln or Arg-Arg or Lys-Arg-Ala-Ala, or a complex transcomplementation mechanism, as discussed (30).

Should this view be borne out in subsequent studies, it would emphasize that the critical element in susceptibility is the strip of helix facing the T-cell receptor and not in the residues facing into the cleft, where they would determine a complementary configuration that influences antigen binding. This latter point would be emphasized by the diverse configuration of the cleft in each of the different alleles, especially with regard to the polymorphic residues contributed to by the first and second diversity regions of the underlying β-pleated sheet structure.

VIII. INFERENCES

In attempting to understand the molecular basis of susceptibility to rheumatoid arthritis, there are three general schemes that relate T-cell help to the initiating event that results in the production of autoantibodies and delayed hypersensitivity type of synovial tissue infiltration with T cells of the CD4 lineage. In the traditional one, we can envision that a specific in situ trimolecular interaction between (1) the α-β T-cell receptor of a CD4 helper T cell, (2) a purely hypothetical antigen fragment "X" to which the immune response that underlies rheumatoid arthritis is directed, and (3) the particular MHC class II allele that, through encoding a conformationally equivalent structure, is capable of presenting antigen "X" to the T cell. According to this speculation, a helper T-cell clone or clones that contain receptors capable of recognizing antigen "X" in the context of the particular MHC class II allele would be necessary. One of the consequences of this interaction is the production of the specific T-cell help for the maturation and expansion of pathogenic B-cell clones such as those manufacturing rheumatoid factors. However, in consideration of the apparent orientation of the crucial strip of helix towards the T-cell receptor, this view would seem less likely.

Alternatively, the role of the class II susceptibility structure could be to act earlier in ontogeny in the formation of the T-cell repertoire through the thymic processes of positive and negative selection. The first process, positive selection, results in a peripheral T-cell population whose repertoire is MHC restricted, i.e., T cells whose receptors respond to antigenic peptides only in the context of self class II molecules (36). The subsequent second process, negative selection, ensures that the repertoire thus constituted does not contain T cells that will respond to self peptides in the context of self class II molecules, i.e., the population is self tolerant (37). An analysis of the potential contribution of either these processes toward the development of a susceptible state must be modified by the known genetics of rheumatoid arthritis. Specifically, the inheritance of the disease appears to be of a dominant nature with regard to DR alleles; the heterozygous individual can manifest the full phenotype. A molecular explanation for this observation may reside in the precise nature of the interaction between the T-cell receptor and class II molecule. It has been hypothesized that the α helices of class II heterodimers interact with the CDR1 and CDR2 regions of the α-β T-cell receptor, which are located on the V segment of the variable region of each chain of the T-cell receptor heterodimer (35). The implication of this interaction during the process of positive selection is that the resultant peripheral T lymphocytes would favor the usage of certain V gene segments. So, for example, the expression of DR molecules in the thymus with the conformationally relevant third diversity region could be seen as positively a biased T-cell population, which in the periphery would be more likely to initiate and perpetuate an autoreactive synovial inflammatory process. Recently, the concept of superantigen has been proposed whereby certain antigens presented in the context of class II molecules (e.g., staphylococcal enterotoxin B) are capable of stimulating all T cells that express a certain V segment (38); an antigenic stimulus of this nature, whether endogenous or exogenous, could be envisaged as initiating a hyperresponsive state in an individual whose T-cell repertoire displays the corresponding V segment at a disproportionately elevated frequency.

Similarly, with regard to negative selection, the maintenance of self tolerance necessarily prohibits the maturation of T cells whose receptors are capable of interacting with self peptides in the context of class II molecules. This deletion creates a "hole in the repertoire" that may result in a T-lymphocyte population that is specifically deficient with regard to its ability to effectively eradicate certain pathogens. This "hole" would also follow a dominant inheritance. In this way, for example, a persistent subclinical viral infection may induce aberrations in immune regulation that eventually result in autoimmune disease. In the special case of rheumatoid arthritis, a functionally evasive pathogen with synovial tropism may initiate a destructive, albeit ineffective, inflammatory response that persists long after the etiologic agent has been eliminated. Fassbender has argued that changes in synovial cells resembling psuedotransformation antedate the appearance of any cells of the immune system (38).

A third possibility derives from current predictions in several laboratories on the nature of peptide conformations that are most efficiently presented by T cells. These include the amphipathic DeLisi-Berzofsky method and the strip-of-helix hydrophobicity algorithm of Humphreys and his colleagues (39,40). In terms of these conformational studies, the third diversity region of the DRβ chain alleles associated with RA susceptibility approaches the criteria of a T-cell presented peptide much more closely than do the other third diversity regions. Taken in concert with notions such as the peptide self hypothesis of Kourilsky and Claverie (41), this would suggest the possibility that the third diversity region itself could be presented as a peptide antigen following an event leading to loss of self tolerance. The implications of each of these three conjectures are different for the T-cell repertoire and should be able to be approached experimentally.

ACKNOWLEDGMENTS

This work was supported in part by NIH grants AI-19411 and AR-35404.

REFERENCES

1. Winchester, R. J. 1981. Genetic aspects of rheumatoid arthritis. *Springer Semin. Immunopathol.*, *4*: 89–102.
2. Stastny, P. 1976. Mixed lymphocyte cultures in rheumatoid arthritis. *J. Clin. Invest.*, *57*: 1148.
3. Gibofsky, A., Winchester, R. J., Patarroyo, M., Fotino, M., and Kunkel, H. G. 1978. Disease associations of the Ia-like human alloantigens. Contrasting patterns in rheumatoid arthritis and systemic lupus erythematosus. *J. Exp. Med.*, *148*: 1728–1732.
4. Gibofsky, A., Winchester, R., Hansen, J., et al. 1978. Contrasting patterns of newer histocompatibility determinants in patients with rheumatoid arthritis and systemic lupus erythematosus. *Arthritis. Rheum.*, *21*: S134–S138.
5. Winchester, R. J. 1977. B-lymphocyte allo-antigens, cellular expression, and disease significance with special reference to rheumatoid arthritis. *Arthritis Rheum.*, *20*: 159s.
6. Stastny, P. 1978. Association of the B-cell alloantigen DRw4 with rheumatoid arthritis. *N. Engl. J. Med.*, *298*: 869.
7. Sacha, J. A., and Kirwan, J. R. 1986. Multiple HLA associations and disease susceptibility. *Disease Markers*, *4*: 13–17.
8. Schiff, B., Mizrachi, Y., Orgad, S., et al. 1982. Association of HLA-Aw31 and HLA-DR1 with adult rheumatoid arthritis. *Ann. Rheum. Dis.*, *41*: 403.
9. Nunez-Roldan, A., Arguer, E., Villechenous, E., and Dela Prada, M. 1982. HLA DR antigens in rheumatoid arthritis. *Rev. Esp. Rheumatol.*, *9*: 9–11.
10. Woodrow, J. C., Nichol, F. E., and Zaviropoulos, G. 1981. DR antigens and rheumatoid arthritis: A study of two populations. *Br. Med. J.*, *283*: 1287.
11. Lang, B., Melchers, I., Urlacher, A., et al. 1990. HLA-DR1 and DRw6 association in DR4 negative rheumatoid arthritis patients. *Rheum. Int.* *10*(4):171–175.
12. Willkens, R. F., Nepom, G. T., Marks, C. R., Nettles, J. W., Nepom, B. S. 1991. Association of HLA-Dw16 with rheumatoid arthritis in Yakima Indians. *Arthritis Rheum.*, *34*:43.
13. Groner, J. P., Watson, A. J., and Bach, F. H. 1983. Dw/LD-related molecular polymorphism of DR4 β chains. *J. Exp. Med.*, *157*: 1687.
14. Reinsmoen, N. L., and Bach, F. H. 1982. Five HLA-D clusters associated with HLA-DR4. *Hum. Immunol.*, *4*: 249.
15. Nepom, G. T., Seyfried, C. E., Holbeck, S. L., Wilske, K. R., and Nepom, B. S. 1986. Identification of HLA-Dw14 genes in DR4+ rheumatoid arthritis. *Lancet*, *2*(8514): 1002.
16. Zoschke, D., and Segall, M. 1986. Dw subtypes of DR4 in rheumatoid arthritis: Evidence for a preferential association with Dw4. *Hum. Immunol.*, *15*: 118–124.
17. Nepom, G. T., Byers, P., Seyfried, C., et al. 1989. HLA genes associated with rheumatoid arthritis. *Arthritis Rheum.*, *32*(1): 15–21.
18. Ollier, W., Carthy, D., Cutbush, S., et al. 1988. HLA-DR4 associated Dw types in rheumatoid arthritis. *Tissue Antigens*, *33*: 30–37.
19. Bjorkman, P. J., Saper, M. A., Samraoui, B., Bennett, W. S., Strominger, J. L., and Wiley, D. C. 1987. Structure of the human class I histocompatibility antigen, HLA-A2. *Nature*, *329*(8 Oct): 506–512.

20. Brown, J. H., Jardetzky, T., Saper, M. A., Samroui, B., Bjorkman, P. J., and Wiley, D. C. 1988. A hypothetical model of the foreign antigen binding site of class II histocompatibility molecules. *Nature, 332*: 845–850.
21. Winchester, R. J. 1989. The major histocompatibility complex. In *Textbook of Rheumatology* (W. N. Kelley, E. D. Harris, S. Ruddy, and C. B. Sledge, eds.). W. B. Saunders Co., Philadelphia, pp. 101–137.
22. Waters, F. J., Winchester, R. J., Nagase, F., Thorbecke, C. J., and Bona, C. A. 1984. Antigen presentation by murine and human cells to a murine T cell hybridoma: Demonstration of a restriction element associated with an MHC class II determinant(s) shared by both species. *Proc. Natl. Acad. Sci. USA, 81*: 7559–7563.
23. Toguchi, T., Burmester, G. R., Nunez-Roldan, A., et al. 1984. Evidence for the separate molecular expression of four distinct polymeric Ia epitopes on cells of DR4 homozygous individuals. *Hum. Immunol., 10*: 69–81.
24. Lee, S. H., Gregersen, P. K., Shen, H. H., Nunez-Roldan, A., Silver, J., and Winchester, R. J. 1984. Strong association of rheumatoid arthritis with the presence of a polymorphic Ia epitope defined by a monoclonal antibody: Comparison with the allodeterminant DR4. *Rheum. Int., 4*(Suppl): 17–23.
25. Matsuyama, T., Winchester, R., Lee, S., Shookster, L., and Nunez-Roldan, A. 1988. Identification of the DRw10 DRβ_1 chain allele as encoding a polymorphic class II MHC epitope otherwise restricted to DRβ_2 molecules of the DRw53 type. *J. Immunol., 140*: 537–543.
26. Gregersen, P. K., Shen, M., Song, Q. L., et al. 1986. Molecular diversity of HLA-DR4 haplotypes. *Proc. Natl. Acad. Sci. USA, 83*: 2642–2646.
27. Merryman, P. F., Crapper, R. M., Lee, S., Gregersen, P. K., Winchester, R. J. 1989. Class II major histocompatibility complex gene sequences in rheumatoid arthritis: The third diversity regions of both DR β1 genes in two DR1, DRw10-positive individuals specify the same inferred amino acid sequence as the DRβ1 and DRβ2 genes of a DR4 (Dw14) haplotype. *Arthritis Rheum., 32*(3): 251–258.
28. Merryman, P., Gregersen, P. K., Lee, S., et al. 1088. Nucleotide sequence of a DRw10 β chain cDNA clone; identity of the third D region with that of the DRw53 allele of the β_2 locus and as the probable site encoding a polymorphic MHC class II epitope. *J. Immunol., 140*: 2447–2452.
29. Merryman, P., Gregersen, P., Matsuyama, T., et al. 1987. Nucleotide sequence of MHC class II region genes in a patient with DR4 negative rheumatoid arthritis (RA) from a multiplex family; simulation of a DR4 haplotype by trans complementation of the HV III regions. *Arthritis Rheum., 30*(4)(supplement): S31 (Abs).
30. Winchester, R. J., and Gregersen, P. K. 1988. The molecular basis of susceptibility to rheumatoid arthritis: the conformational equivalence hypothesis. *Springer Semin. Immunopathol., 10*: 119–139.
31. Gregersen, P. K., Silver, J., and Winchester, R. J. 1987. The shared epitope hypothesis—an approach to understanding the molecular genetics of rheumatoid arthritis susceptibility. *Arthritis Rheum., 30*: 1205–1213.
32. Spies, T., Sorrentino, R., Boss, J. M., Okada, K., and Strominger, J. L. 1985. Structural organization of the DR subregion of the human major histocompatibility complex. *Proc. Natl. Acad. Sci. USA, 82*: 5165–5169.

33. Bignon, J. D., Semana, G., Tiercy, J. M., Simons, M, Lalouel, J. M., and Cohen, D. 1989. DNA-RFLP analysis: HLA-DR beta workshop report. In *Immunobiology of HLA*. Volume I: *Histocompatibility Testing 1987* (B. Dupont, ed.). Springer-Verlag, New York, pp. 851–860.
34. Gorski, J., and Mach, B. 1986. Polymorphism of human Ia antigens: Gene conversion between two DR B loci results in a new HLA-D/DR specificity. *Nature, 322*: 67–70.
35. Davis, M. M., and Bjorkman, P. J. 1988. T-cell antigen receptor genes and T-cell recognition. *Nature* [NSC], *334*: 395–402.
36. Bevan, M. J. 1977. In a radiation chimera, host H-2 antigens determine immune responsiveness of donor cytotoxic cells. *Nature, 269*: 417–418.
37. Kappler, J. W., Roehm, N., and Marrack, P. 1987. T cell tolerance by clonal elimination in the thymus. *Cell, 49*: 273–280.
38. Fassbender, H. G., and Simmling-Annefeld, M. 1983. The potential aggressiveness of synovial tissue in rheumatoid arthritis. *J. Pathol., 139*: 399–406.
39. DeLisi, C., and Berzofsky, J. A. 1985. T-cell antigenic sites tend to be amphipathic structures. *Proc. Natl. Acad. Sci. USA, 82*: 7048–7052.
40. Stille, C. J., Thomas, L. J., Reyes, V. E., and Humphreys, R. E. 1987. Hydrophobic strip-of-helix algorithm for selection of T cell-presented peptides. *Molec. Immunol., 24*: 1021–1027.
41. Kourilsky, P., and Claverie, J.-M. 1986. The peptidic self model: a hypothesis on the molecular nature of the immunological self. *Ann. Inst. Pasteur, 137D*: 3–21.

12

Functions and Structures in a Regulatory Network for Self-Reactivity

Maurizio Zanetti, Maurizio Sollazzo, and Rosario Billetta
University of California at San Diego, San Diego, California

I. INTRODUCTION

The relationship between the external world, the environment, and the organism is a complex phenomenon mediated by many different types of receptors converging into main regulatory systems, e.g., the nervous, the immune, and the endocrine systems, to name a few. Fluctuations within the normal regulatory activity of one system are part of the homeostatic balance. Deviation from homeostasis yields dysregulation often associated with pathology. The organism and the species have learned, and continue to learn, how to adapt to external forces on the basis of autonomous internally regulated mechanisms. The sum of these two orders of interactive forces, internal and external, are reflected in ontogeny and phylogeny.

Nature as a whole and organisms as individuals do not produce innovation from scratch, rather they may be seen as part of an evolving process that acquire new functions by combining multiple systems to produce more complex ones, a process that may well be called integration. The immune system is subject to the same set of general rules. We can only speculate how simple the immune system could have been at the beginning of phylogeny. The scientific method allows us to make predictions about known functions of a given regulatory system and guesses on the evolution of the same functions. Both are by necessity limited to the method of analysis on the one hand and the ability to overcome our ignorance of their understanding on the other.

The idea that the immune system is regulated through the dynamic interaction between discrete structural sites of the immunoglobulin (Ig) fold of antibody variable (V) regions and B- and T-cell receptors (1) has been proven experimentally and is now a widely accepted concept in immunology. An aspect yet to be fully demonstrated is how the system of binary interactions predicted by the network theory can account for the response to self antigens and regulation thereof. We have dealt with this issue on several occasions in the past (2–4) and will not discuss in detail the same points in this chapter. Rather, we will focus briefly on the existing evidence that the immune system has evolved to encompass a set of regulatory mechanisms based on self recognition (the autoimmune network) (5) and on the relationship between the function of the latter and the structures that might be implicated.

II. AUTOIMMUNE NETWORK: A SELF-REFERENTIAL MODUS OPERANDI WITH RELEVANCE TO REGULATION AND PATHOLOGY

The latent state of activation of the immune system as well as the maintenance of tolerance to self components are likely to depend upon a delicate equilibrium among various elements of the internal environment, namely autoantigens, idiotypes, and anti-idiotypes. This finely tuned homeostatic mechanism can be perturbed by (1) changes in the relative concentration of any of these three elements, and (2) the interaction between antibodies and receptors on cells of either the immune system or other systems in the organism. Balance within such a self-centered immune system is, therefore, a highly complex phenomenon, and self-reactivity as an autonomous *modus operandi* is directly implicated in the physiology and pathology of the immune system. At one end there are aspects of a merely regulatory nature, at the other conditions that more directly pertain to pathology. These are summarized in Figure 1.

It is necessary to realize that a distinction between the two poles may at times be difficult to make. Moreover, it is still not clear how this may be realized effectively and what the structures ensuring this distinction at the functional level might be. The distinction implied in Figure 1 may be highly speculative, and only the identification of structures and pathways, and their functional analysis in experimental systems, will provide a firmer viewpoint.

Let us review some experimental facts that have emerged during the past decade that support the idea that the relationship between immunity and self antigens is internally connected and regulated. These are as follows:

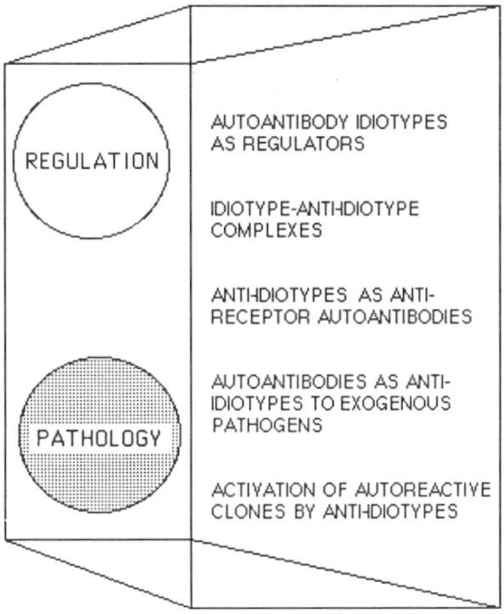

FIGURE 1 A schematic view of the relationship between a regulatory network and pathology based on idiotypic complementarity interactions. The functional events listed have been experimentally demonstrated to be associated with either regulation or pathology. (For details, see Ref. 3.)

1. The immune response to self antigens in vivo can be suppressed by anti-idiotypic antibodies administered before immunization with self antigen (reviewed in Ref. 3).
2. The humoral and cellular responses to self can be suppressed in vivo by active immunization with the idiotype on autoantibodies to the same self antigen (3,6).
3. Humoral and cellular responses to self can be suppressed in vivo by active immunization with antigen-reactive (and idiotype-positive) T cells (7,8).
4. The humoral response to self can be suppressed in vivo by passive transfer of idiotype-primed T cells (9,10).
5. Self-reactive antibodies can be induced in naive animals by active immunization with anti-idiotypic antibodies (1,12).
6. Immunization with a self antigen may induce antireceptor autoantibodies via an idiotypic mechanism (13,14).
7. The T-cell receptor (TcR) repertoire of antiself responses is, at least in some instances, characterized by a single idiotype encoded by a particular combination of V genes (15).
8. Active immunization with a synthetic peptide of the TcR common idiotype leads to prevention of T-cell–mediated autoimmune disease (16,17).

The arguments listed above are summarized in the schema shown in Figure 2. Thus, interactions based on molecular complementarity having direct functional impact can be divided into two groups, one pertaining to B and the other to T lymphocytes. Although the two groups are separate, and may in fact develop

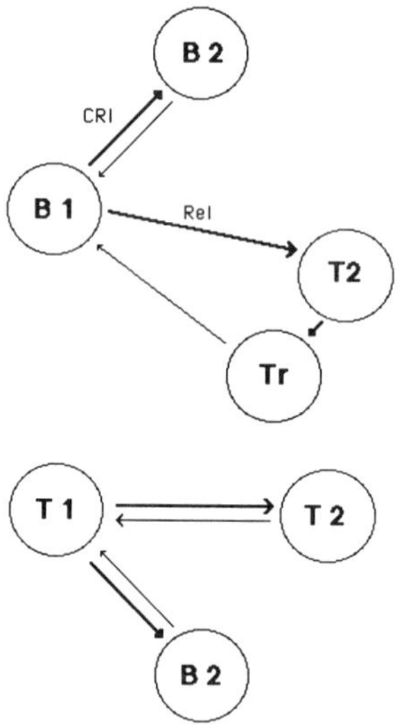

FIGURE 2 A schema of the hypothetical pathways for the regulation of the autoimmune network is shown. B1 and T1 represent the first set of B and T lymphocytes activated by antigen or antigen plus MHC, respectively. Two mutally nonexclusive pathways are then activated. Complementary anti-idiotypic B lymphocytes (B2) could be responsible for antibody-mediated downregulation of the B1 and T1 sets, respectively. Although it is possible that the anti-idiotypic response is directed against many idiotypic determinants on either antibody or TcR, it is likely that cross-reactive idiotypes (CRI) are primarily involved in this event. Anti-CRI antibodies may inactivate the respective clonotype by either modulation of the surface Ig, complement-mediated lysis, or antibody-dependent cytotoxicity. A second regulatory pathway involves complementary T cells. In the upper part of the schema it is indicated that their activation is promoted by regulatory idiotype (ReI) as those structurally conserved elements that exert their function by recruiting T cells. It is unclear whether the overall effect solely depends upon the interaction between T2 and B1 cells or rather requires the additional activation of regulatory T cells (Tr), which then produce feedback on the B1 clonotype. (For details see Refs 4 and 5.) In the lower part of the schema the downregulation of the T1 set of self-reactive cells is realized primarily through the direct effect of anti-idiotypic T cells via a receptor–antireceptor interaction based on structural complementarity. The TcR idiotope that activates this regulatory T-T pathway can be compared to ReI, i.e., a highly conserved germline-encoded element. (▬▬) activation; (——) suppression.

independently, interdigitations are possible, e.g., T-cell regulation of B-cell responses and vice versa and antibody modulation of T-cell responses.

A functional autoimmune network at the level of antibodies and B cells relies on the fact that autoantibodies to the same self antigen possess cross-reacting idiotypes (CRI) and regulatory idiotype (ReI) (5,18). The first are in principle subject to regulation by sets of homologous anti-idiotypic antibodies. How efficient this mode of regulation may be is not entirely known. On an a priori ground one could argue that the immune system cannot engage in the regulation of all possible idiotypes that are generated. Preferably, among those amenable to a feedback regulation by complementary anti-idiotype would be antibodies "connected" within the immune system under physiological conditions (18). On the other hand, ReI ensure their regulatory function on their ability to recruit complementary T cells (10).

Over the past decade several reports have also appeared to indicate the occurrence of naturally occurring auto-anti-idiotype antibodies specific for autoantibodies (Table 1). The first demonstration was the presence of antibodies which would specifically block the binding of DNA-autoantibodies to DNA in the serum of lupus patients taken during an inactive phase (19). The activity was best evidenced when the serum was first depleted of anti-DNA antibodies as well as DNA. In NZB mice with lupus-like syndrome, it was shown that F_1 hybrids of the NZB strain and several normal strains which produce low quantities of antierythrocyte (Coombs) autoantibodies spontaneously develop auto-anti-idiotypes which agglutinate erythrocytes from Coombs-positive NZB mice (20). The occurrence of auto-anti-idiotype antibodies has also been documented in patients with myasthenia gravis (21,22) and in a single patient after a pneumococcal bacteremia with specificity for a rheumatoid factor monoclonal IgM gammopathy (23). Of a similar nature is the report of circulating auto-anti-idiotypic in patients with acquired C1-inhibitor deficiency associated with B-cell lymphoma and angioedema (24,25), and in a patient with antihemophilic factor (Factor VII) autoantibodies (26). Naturally occurring anti-idiotypes have also been found among human myeloma proteins reacting with human autoantibodies to thyroglobulin (26).

A role for network interactions in the physiological regulation of the immune system is supported by the following observations. It was shown long ago that loss of immune competence with age could be due to increase control of the B-cell repertoire by anti-idiotype antibodies (27). More recently, the existence in vivo of a functional idiotypic network among natural, "connected" antibodies was demonstrated in adult animals (18). Experiments from this laboratory demonstrate that ReI are present within the natural repertoire at the beginning of ontogeny, i.e., at the time when regulatory pathways in the developing immune system are set in place, and may be germline encoded (28).

Evidence for the B-cell repertoire propensity to form both idiotypic and anti-idiotypic antibodies, i.e., the immune system is formed of sets of complementary

TABLE 1 Evidence for Naturally Occurring Anti-idiotypes to Autoantibodies

Anti-idiotype specificity	Clinical association	Species	Ref.
Autoantibodies to DNA	SLE	Human	19
Anti-erythrocyte antibodies	SLE	Mouse	20
Autoantibodies to ACh receptor	Myasthenia gravis	Human	21,22
Rheumatoid factor	Pneumococcal bacteremia	Human	23
Autoantibodies to monoclonal gammopathy	Acquired angioedema	Human	24
Autoantibodies to factor VIII	Acquired hemophilia	Human	25
Autoantibodies to thyroglobulin	Myeloma	Human	26

antibodies, comes from the demonstration that therapeutic (commercial) pools of immunoglobulin contain anti-idiotypic antibodies to human autoantibodies. For instance, anti-idiotypes have been documented for autoantibodies to factor VIII, anti-DNA, and anti-thyroglobulin antibodies (29). Although the exact significance of this finding remains to be firmly established, this observation corroborates the notion that the immune system is not only programmed but also de facto providing anti-idiotype antibodies to self-reactive antibodies. All this complies with the notion of autoimmune network.

III. PRINCIPLES OF IDIOTYPY

The Fab fragment of immunoglobulin is responsible for antigen binding and idiotype expression. The Fc fragment determines the isotype and several effector functions, e.g., complement fixation, binding to Fc receptors, etc. Most idiotypes mapped to date are localized in discrete areas of variability within antibody V regions, hypervariable (HV), or complementarity determining regions (CDR). The three-dimensional structure of antibody and the topology of sequence conservation have indicated that HV loops are regularly interspersed between framework regions (FR). Within this overall organization HV loops can drift in sequence and conformation with little effect on the structure of FR. These are arranged in β-pleated sheets filled with hydrophobic side chains and an invariant disulfide bond linking two β sheets together (the "Ig fold"). The constraints on the side chains necessary to preserve the Ig fold are sufficiently stringent to explain the sequence conservation of FR (30).

Residues from the six CDR of both heavy (H)- and light (L)-chain V domains cluster at the surface of the molecule to form a large contact area including the binding site. Of this an area of about 1800 Å^2 is buried between the two V domains. Approximately three quarters of this interface is formed by the packing of V_L and V_H β sheets in the conserved frameworks and one quarter from contacts between CDR (31,32). Although these contacts are considered to be important for the assembly and interactions of V_H and V_L domains, nonconservative mutations in the D region of the V_H domain do not affect assembly (41). Because somatic recombination mechanisms (33) produce larger sequence variations in the H chain than in the L chain (particularly the D region), the H chain offers a greater contact area than the L chain in and around the central region of the CDR cluster.

In protein–protein interactions, contact residues play a critical role in the formation of a stable complex. In the Ig V region, epitopes may involve both CDR and FR residues, and only about 25% of the CDR residues are strongly antigenic. The antigenically active loops of the V domain form large, almost contiguous areas on the surface of the domain (34). Whereas the binding site recognizes a surface of approximately 700 Å^2, some of the experimentally defined idiotype may overlap sites from both the L and H chains (35) or the V and C domains.

The characterization of idiotypes has proven difficult in most systems, and with rare exceptions the structure/function correlate of idiotype remains poorly understood. In part the problem is due to the fact that idiotypes are antigenic determinants defined by other antibodies (anti-idiotypes), i.e., the power of resolution is the one allowed by the binding site of an antibody molecule. As for other protein antigens, idiotypes can be divided into two categories, continuous and discontinuous. The former are composed of amino acid residues contiguous in the primary structure. The latter originate from amino acid residues contributed by different regions of the molecule that come together during the folding of native polypeptide. Idiotypes have been localized on the H and the L chain as well as on both chains (reviewed in Refs. 36 and 37). Within these categories, examples have been described where idiotypy is contributed predominantly by one chain with an additive effect by the other chain.

As mentioned above, the instances in which idiotypy in one chain has been mapped to a precise region are limited. Although the cumulative data are as yet scarce, it appears that residues in the CDR3 of the H chain contribute most often to idiotype expression, albeit the CDR2 of both the H and L chains have also been implicated (36,37). From crystallographic studies it appears that the CDR3 loop protrudes from the supporting FR sheet and is both accessible to solvent, i.e., hydrophilic, and mobile (38).

Several factors may influence idiotype expression. Among these are the size, the shape, the presence of contact residues, the flexibility of the polypeptide chain, and the relative mobility of one polypeptide chain with respect to the other. In general, idiotypes may be seen as convex sites with large polar side chains hallmarked by the ability to provide contact bonds for receptors, ligands, and anti-idiotypic antibodies. It cannot be excluded that concave idiotypes may also exist, although it is difficult to envision their interaction with the surrounding molecular environment. All these factors, alone or in combination, determine the extent to which idiotypes as protein surface determinants are subjet to molecular recognition and determine the immune function.

IV. STRUCTURAL DEFINITION OF REGULATORY STRUCTURES OF THE AUTOIMMUNE NETWORK

In this section we will review a molecular characterization of the autoimmune network and its regulatory structure, i.e., idiotypy of autoantibodies and TcR, respectively. First we will discuss a prototypic ReI studied in this laboratory for the past decade focusing on new insights concerning its molecular structure. Then we will comment on recent reports addressing TcR idiotypy and the use of synthetic TcR idiotopes to modulate autoimmunity.

A. ReI Function and Structure

As a model system to explore ReI function, we used the idiotype borne on murine autoantibodies to thyroglobulin termed Id62 (39). This is a recurrent, nondominant component (<2%) of the autoantibody response to thyroglobulin in BALB/c mice and is autoimmunogenic for B and T cells (see below). Both Id62$^+$/antigen-binding and Id62$^+$ antibodies can be found in the spleen cells of adult immunized mice as well as unmanipulated neonatal BALB/c mice (28). In a series of in vivo studies we assessed the relative importance of cellular vs. humoral events in the suppression of autoreactivity (10). We found that (1) autologous idiotype activates both the B- and T-cell compartments, and (2) specific suppression by idiotype immunization best correlates with the activation of idiotype-recognizing T cells. For instance, a challenge with a low dose of self antigen in adjuvant subsequent to elicitation of high titer circulating anti-idiotype antibodies was followed by a marked suppression of autoantibody production. By adoptively transferring separate T- and B-cell populations, we found that idiotype-primed B lymphocytes could transfer the ability of making auto-anti-idiotype but not suppression of autoreactivity. In contrast, idiotype-primed T lymphocytes could transfer suppression of autoantibody production.

1. *Idiotype Expression of Isolated H-Chain: Analysis with Recombinant Molecules*

The V_H62 rearrangement was cloned from a library constructed from 2–2.5 kb size-selected fragments generated by EcoRI digestion of parental hybridoma 62

DNA (40). The genomic DNA rearrangement encoding the L-chain variable (V) region was also cloned from the unrelated MOPC21 myeloma cell. Expression vectors coding for H- and L-chain were constructed and used in transfection experiments to yield Igs with different L-chain combinations. The H-chain plasmid vector (pN$\gamma_1$62), which encodes for V_H62 and the human γ_1 constant (C) region, was electroporated in one instance into J558L myeloma cells, which express a γ1 L chain, and in the other into P3X3 Ag8 cells together with the MOPC 21 L-chain vector (pSVCkVkM21). The expressed recombinant Igs were tested for Id62 expression and antigen binding. The results summarized in Table 2 indicate that Id62 is expressed on V_H62 independently from the associated L chain. On the other hand, antigen-binding specificity could not be recreated by these chain-recombination experiments and appears, therefore, to require the association of V_H62 with the parental V_K62 polypeptide chain.

2. *Primary Sequence Analysis*

The complete nucleotide sequence of V_H62 was determined by subcloning into the M13 vector. We found that this V region belongs to the most J-proximal V_H7183 gene family in the murine V_H gene locus (40). The D segment is only 50% homologous to published murine D segments. The J segment utilized is JH4 in its germline configuration. Figure 3 shows the primary structure of V_H62 in comparison to that of other closely related antibodies whose V_H are also encoded by genes of the murine V_H7183 family. Excluding differences in the D region, V_HB13, A26, and 62 differ by only one amino acid residue at position 31. Because neither MAbB13 nor A26 express Id62, we excluded a direct involvement of FR residues in Id62 specificity, hence indicating that the latter must be due to residues located in the CDR. This prompted the study of idiotype mapping described below.

3. *Idiotype Analysis by Constructing Id62 Mutants*

Mutants of the V_H62 domain were constructed by oligonucleotide site-directed mutagenesis (41). The mutated domains were joined, at the gene level, to the human γ_1 H-chain C region. Nonconservative mutants of solvent-exposed residues of the V_H domain were designed, and vectors for expression in myeloma cells constructed using the plasmid pNγ_1 coding for a human γ_1 C-region gene. H-chain mutant DNA constructs were introduced by electroporation into the murine myeloma cell line J558L. Purified engineered antibodies were analyzed for idiotype expression.

We first shortened the CDR1 loop by engineering Δ33/34YM in which CDR1 amino acid residues Tyr33 and Met34 were deleted. Because of this deletion the molecule lost Id62 expression. The amino acid substitution of the solvent-exposed Tyr33→Sr (Y33S) did not affect Id62 specificity. We then engineered the mutation M34K where the highly conserved hydrophobic amino acidiotype Met34

TABLE 2 Idiotype and Antigen Specificity of Recombinant Antibodies

Antibody	Heavy chain	Light chain	Id62 expression	Antigen binding
WT	V_H62	$V\lambda_1$	+	–
$\gamma_1 V_k M$	V_H62	V_kMOPC21	+	–
MAb62	V_H62	V_k62	+	+

was replaced with a positively charged Lys residue. This resulted in loss of Id62 expression. Although this could argue that CDR1 is critical for idiotype expression, an atomic model of the V_H62 domain predicted on the basis of its primary structure suggests that Met34 is essential for the maintenance of the V_H fold (Fig. 4). Therefore, by substituting Met34 with a positively charged amino acid, we likely perturbed the domain's fold and consequently the reactivity with the anti-idiotype antibodies.

```
                                        CDR1
                                         30
62       DVKLVESGGGLVKLGGSLKLSCAASGFTFSRYYMSWVRQTPEKRLELVA
A26      ------------------------------S------------------
B13      ------------------------------S------------------
MOPC21   --Q---------QPRE--------------SFG-H----A---G---W-
66E-3    E-M------V-MEP------------------A--------------W-

             CDR2
                  60                            90
62       AINSNGGSTYYPDTVKGRFTISRDNAKNTLYLQMSSLKSEDTALYYCAR
A26      -------------------------------------------------
B13      -------------------------------------------------
MOPC21   Y-S-GSSTLH-A-------------P----F---T--R-----M-----
66E-3    T-S-G-S-HLPSRQCE---------------------R-----M-----

             CDR3                                     Id

62       KAYSHG    MDYWGQGTS                          +
A26      HELTGTALFA---------LV                        -
B13      QALLSIHYFA---------TL                        -
MOPC21   WGNPYYA   ---------                          -
66E-3    PPLSLLDAYA---------                          -
```

FIGURE 3 The amino acid sequence of V_H62 and, by comparison, of three hybridoma antibodies (mAB A26, B13, and 66E-3) and a myeloma MOPC21 that share >80% identity with the V_H62 sequence. None of these $\gamma1$ proteins share the same antigen binding or expresses Id62. (For details see Ref. 40.)

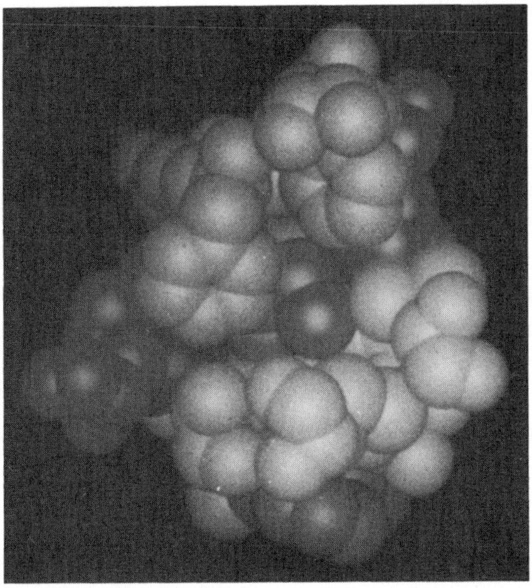

FIGURE 4 Space-filling model of the residues surrounding Met34.

To investigate the role played by CDR2 residues, we constructed two nonconservative mutants in this region, mutant N53I, in which the solvent exposed Asn53 residue was substituted with the hydrophobic amino acid Ile, and mutant Y58D, in which the surface residue Tyr58 was replaced with a negatively charged Asp residue. Both CDR2 mutants maintained Id62 expression. Thus, based on mutant analysis of the first and second CDR, we could rule out the contribution of these regions in determining Id62 specificity.

The role of the CDR3 (D region) was investigated next. The first mutant A96V/P carries an amino acid substitution (Ala96 → Val) plus the insertion of a Pro residue between Val96 and Tyr97. This mutation, by altering the conformation of the loop, severely affected idiotype expression. To confirm this result we designed another mutant Y97N where the exposed amino acid residue Tyr97 was replaced with Asn. Such a substitution was sufficient to dramatically alter Id62 specificity. Altogether, these results indicate that the D region of V_H62 domain is the structural correlate of Id62 and suggest that Tyr97 plays a key role in stabilizing the conformation of the loop where Id62 is expressed. This conclusion is also consistent with the atomic model of the V_H62 domain that suggest that the D region is protruding from the surface of the molecule, hence accessible to interact with anti-idiotype. Mutants bearing large insertions (3–15 amino acids) in the D region also caused loss of idiotype expression and confirmed that the structural correlate of this murine ReI is the D region. Table 3 summarizes the nature of the mutations and the way they affected idiotype specificity.

B. TcR Idiotope Structure and Function

Recent data indicate that the encephalitogenic T cells from mice and rats share germline TcR genes despite differences in peptide specificity. As mentioned above, vaccination with autoantigen-reactive T cells provided indirect evidence that an autoimmune recognition of TcR epitopes could protect against the induction of autoimmune disease (7,8). More recently the TcR structures involved in this regulatory process have been not only identified but also used to prove that they can effectively perturb the autoimmune network and prevent a defined disease process (16,17).

In the experimental allergic encephalomyelitis (EAE) model, two groups demonstrated that active immunization with synthetic peptides of TcR primary structures considered disease- and antigen-associated could protect from the subsequent induction of disease (16,17). It is interesting to note that at least in one report the sequence used corresponded to the VDJ junction (17). Suppression of disease induction could also be passively transferred by T cells propagated in vitro by stimulation with TcR peptides (16), further strengthening the regulatory role of idiotype–anti-idiotype interactions among T cells. It is interesting to note that regulation by anti-idiotype T cells had been proposed in the past relative to suppression of the graft-versus-host reaction in the rat (43). Interestingly, natural "regulatory" T cells were functionally identified as exerting their suppressive action on T cells sharing identical allospecificity and cross-reactive idiotypy in spite of the different MHC haplotype (44).

TABLE 3 Mutations in CDR of Heavy Chain and Idiotype Expression

Antibody	Site mutation	Type mutation	aa Change	Position	Id specificity[a]
wt	none	none	none	none	+
YMΔ33/34	CDR1	deletion	two aa	33–34	–
Y33S	CDR1	substitution	Y → S	33	+
M34K	CDR1	substitution	M → K	34	–
N53I	CDR2	substitution	N → I	53	+
Y58D	CDR2	substitution	Y → D	58	+
A96V/P	CDR3	subst/insert	A → V/+P	96	–
Y97N	CDR3	substitution	Y → N	97	–

[a]Id62 expression was assessed by completion of the ELISA binding of Id62 (monoclonal antibody 62) and WT to anti-Id62.

V. CONCLUSIONS

In this article we reviewed some concepts and experimental work from several laboratories, including our own, in support of the idea proposed some time ago (5) that immunity to antigens of the internal environment is part of a network dynamics referred to as the autoimmune network. The evidence provided herein, albeit limited, is consistent with the idea that network dynamics is dependent upon antibody or TcR V-region structures that appear to have the following two characteristics: they are borne on single polypeptide chains and are likely to be germline encoded.

The implications of these assumptions are best understood in the context of a necessary integrated view of the immune function encompassing soluble antibodies and B- and T-cell receptors. Although many different facets of immune function could be discussed, we will focus on one rather seminal concerning T-cell recognition of V regions of antibodies or T-cell receptors.

Several lines of evidence indicate that Ig V_H-linked genes influence the development of helper, cytotoxic, and suppressor T cells (45–47). Because idiotype sharing between T and B lymphocytes is a remote eventuality and it is well accepted that T cells do not rearrange functional Ig V genes, an innate characteristic of the immune system is the parallel development of idiotypic polymorphism in the B- and T-cell compartments. This implies that the T-cell repertoire is selected on the basis of its ability to interact with both MHC and endogenous Ig V regions. For instance, treatment early in life with anti-μ antibodies abrogates genetically restricted and Ig V_H-linked interactions, while leaving unaffected other T-cell functions (reviewed in Ref. 47). This validates the notion that the B-cell compartment influences the development of T cells and the selection of the T-cell repertoire from the early phases of ontogeny (48).

T lymphocytes predominantly recognize soluble foreign proteins associated with membrane-bound MHC products (49) that would have the role of holding processed peptides in a favorable conformation for recognition. Do the same rules apply to V-region idiotypes? The ideas in this regard are quite divided (reviewed in Ref. 45). Because T cells are required for anti-idiotype antibody response and other regulatory functions within the immune network, an integrated understanding of how molecular recognition influences immune function is necessary.

Accessibility computations have indicated the existence of about 40 distinct determinants on the V regions of a single Ia molecule (50). It is highly unlikely that every idiotype is target of regulation via network interactions. How is, therefore, regulation actualized without generation of chaos? Is there a common trend to it that enables functions to occur in keeping with specificity? Using our model of ReI, a modulator of a bona fide antiself response, we found that its regulatory structural element is localized on a germline V_H domain expressed independently from the association with the L chain. (The term domain refers to a portion of the tertiary structure of a polypeptide chain that forms a spatially distinct folding.) Similarly, the TcR sequence able to modulate EAE is germline encoded.

These considerations are important in light of the current paradigm on antigen processing and presentation. In fact, if both events were necessary for idiotype recognition by T cells, how could this phenomenon be possible for conformational idiotypic determinants contributed by the interaction between H and L chains? How could they survive the action of intracellular proteolytic enzymes? The only obvious solution is that regulatory structures are expressed on single polypeptide chains. As previously indicated the development of network dynamics during the early ontogeny is likely to be based on such a principle (4,51).

The molecular aspects of the phenomenon involving presentation of idiotypes to T cells can be discussed further. A series of elegant experiments (52,53) and the recently proposed *peptidic self* model (54) argue that antibody, and possibly TcR V regions, are handled, i.e., processed and presented in the context of MHC molecules, as the nonself antigen counterpart. This implies that regulatory structures are in fact borne on single polypeptide chains and possess sufficient affinity for MHC molecules. This, however, does not seem to explain (1) a non–MHC-restricted anti-idiotype responses (reviewed in Refs. 55,56), (2) non–MHC-restricted cellular responses to a variety of classical autoantigens in humans (reviewed in Ref. 57), and (3) the ability of certain synthetic peptides to elicit a T-cell response in various MHC haplotypes (58,59). More importantly, it requires that various types of antigen-presenting cells (macrophages, dendritic cells, and B cells) from different individuals are endowed with identical sets of proteolytic enzymes, an unlikely eventuality.

An alternative possibility is that solvent-accessible idiotypic determinants can instruct T cells directly, without being processed. This view may require a deeper understanding of the basis of physical chemical rules for complementarity between protein surfaces both at the structural and functional levels, and a better knowledge of the possible role of accessory molecules on T-cell function. For instance, along this line we recently identified an interaction between Ig and CD4 (60). Future studies in these directions may elucidate this aspect of the immune system.

ACKNOWLEDGMENTS

This work was supported in part by grants No. 2124 from the Council for Tobacco Research, U.S.A., Inc. and from the National Institutes of Health AI23871. The authors are thankful to Dr. Anna Tramontano for the molecular model V_H62, and Ms. Caroline Lockhart for the help provided in the preparation of the manuscript.

REFERENCES

1. Jerne, N. K. 1974. Towards a network theory of the immune system. *Ann. Immunol. Inst. Pasteur* (Paris), *125*: 373–389.
2. Zanetti, M., and Katz, D. H. 1985. Self recognition, autoimmunity and internal images. In *Current Topics in Microbiology and Immunology*, Volume 119. (H. Koprowski and F. Melchers, eds.). Springer-Verlag, Heidelberg, pp. 112–125.
3. Zanetti, M. 1986. Idiotypic regulation of autoantibody production. *CRC Crit. Rev. Immunol.*, *6*: 151–183.
4. Zanetti, M. 1988. Self immunity and the autoimmune network: A molecular perspective to ontogeny and regulation of the immune system. *Ann. Immunol. Inst. Pasteur* (Paris), *139*: 619–631.
5. Zanetti, M. 1985. The idiotype network in autoimmune processes. *Immunol. Today, 6*: 299–302.
6. Zouali, M., Jolivet, M., LeClerc, C., Ravisse, P., Audibert, F., Eyquem, A., and Chedid, L. 1985. Suppression of murine lupus autoantibodies to DNA by administration of muramyl dipeptide and syngenetic anti-DNA IgG. *J. Immunol.*, *135*: 1091–1096.
7. Neilson, E. G., and Phillips, M. S. 1982. Suppression of interstitital nephritis by auto-anti-idiotypic immunity. *J. Exp. Med.*, *155*: 179–189.
8. Lider, O., Reshef, T., Beraud, E., Ben-Nun, A., and Cohen, I. R. 1988. Anti-idiotypic network induced by T-cell vaccination against experimental autoimmune encphalomyelitis. *Science, 239*: 181–183.
9. Neilson, E. G., McCafferty, E., Phillips, S. M., Clayman, M. D., and Kelly, C. J. 1984. Anti-idiotypic immunity in intersstitial nephritis.—II. Rats developing anti-tubular basement membrane disease fail to make an anti-idiotypic regulatory response: The modulatory role of an RT7.1+, OX8-suppressor T cell mechanism. *J. Exp. Med.*, *159*: 1009–1026.
10. Zanetti, M., Glotz, R., and Rogers, J. 1986. Perturbation of the autoimmune network. II. Immunization with isologous idiotype induces auto-anti-idiotypic antibodies and suppresses the immune response elicited by antigen. *J. Immunol.*, *137*: 3140–3146.
11. Zanetti, M., Rogers, J., and Katz, D. H. 1984. Induction of autoantibodies to thyroglobulin by anti-idiotypic antibodies. *J. Immunol.*, *133*: 240–243.
12. Essani, K., Srinivasappa, J., McClintok, R., Prabhakar, B. S., and Notkins, A. L. 1986. Multi-organ reactive IgG antibody induced by antiidiotypic antibody to a human monoclonal IgM autoantibody. *J. Exp. Med.*, *163*: 1355–1360.
13. Shechter, Y., Maron, R., Elias, D., and Cohen, I. R. 1982. Autoantibodies to insulin receptor spontaneously develop as anti-idiotypes in mice immunized with insulin. *Science, 216*: 542–545.
14. Wasserman, N. H., Penn, A. S., Freimuth, P. I., Treptow, N., Wentzel, S., Cleveland, W. L., and Erlanger, B. F. 1983. Anti-idiotypic route to anti-acetylcholine receptor antibodies and experimental myasthenia gravis. *Proc. Natl. Acad. Sci. USA, 79*: 4810–4814.
15. Owhashi, M., and Heber-Katz, E. 1988. Protection from experimental allergic encephalomyelitis conferred by a monoclonal antibody directed against a shared

idiotype on rat T cell receptors specific for myelin basic protein. *J. Exp. Med., 168*: 2153–2164.
16. Vandenbark, A. A., Hashim, G., and Offner, H. 1989. Immunization with a synthetic T-cell receptor V-region peptide protects against experimental autoimmune encephalomyelitis. *Nature, 341*: 541–544.
17. Howell, M. D., Winters, S. T., Olee, T., Powell, H. C., Carlo, D. J., and Brostoff, S. 1989. Vaccination against experimental allergic ancephalomyelitis with T cell receptor peptides. *Science, 246*: 668–672.
18. Lundkvist, I., Coutinho, A., Varela, F., and Holmberg, D. 1989. Evidence for a functional idiotypic network among natural antibodies in normal mice. *Proc. Natl. Acad. Sci. USA, 86*: 5074–5078.
19. Abdou, N. I., Wall, H., Lindsley, H. B., Halsey, J. F., and Suzuki, T. 1981. Network theory in autoimmunity. In vitro suppression of serum anti-DNA antibody binding to DNA by anti-idiotypic antibody in systemic lupus erythematosus. *J. Clin. Invest., 67*: 1297–1304.
20. Cohen, P. L., and Eisenberg, R. A. 1982. Anti-idiotypic antibodies to the Coombs antibody in NZB F_1 mice. *J. Exp. Med., 156*: 173–180.
21. Dwyer, D. S., Bradley, R. J., Urquhart, C. K., and Kearny, J. F. 1983. Naturally occurring anti-idiotypic antibodies in myasthenia gravis patients. *Nature, 301*: 611–614.
22. Lefvert, A.-K., James, R. W., Alliod, C., and Fulpius, B. W. 1982. A monoclonal anti-idiotypic antibody against anti-receptor antibodies from myasthenic sera. *Eur. J. Immunol., 12*: 790–792.
23. Abe, T., Takeuchi, T., Kiyotaki, M., Koide, J., Hosono, O., Homma, M., Otake, T., and Kano, S. 1984. Anti-idiotypic antibodies in a patient with monoclonal rheumatoid factor after pneumococcal bacteremia. *J. Immunol., 132*: 2381–2385.
24. Geha, R. S., Quinti, I., Austen, K. F., Cicardi, M., Sheffer, A., and Rosen, F. 1985. Acquired C1-inhibitor deficiency associated with autoantiidiotypic antibody to monoclonal immunoglublins. *N. Engl. J. Med., 312*: 534–540.
25. Sultan, Y., Rossi, F., and Kazatchkine, M. D. 1987. Recovery from anti-VIII:C (antihemophilic factor) autoimmune disease is dependent on generation of antiidiotypes against anti-VIII:C autoantibodies. *Proc. Natl. Acad. Sci. USA, 84*: 828–831.
26. Zouali, M., Fine, J-M., and Eyquem, A. 1984. A human monoclonal IgG_1 with anti-idiotypic activity against anti-human thyroglobulin autoantibody. *J. Immunol., 133*: 190–194.
27. Szewczuk, M. R., and Campbell, R. J. 1980. Loss of immune competence with age may be due to auto-anti-idiotypic antibody regulation. *Nature, 286*: 164–166.
28. Glotz, D., and Zanetti, M. 1986. Detection of a regulatory idiotype on a spontaneous neonatal self-reactive hybridoma antibody. *J. Immunol., 137*: 223–227.
29. Rossi, F., Dietrich, G., and Kazatchkine, M. 1989. Anti-idiotypes against autoantibodies in normal immunoglobulins: Evidence for network regulation of human autoimmune responses. *Immunol. Rev., 110*: 135–149.
30. Alzari, P. M., Lascombe, M-B., and Poljak, R. J. 1988. Three-dimensional structure of antibodies. *Ann. Rev. Immunol., 6*: 555–580.
31. Chothia, C., Novotny, J., Bruccoleri, R., and Karplus, M. 1985. Domain association

in immunoglobulin molecules. The packing of variable domains. *J. Mol. Biol.*, *186*: 651-663.

32. Poljak, R. J., Amzel, L. M., Avey, H. P., Chen, B. L., Phizackerly, R. P., and Saul, F. 1973. Three-dimensional structure of the Fab-fragment of a human immunoglobulin at 2.8 A resolution. *Proc. Natl. Acad. Sci. USA*, *70*: 3305-3310.
33. Honjo, T. 1983. Immunoglobulin genes. *Ann. Rev. Immunol.*, *1*: 499-528.
34. Jeske, D., Milner, E. C. B., Leo, O., Moser, M., Marvel, J., Urbain, J., and Capra, J. D. 1986. Molecular mapping of idiotopes of anti-arsonate antibodies. *J. Immunol.*, *136*: 2568-2574.
35. Haba, S., Lascombe, M-B., Poljak, R., and Nisonoff, A. 1989. Structure of idiotopes associated with antiphenylarsonate antibodies expressing an intrastrain crossreactive idiotype. *J. Exp. Med.*, *170*: 1075-1090.
36. Rudikoff, S. 1983. Immunoglobulin structure-function correlates: Antigen binding and idiotypes. *Cont. Top. Mol. Immunol.*, *9*: 169-209.
37. Borden, P., and Kabat, E. A. 1988. The specificities of polyclonal and monoclonal anti-idiotypes to anti-(1-6)dextrans; possible correlations of idiotype with amino acid sequence. *Mol. Immunol.*, *25*: 251-262.
38. Davies, D. R., Sheriff, S., Padlan, E. A., Silverton, E. W., Cohen, G. H., and Smith-Gill, S. J. 1989. Three-dimensional structures of two Fab complexes with lysozyme. In *The Immune Response to Structurally Defined Proteins. The Lysozyme Model* (S. Smith and E. Sercarz, eds.). Academic Press, pp. 125-132.
39. Zanetti, M., DeBaets, M., and Rogers, J. 1983. High degree of idiotypic cross-reactivity among murine monoclonal antibodies to thyroglobulin. *J. Immunol.*, *131*: 2452-2457.
40. Sollazzo, M., Hasemann, C. A., Meek, K. D., Glotz, D., Capra, J. D., and Zanetti, M. 1989. Molecular characterization of the V_H region of murine autoantibodies from neonatal and adult BALB/c mice. *Eur. J. Immunol.*, *19*: 453-457.
41. Sollazzo, M., Castiglia, D., Billetta, R., Tramontano, A., and Zanetti, M. 1990. Structural definition of an idiotypic determinant by antibody engineering. *Prot. Eng.*, *3*: 531-539.
42. Heber-Katz, E., and Acha-Orbea, H. 1989. The V-region disease hypothesis: Evidence from autoimmune encephalomyelitis. *Immunol. Today*, *10*: 164-169.
43. Wilson, D. B. 1984. Idiotypic regulation of self-reactive and alloreactive T cells in autoimmunity and graft-versus-host disease. *Immunol. Today*, *5*: 228-230.
44. Bellgrau, D., and Wilson, D. B. 1979. Immunological studies of T-cell receptors. *J. Exp. Med.*, *149*: 234-243.
45. Janeway, C. A. 1984. The role of idiotype and of immunoglobulin in T-cell differentiation and function. In *The Biology of Idiotypes* (M. I. Greene and A. Nisonoff, eds.). pp. 349-363.
46. Sherman, L. A., and Riblet, R. 1985. Comparison of the H-2K^b-specific cytolytic T lymphocyte receptor repertoire in IgH recombinant strains. *J. Immunol.*, *134*: 3569-3573.
47. Hayglass, K. T., Benacerraf, B., and Sy, M-S. 1986. The influence of B-cell idiotypes on the repertoire of suppressor T cells. *Immunol. Today*, *7*: 179-182.
48. Martinez, A. C., Bernabe, R. R., de la Hera, A., Pereira, P., Cazenave, P. A.,

and Coutinho, A. 1985. Establishment of idiotypic helper T-cell repertoires early in life. *Nature, 317*: 721–723.

49. Berzofsky, J. A. 1988. Structural basis of antigen recognition by T lymphocytes. *J. Clin. Invest., 82*: 1811–1817.
50. Novotny, J., Handschumacher, M., and Bruccoleri, R. 1987. Protein antigenicity: A static surface property. *Immunol. Today, 8*: 26–31.
51. Fougereau, M., and Schiff, C. 1988. Breaking the first circle. *Immunol. Rev., 105*: 69–84.
52. Bogen, B., Malissen, B., and Haas, W. 1986. Idiotype-specific T cell clones that recognize syngeneic immunoglobulin fragments in the context of class II molecules. *Eur. J. Immunol., 16*: 1373–1378.
53. Weiss, S., and Bogen, B. 1989. B-Lymphoma cells process and present their endogenous immunoglobulin to major histocompatibility complex-restricted T cells. *Proc. Natl. Acad. Sci. USA, 86*: 282–286.
54. Kourilsky, P., Chaouat, G., Rabourdin-Combe, C., and Claverie, J-M. 1987. Working principles in the immune system implied by the "peptidic self" model. *Proc. Natl. Acad. Sci. USA, 84*: 3400–3404.
55. Ertl, H. C. J., Homans, E., Tournas, S., and Finberg, R. W. 1984. Sendai virus-specific T cell clones, V. Induction of a virus-specific response by antiidiotypic antibodies directed against a T helper cell clone. *J. Exp. Med., 159*: 1778–1783.
56. Sharpe, A. H., Gaulton, G. N., McDade, K. K., Fields, B. N., and Greene, M. I. 1984. Syngeneic monoclonal antiidiotypic can induce cellular immunity to reovirus. *J. Exp. Med., 160*: 1195–1205.
57. Boitard, C., and Bach, J. F. 1986. Cell-mediated versus humoral immunity in autoimmune diseases and their pharmacologic control with particular reference to type I diabetes mellitus. *Concepts Immunopathol., 3*: 193–224.
58. Sinigaglia, F., Guttinger, M., Kilgus, J., Doran, D. M., Matile, H., Etlinger, H., Trzeciak, A., Gillessen, D., and Pink, J. R. L. 1988. A malaria T-cell epitope recognized in association with most mouse and human MHC class II molecules. *Nature, 336*: 778–780.
59. Panina-Bordignon, P., Tan, A., Termijtelen, A., Demotz, S., Corradin, G., and Lanzavecchia, A. Universally immunogenic T cell epitopes: Promiscuous binding to human MHC class II and promiscuous recognition by T cells. *E. J. Immunol., 19*: 2237–2242.
60. Lenert, P., and Zanetti, M. CD4 has a binding site for immunoglobulin. 1990. *Science, 248*: 1639–1643.

13

Molecular Mimicry of Self-Antigens

Constantin A. Bona
Mount Sinai School of Medicine, New York, New York

I. INTRODUCTION

Molecular mimicry defines similar but not identical molecules, products of dissimilar genes which can interact with other molecules represented by an immunological reagent, a cell receptor, or a biologically active substance.

Mimicking a portion of a macromolecule, which for the sake of simplicity one may call "mimicking epitope," should necessarily involve a surface exposed determinant which could be either a linear or a conformational structure. The phenomenon of molecular mimicry of autoantigens by foreign substances can be particularly important for the pathogenesis of autoimmune diseases, since one may imagine that a genetically programmed silent or tolerized self-reactive clone can be activated by a foreign antigen mimicking a self-antigen. The molecular mimicry concept implies that two dissimilar molecules should share some contacting residues or chemical groups involved in the interaction with a third molecule.

X-ray crystallographic studies of antibody–antigen complexes showed that limited surfaces of 30–50 square Å (1) involving only a few contacting residues borne by variable regions of the antibody interact with functional groups of the antigen (2). The binding of a hapten to an antibody is based on a structural complementarity with minimal structural adaptation because only a few contacting residues of the interacting molecules are involved. Molecular mimicry should be explained at the level of three major receptors of the immune system involved in antigen recognition: MHC gene products expressed on the surface of antigen presenting cells, TCR of T cells, and immunoglobulin receptors of B cells.

Class I antigens are encoded in humans by alleles located in three loci (A,B,C) and class II antigens by alleles located in three other loci (DR, DP, and DQ) indicating that in a heterozygous individual a maximum of six alleles can encode class I or class II antigens. The specificity of interaction of the MHC products with a multitude of foreign peptides (10^8–10^9) should be very low. Therefore, it appears that because of limited polymorphism of MHC gene products and limited structural variability, there are no major constraints in the interaction between MHC antigens and two dissimilar substances which share some identical contacting residues.

TCR recognizes the tertiary complex resulting from the binding of peptides to MHC gene products. TCR is a heterodimer molecule encoded by three gene segments for β chain and two for α chain. The diversity of T-cell receptors results from the recombination of β and α genes and N-diversity generated during rearrangement of germline genes (3).

It is generally accepted that the contacting residues of peptides involved in the binding to MHC are different from those involved in the binding to TCR. This suggests that mimicking epitopes recognized by T cells requires sharing of additional contacting residues involved in the binding of MHC–peptide complexes to TCR.

The recognition of antigens by B cells is more specific because of the exquisite specificity of immunoglobulins derived from their vast diversity. The diversity of Ig receptors results not only from the recombination of V_HD and J_H and V_L and J_L gene segments but also from N-diversity during joining of these segments and somatic mutations (4).

Guide the interaction between antigen and antibody is highly specific and involves a large number of contacting residues (2), the constraints of molecular mimicry at the level of interaction with antibody should be very high.

The interaction between minicking epitopes and antibodies should be distinguished from multispecificity of some antibody molecules. During the last decade it was documented that there are antibodies that can bind to a multitude of dissimilar epitopes (5). This binding is characterized by low affinity interactions. Little is known about the affinity constant that characterize the interaction of mimicking epitopes with MHC antigens, TCR, and immunoglobulin receptors.

II. MOLECULAR MIMICRY OF SELF-ANTIGENS BY BACTERIAL ANTIGENS

One of the first well-documented examples of molecular mimicry originates from a clinical observation made by van de Rijin et al. (6), who showed that heart-reactive antibodies occurring in patients with acute rheumatic fever reacted with streptococcal membrane antigens. Later it was shown that antistreptococcal antibodies could bind not only to heart tissue but also to fibroblasts (7), brain (8), thymus (8), and skeletal muscle (9).

The binding of such antibodies to fibroblasts could be inhibited by streptococcal peptides (10). These observations strongly suggested that streptococcal antigens can mimic antigens borne by mammalian cells. Indeed, the immunization of rabbits with group A streptococci elicited the production of antibodies which bind to heart tissue (11). Since it was known that strains of *Streptococcus pyogenes* are the causative agent of rheumatic heart disease, a series of studies were undertaken to determine which microbial antigens cross-react with human heart tissue. The identification of such antigens has been facilitated by preparation of monoclonal antibodies. For example, Cunningham and Swerlick (12) showed that two MAbs bound to streptococcal M protein and two polypeptides of 62 and 67 kD of *S. pyogenes* membranes as well as to cardiac and skeletal muscle myosin. Monoclonal antibodies produced against *S. pyogenes* M type 5 bound to myosin. These antibodies probably recognize a conformational determinant of dimeric form of a M 5 protein. This molecular mimicking is related to the structural resemblance between type 5 M protein and myosin. Fischetti and Manjula (13) have shown that the structure of M protein, i.e., α helical coiled-coil type with seven amino acid residues periodicity, is similar to that of myosin, tropomyosin, and desmin, or keratin, which explains why antistreptococcal antibodies bind not only to heart or skeletal muscle but also to skin.

Based on this molecular mimicry, it appears that antibodies produced by clones expanded by microbes such as streptococci can become self-reactive and can even be responsible for the pathogenesis of the diseases associated with such infections. Another interesting example is represented by molecular mimicry between the uveitopathogenic site of retinal S-antigen and an *E. coli* protein. An experimental autoimmune uveitis can be induced by injection in various susceptible strains of animals of minute amounts of soluble retinal proteins designated as antigen-S. This experimental disease resembles human uveitis (14). The disease is mediated by T cells responsible for the inflammatory processes that occur in the eye, particularly in the retina and uveal tract (iris, ciliary body, and choroid).

Donoso et al. (15) showed that the most potent peptide corresponding to amino acid residues 521–540 of human interstitial retinoid-binding protein is able to induce autoimmune uveitis in primates and in Lewis rats. Other studies showed that 12 amino acid residues on the amino terminal portion of peptide 7 of

S-antigen is important for pathogenicity. Singh et al. (16) found that E-116 *E. coli* protein shares six identical amino acid residues with M-peptide of S-antigen. Two peptides sharing these six common amino acid residues were able to induce the disease in Lewis rats. These data strongly indicate that mimicking epitopes can activate self-reactive clones.

There are human diseases in which molecular mimicry can play a role. For example, it is well established that there is a high risk association between HLA-B27 antigen and ankylosing spondilitis. Six amino acid residues of the variable region of B27 are identical with a region of the nitrogenase of *Klebsiella pneumoniae* (17).

III. MOLECULAR MIMICRY BETWEEN VIRAL ANTIGENS AND SELF-ANTIGENS

Encephalitis, myelitis, and neuritis are complications of viral diseases which often involve an autoimmune reaction. Such complications occur even after vaccination with attenuated or killed viral vaccines. These clinical observations have stimulated a search for the existence of molecular mimicry between viral and host antigens in order to explain the activation of self-reactive clones.

Indeed, subsequent to the development of hybridoma technology, it was observed that antibodies specific for viral proteins can bind to mammalian cells. Thus, it was shown that MAb specific for coxsackievirus also interacts with heart muscle. Coxsackievirus was associated with mycorditis. Furthermore, a monoclonal antibody specific for neutralizing epitope of Theiler's virus reacted with galactocerebroside, one of the components of the oligodendrocyte surface. Infection with this virus can be associated with demyelination processes, and oligodendrocytes play an important role in myelinogenesis (20). Janke et al. (18) carried out a database search to identify the homology of viral sequences with host protein sequences. A homology was found between measles nucleopeptide and P_2 protein, which can induce neuritis in rabbits. Some homology was also found with some influenza type A viruses, which also can induce neuritis in rabbits. The possible pathogenic role of minicking epitopes of influenza virus is strongly supported by data which showed that the immunization of rabbits with certain neurotropic strains such as NWS/33 resulted in the production of autoantibodies which bind to a brain-specific 37 kD protein (19). This protein is a neuronal antigen.

There are data that show sequence homology between myelin basic protein and viral protein, such as between the encephalitogenic site of rabbit HBP and hepatitis B polymerase (20).

Other homologies were found between autoantigens and retroviral proteins, such as between topoisomerase and p35 gag mammalian retroviruses (21). Antitopoisomerase antibodies are found in patients with scleroderma but not with other autoimmune diseases. The appearance of such autoantibodies is considered as an epiphenomenon, and no pathogenic role for such autoantibodies has been demonstrated. Comparison of the sequence of topoisomerase I with mammalian p30 gag proteins showed that six amino acid residues matched a sequence of feline sarcoma virus. Antitopoisomerase autoantibodies from patients with scleroderma bind to synthetic peptide corresponding to p30 gag protein.

Taken together, these results indicate that mimicking epitopes of viral proteins can activate self-reactive clones and therefore can contribute to the occurrence of both pathogenic or non–organ-specific autoantibodies.

IV. ACTIVATION OF SELF-REACTIVE CLONES BY IDIOTYPES MIMICKING FOREIGN ANTIGENS

Lindemann (22) and Jerne (23), in the early 1970s, developed the concept of internal image of antigens, which suggested that the idiotype of the variable region of lymphocytic receptor, can mimic antigens. Indeed, if we accept that the idiotypes associated with the combining site represent the negative imprint of the antigen, then the idiotpye of anti-idiotype antibody should represent the positive imprint and resemble antigen. Sege and Pete (24) demonstrate the validity of this concept by showing that an anti-Id antibody against antiinsulin antibody mimicked insulin since it was able to bind to insulin receptor.

In subsequent years additional studies have clearly demonstrated that anti-Id antibodies can mimic bacterial, parasite, viral, and tumor antigens, as well as biologically active ligands (25–27). However, there is no information that mimicking epitopes may be resonsible for the activation of self-reactive clones.

A few years ago we showed that some monoclonal antibodies specific for self antigens also reacted with foreign antigens such as bacterial antigens, lysozyme, arsonate hapten, and synthetic peptide polymers (28). In this study, we found that some autoantibodies specific for glutamic acid, alanine, tyrosine (GAT) terpolymer expressed cGAT IdX of anti-GAT antibodies. Based on this observation, we conducted a study to determine whether a monoclonal anti-IdX antibody could stimulate the activation of self-reactive clones. We chose an anti-Id antibody specific for IdX of anti-GAT and GT antibodies since this antibody shares in D segment, a GTT tripeptide, and therefore structurally carried the internal image of the antigen. This MAb is called HP20.

Immunization of 1-month-old MRL/lpr mice, a strain prone to develop a lupus- and arthritis-like syndrome, with monoclonal HP20 induces a significant titer of anti-DNA, Sm, and RF antibodies. These self-reactive antibodies are associated with lupus and rheumatoid arthritis.

Immunization of C_3H/HeJ mice, with HP20 (a normal strain which shares the same V_H haplotype with MRL/lpr) was associated with an increase of only the RF titer (29). These results suggested that an antibody carrying the internal image of a foreign antigen was able to activate clones producing multireactive antibodies specific for foreign and self antigens. In order to strengthen this interpretation, we produced hybridomas from MRL/lpr and C_3H/HeJ mice immunized with HP20 MAb or from BALB/c mice immunized with a synthetic peptide corresponding to the D segment of HP20 antibody.

The immunochemical analysis of these monoclonal antibodies showed that:

1. The frequency of multispecific antibodies which bind to GT homopolymer and to self antigens was higher in MRL/lpr mice immunized with HP20 MAb than in MRL/lpr mice immunized with 63-4, MAb specific for Id of anti-influenza virus antibody or of C_3H/HeJ mice immunized with HP20 MAb.
2. The affinity constant of MAb binding to GT was similar to that of DNA, Sm, or IgG_2, varying between 10^6 and 10^7.
3. An important fraction of these antibodies share the IdX of anti-GT antibodies or anti-DNA, Sm, and RF antibodies (29).

In conclusion, our data demonstrate that B-cell clones producing antibodies able to interact with a similar affinity constant with a foreign and self-antigen may be expanded by the foreign antigen or an anti-Id antibody carrying the internal image of the foreign antigens. It appears, therefore, that autoreactive clones can be activated by foreign antigens or anti-Id antibodies produced in response to immunizations or infections and that such autoantibodies could be involved in the pathogenesis of autoimmune disease.

The observations discussed in this chapter clearly indicate that mimicking epitopes can contribute to the activation of self-reactive clones and thus that molecular mimicry may be an important factor in the pathogenesis of autoimmune diseases.

REFERENCES

1. Huber, R. 1986. Structural basis for antigen-antibody recognition. *Science, 233*: 702–703.
2. Amit, A. G., Mariuzza, R. A., Phillips, S. E. V., and Poljak, R. G. 1986. Three dimensional structure of an antigen-antibody complex at 2.8 Å resolution. *Science, 233*: 747–753.
3. Chien, Y., Gascoigne, N. R. J., Kavaler, J., Lee, N. E., and Davis, M. M. 1984. Somatic recombination in a murine T-cell receptor gene. *Nature, 309*: 322–326.
4. Alt, F. W. 1985. Expression of cloned immunoglobulin genes in hybridoma technology. In *The Biosciences and Medicine* (T. S. Springer, ed.). Plenum Publ. Corp., pp. 117–137.
5. Avrameas, S., ed. 1988. Multispecific antibodies. *International Rev. Immunology, 3*: 1–133.
6. van de Rijin, I., Bleiveis, A. S., and Zabriskie, J. B. 1976. Antigens in streptococcus mutants cross-reactive with human heart muscle. *J. Dent. Res., 55C*: 59.

7. Zabriskie, J. B., Hsu, K. C., and Segal, B. C. 1970. Heart reactive antibody associated with rheumatic fever: Characterization and diagnostic significance. *Clin. Exp. Immunol., 7*: 147–154.
8. Husby, G., van de Rijin, I., Zabriskie, J. B., Abdin, Z. H., and Williams, R. C. 1976. Antibodies reacting with cytoplasm of subthalamic and caudate nuclei neurons in chorea and acute rheumatic fever. *J. Exp. Med., 144*: 1094–1099.
9. Zabriskie, J. B., and Freimer, E. H. 1986. An immunological relationship between the group A streptococcus and mammalian muscle. *J. Exp. Med., 124*: 661–672.
10. Kaplan, M. H. 1980. Streptococcal cross-reactions with tissue antigens: cardiac, myofibers, smooth muscle and heart valve fibroblasts. In *Streptococcal Diseases and the Immune Response* (S. G. Read and J. B. Zabriskie, eds.). Academic Press, New York, p. 625.
11. Dale, J. B., and Beachey, E. H. 1982. Protective antigenic determinant of streptococcal M protein shared with sarcolema membrane protein of human heart. *J. Exp. Med., 156*: 1165.
12. Cunningham, M. W., and Swerlick, R. A. 1986. Polyspecificity of antistreptococcal murine monoclonal antibodies and their implications in autoimmunity. *J. Exp. Med., 164*: 998–1012.
13. Fischetti, V. A., and Manjula, B. N. 1982. Biologic and immunologic implications of the structural relationship between streptococcal M protein and mammalian tropomyosin. *Semin. Infect. Dis., 4*: 411.
14. Horose, S., Kuwabara, T., Nussenblatt, R. B., Weigert, B., Redmond, T. M., and Gery, I. 1986. Uveitis induced in primates by interphotoreceptor retinoid-binding protein. *Arch. Dyhte Mol., 104*: 1698.
15. Donoso, L. A., Merryman, C. F., Sery, T., Sanders, R., Vrabee, T., and Fong, S-L. 1989. A potent uveitopathogenic agent for the induction of experimental autoimmune uveitis. *J. Immunol., 143*: 79–83.
16. Singh, V. K., Yamaki, K., Abe, T., and Shinohara, T. 1989. Molecular mimicry between uveitopathogenic site of retinal S-antigen and *E. coli* protein: Induction of experimental autoimmune uveitis and lymphocyte cross-reaction. *Cell. Immunol., 122*: 262–273.
17. Oldstone, M. B. A. 1987. *Cell, 50*: 819.
18. Janke, U., Fischer, E. H., and Alvord, E. C. 1985. Sequence homology between certain viral proteins and proteins related to encephalomyelitis and neuritis. *Science, 119*: 282–289.
19. Laing, P., Knight, J. G., Hill, J. M., Harris, A. G., Oxford, J. S., Webster, R. G., Markwell, M. A. K., Paul, S. M., and Pert, C. B. 1989. Influenza viruses induce autoantibodies to a brain-specific 37 kd, a protein in rabbit. *Proc. Natl. Acad. Sci., 86*: 1998–2002.
20. Oldstone, M. B. A. 1989. Molecular mimicry. In *Concepts in Viral Pathogenesis* (A. L. Notkins and M. B. A. Oldstone, eds.). Springer-Verlag, New York, p. 22.
21. Maul, G. G., Jimenez, S. A., Riggs, E., and Ziemnicka-Kolula, D. 1989. Determination of an epitope of the diffuse systemic sclerosis marker antigen DNA topoisomerase I: Sequence similarity with retroviral p30 gag protein suggests a possible cause for autoimmunity in systemic sclerosis. *Proc. Natl. Acad. Sci., 86*: 8432–8436.

22. Lindemann, J. 1979. Homobodies: Do they exist? *Ann. Immunol. (Inst. Pasteur), 130C*: 311–318.
23. Jerne, N. K., Roland, J., and Cazenave, P. A. 1982. Recurrent idiotopes and internal images. *The EMBO J., 1*: 243–247.
24. Sege, K., and Pete, P. A. 1978. Antiidiotypic antibodies against anti-Vitamin A. transporting protein react with prealbumin. *Nature* (London), *271*: 167–168.
25. Bona, C., and Moran, T. 1985. Idiotype vaccines. *Ann. Immunol. (Inst. Pasteur), 136C*: 299–312.
26. Ertl, H. C. J., and Bona, C. 1988. Criteria to define antiidtiotypic antibodies carrying the internal image of an antigen. *Vaccine, 6*: 80–84.
27. Hiernaux, J. 1988. Idiotype vaccines and infectious diseases. *56*: 1407–1413.
28. Monestier, M., Bonin, B., Migliorini, P., Dang, H., Datta, S., Kuppers, R., Rose, N., Maurer, P., Talal, N., and Bona, C. 1987. Autoantibodies of various specificities encoded by genes from the V_H J588 family bind to foreign antigens and share idiotopes of antibodies specific for self and foreign antigens. *J. Exp. Med., 166*: 1109–1124.
29. Bailey, N. C., Fidanza, V., Mayer, R., Mazza, G., Fougereau, M., and Bona, C. 1989. Activation of clones producing self-reactive antibodies by foreign antigens and antiidiotype antibody carrying the internal image of the antigen. *J. Clin. Invest., 84*: 744–756.

14

Immunodominant Determinants of Thyroglobulin Associated with Autoimmune Thyroiditis

Rudolf C. Kuppers, Herbert S. Bresler,* C. Lynne Burek, Shannon L. Gleason,† and Noel R. Rose

The Johns Hopkins School of Hygiene and Public Health, Baltimore, Maryland

I. INTRODUCTION

Autoimmune phenomena in thyroid disease were initially described in 1956 by two independent groups of investigators. Rose and Witebsky observed autoantibodies to thyroglobulin (Tg) and thyroid lesions in rabbits immunized with extracts from normal rabbit thyroids as well as in humans with chronic nonspecific forms of thyroiditis (1,2). At the same time Roitt, Doniach, and colleagues demonstrated that the serum from patients with Hashimoto's disease precipitated constituents of normal human thyroid, principally Tg (3). Autoimmune involvement in chronic lymphocytic thyroiditis (CLT) has since been unequivocally established. Autoimmune thyroid diseases remain the subject of numerous investigations, both clinical and experimental, to explore the various factors influencing their development. They are, furthermore, the prototype of a large number of organ-specific autoimmune diseases including insulin-dependent diabetes and pernicious anemia.

*Present affiliation: Biotronic Systems Corporation, Rockville, Maryland
†Present affiliation: Dow Chemical Company, Midland, Missouri

The purpose of this chapter is to review the present state of our knowledge of the autoantigenic sites on Tg as well as the genetic diversity of thyroid autoantibodies produced by patients with CLT and mice developing experimental autoimmune thyroiditis (EAT) following immunization with mouse Tg (mTg).

II. THE Tg MOLECULE

Tg is the dominant protein produced by the thyroid gland, representing approximately 75% of the protein in mammalian thyroids (4,5). Its function is to act as a storage form for thyroid hormones, and its metabolism is essential to thyroid hormone synthesis.

While Tg's large size, a dimer of two 330 kD peptides, total MW 660 kD, and abundance in thyroid has allowed it to be isolated rather easily, the characterization of the molecule has been difficult. The major question was whether the protein was a true heterodimer or a homodimer, whose apparent heterogeneity were due to modifications occurring after synthesis. Natural thyroid cathepsins are known to cut the polypeptide chains in vivo creating apparent size heterogeneity between the chains. In addition, these proteolytic events lead to the generation of several fragments upon chemical reduction of the molecule creating a problem determining the true structure of the molecule. Further, confounding the problem was the large number of posttranslational modifications including iodination and differential glycosylation which were known to occur and may not occur symmetrically on each chain.

New studies in understanding the basic structure of Tg have come from the application of molecular genetic techniques to the problem. Tg cDNA has now been cloned from several species (6–11) with the realization that there is a single Tg gene that encodes for a homodimeric protein.

In man, the single Tg gene covers a genomic area of about 300 kilobases and contains at least 37 exons (12–14). It is localized to chromosome 8, region 8q242 to 8q243 (15–17). In rat, the gene is smaller, approximately 170 kilobases containing 42 exons. It has been localized to chromosome 7 in rat (18) and to chromosome 15 in mouse (19). In mouse, there appear to be at least 8 allelic forms of the Tg gene as defined by restriction fragment length polymorphism (19). Protein heterogeneity resulting from allelic differences has not been documented, but this finding raises the possibility that allelic differences may play a role in the immunogenicity of Tg in experimental thyroiditis.

The size of the messenger RNA encoded by the Tg gene is approximately 8500 base pairs (20–23) (personal communication with Dr. Roberto DiLauro). It seems of fairly uniform size in mammalian species. Of the 8500 base pairs, 8,301 encode for the protein in humans, and 8,307 in cattle. Of the sequences published, it has been found that 80% sequence homology exists between human and ovine mRNA and 81% between human and bovine in the coding area. These homologies are spread over the entire coding region.

Molecular cloning has also led to a determination of the primary amino acid structure of the molecule, which was virtually impossible by standard protein-sequencing techniques. The peptide encoded by the human thyroglobulin (huTg) mRNA is 2767 amino acids. At the protein level 77.2% homology is seen between human and bovine Tg. Analysis of the primary structure of huTg shows three types of internal homologies (20). In the amino-terminal half of the peptide, 10 domains of about 60 amino acids were found. The presence of cystine, proline, and glycine residues in varying positions in these domains suggests that these regions may be involved in forming the rigid three-dimensional structure necessary for hormone production. A second domain consists of three consecutive segments encoding for a 14–17 amino acid piece, which are found in the central portion of the molecule. Five other domains show a third type of homology. These share a degree of homology in their organization and the presence of cystine and certain other residues. When the amino acid sequence of Tg is compared to other proteins three homologies have been found. One at the C-terminal portion of Tg is related to the acetylcholinesterase of *Torpedo*, the molecules reaching 60% homology in certain regions (24). The 10 type I repetitive domains in the N-terminal portion of Tg have homology with the cytoplasmically expressed piece of the invariant chain of the Ia protein (25). The significance of this homology with the histocompatibility system is of potential interest, although so far the significance of this homology to autoimmune disease is unknown. Homology between Tg and thyroid peroxidase, an enzyme involved in the iodination of the molecule, has also been found (26,27).

The Tg monomer undergoes several posttranslational modifications. These include glycosylation, iodination, phosphorylation, and sulfation. The carbohydrate moiety of Tg may represent up to 10% of its mass. Glycosylation consists of 20–30 N-linked carbohydrate units, of which 5–8 are of the high mannose type, 13–22 complex units, and an unknown number of O-linked glycosylations (18). Based on the amino acid sequences of human and bovine Tg, the potential number of N-glycosylation sites is perhaps 20 per monomer (20), although only 15 have been characterized. In addition to N-linked carbohydrate moieties, huTg contains two types of glycosidic units: a sulfate glucosaminoglycan-like chain and a mucin-like chain (28).

In addition to glycosylation, there are numerous sulfate residues found in the molecule. Of approximately 13 sulfates per molecule, 9 appear to be linked to tyrosine, and the others to a high mannose type chain (29). Phosphorylation of Tg is also thought to occur. The presence of phosphoserine (30–32) and phosphotyrosine (32) have been reported. There is, at present, no consensus as to whether phosphorylated mannose residues are present on Tg as they have been reported by some, but not all, laboratories (31–34).

The major function of Tg is to store thyroid hormones. Tg contains iodine in the form of either mono- or di-iodotyrosine. Iodothyroxines such as thyroxine (or T4) and tri-iodothronine (or T3) are synthesized by intramolecular coupling between two iodotyrosine residues by mechanisms not totally understood. The iodination of tyrosine is mediated by a membrane-bound thyroid peroxidase, which has also been recently isolated and sequenced (35–37). It is also thought to be the so-called microsomal antigen to which antibodies occur in many thyroiditis patients.

In the Tg molecule there are 130 tyrosine residues of which only 25–40 appear capable of being iodinated to iodotyrosines (6–11,38–44). Of these, only a few, maybe 4–6, participate in the coupling reaction leading to the formation of thyroid hormone.

The iodotyrosines involved in the coupling reaction appear to be found in unique regions of the molecule (45–47). The amino acid structure around these hormone residues has been studied and shows a certain degree of homology from site to site. The hormonogenic site in the N-terminal part of the molecule appears to be a preferred site for hormonogenesis in huTg (48), and it is at this site that T4 formation appears to occur preferentially. Conformational constraints appear to be important for thyroid hormone synthesis. Synthesis is diminished or does not occur if Tg has been partially denatured (49,50), indicating that the orientation of iodotyrosines contributing to hormone synthesis is important.

Serologic studies have shown that there are multiple antigenic determinants recognized by heterologous antiserum to Tg. At least 40 antigenic determinants have been suggested on the huTg molecule (51). Many laboratories have generated monoclonal antibodies (MAbs) to Tg in order to better understand the antigenic diversity of the Tg molecule (52–55). While many of these MAbs recognize distinct epitopes, for the most part the exact locations of these epitopes are unknown. It appears that most of these antibodies recognize peptide moieties and many are reactive with conformational determinants of the Tg molecule. Anti-T4 antibodies have been found in autoimmune sera which react with Tg suggesting these sites are exposed and are antigenic (56). No MAbs against the glycan moiety have been specifically demonstrated, though in work described later, the reactivity of some MAbs with huTg can be affected by periodate treatment of Tg.

Many laboratories are developing strategies designed to characterize the epitopes recognized by these MAbs. One approach is to look at the ability of these antibodies to react to fragments of the Tg molecule. A second approach is that of generating peptides through the use of expression vectors containing various Tg cDNA segments. The use of the cDNA approach has advantages in that defined peptides can be produced without having to deal with extensive peptide separations. This may allow for identification of sequential or conformational epitopes on portions of the molecule. The disadvantage is that posttranslational modifications will not have occurred. Iodination of the molecule may have significant effects on its conformation, as well as being involved as antigenic determinants themselves. We have generated two separate series of MAbs against human Tg and mTg. The characteristics of these MAbs, in particular specificity and epitopic recognition patterns, will be discussed in the following sections.

III. STUDIES OF MURINE EXPERIMENTAL AUTOIMMUNE THYROIDITIS

A. Epitope Recognition in Experimental Autoimmune Thyroiditis in the Mouse

Several laboratories have attempted to identify the number of epitopes that are recognized in an autoantibody response. All of these studies have indicated a small number. Most suggest that four to six antigenic determinants are recognized by human thyroiditis patients' autoantibodies (51,57,58) and five to eight autoepitopes on mTg (53,59). This contrasts with 40 or more antigenic determinants which may be recognized in a heterologous response against Tg (51). Allogeneic differences between Tgs have been looked for, but at the antibody (Ab) level none have been conclusively shown (53,59). In terms of antigenicity, Tg from poor responder mice has been shown to have low antigenicity, whereas Tg from high responder mice appears to have high antigenicity as reflected in Ab titer and pathogenesis during EAT (60). Whether this in fact is a reflection of differences in the Tg at the genetic level, reflected by peptide sequence heterogeneity or by posttranslational modification, is not clear.

Studies of MAbs prepared in mice against mTg have shown several interesting features. First, immunization with autologous Tg or homologous Tg (from a different mouse strain) leads to MAbs that recognize a restricted number of epitopes or determinant regions. Kotani et al. have identified six dominant regions (59). In our earlier studies, we found that eight different determinants were recognized by species-restricted sites by means of a panel of 11 MAbs (53). Reported here is the characterization of another set of 16 mouse anti-mTg MAbs.

The specificity of these antibodies have been examined as to their reactivity to Tg, thyroid hormones, and other antigens. Testing with seven different Tgs isolated from various mammalian species, the great majority of the antibodies recognize only mouse or rat Tg (Fig. 1). The reactivity of most is clearly stronger to mouse than any other Tg. It is interesting that such a large number shows a high degree of autospecificity. This suggests that autoepitopes are preferred in the response to this self-antigen. This finding is consistent with other reports in mouse showing species-restricted responses (59) and reports in humans showing a similar phenomenon (52). There is, in contrast, a subset of antibodies that appear to recognize Tg from any or all species. These results demonstrate that autoimmunization of mice leads to a high frequency of Abs to immunodominant,

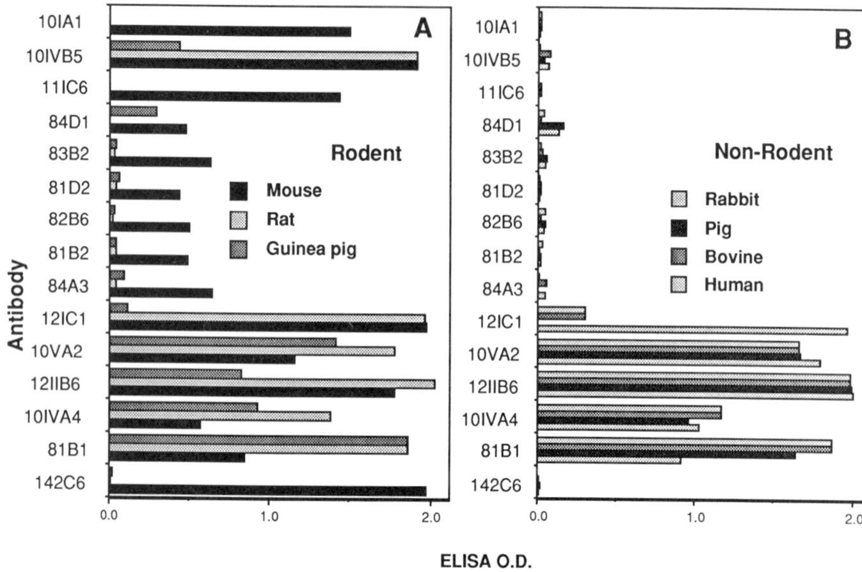

FIGURE 1 Thyroglobulin specificity of mouse Tg autoantibodies. MAbs containing culture supernatants were tested in an ELISA assay for binding to Tgs from the indicated sources. The optical density generated by each is given A) for rodent Tgs and B) for other Tgs.

species-specific epitopes expressed on mTg, as well as less common Abs reactive to phylogenetically conserved regions of the molecule.

We have further characterized these antibodies for their fine specificity by generating a reactivity map. A reciprocal inhibition assay was performed in which the binding of one MAb was inhibited by another. The MAbs fall into distinctive reactivity groups based upon their ability to inhibit or to be inhibited by other MAbs. Strong reciprocal inhibition was the primary criterion for assigning an Ab to a reactivity group. Based on this, the panel of MAbs was arranged into seven groups (Fig. 2). It must be noted that one-way and partial inhibitions have also been included in this figure, although they were not a primary criterion for assigning an Ab to a reactivity group. The antibodies in groups I through IV show rodent specificity; however, they are not necessarily highly restricted to mouse, whereas those antibodies in group V all appeared to be very specific for mTg with little cross-reactivity to rat. The antibodies in group V are all mutually inhibitory, suggesting that the determinants recognized by the antibodies within this group are spatially close together. These results strengthened the argument

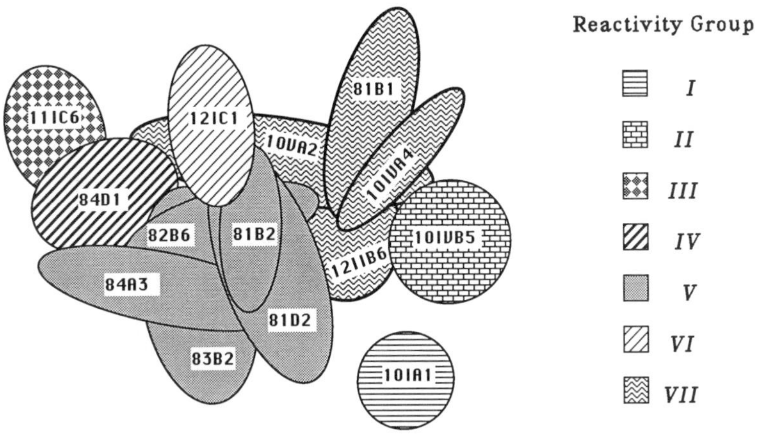

FIGURE 2 Reciprocal inhibition of the binding of mouse MAbs to mTg. The binding of labeled MAbs to mTg was tested in an ELISA for its ability to be inhibited by unlabeled MAbs. The ability of MAbs to inhibit one another is represented in this Venn diagram, including one-way and partial inhibitions. Based upon the ability of one Ab to strongly inhibit another, reactivity groups were assigned.

that there exists a major immunodominant mouse-specific region of Tg which is recognized by the mouse in its response to immunization with mTg.

The MAbs in groups VI and VII are reactive to a variety of Tgs, whether homologous or heterologous. These multireactive antibodies are also cross-inhibitory among themselves; that is, they inhibit each other from binding to Tg, but they do not strongly inhibit nor are strongly inhibited by the other MAbs. This indicates that the sites to which the multireactive antibodies bind are distinct from the mouse-specific epitopes.

We have further characterized these MAbs as to their reactivity to other antigens. It is known, for instance, that many of the natural or polyreactive type of antibodies are capable of binding to Tg. In order to test for polyreactivity, the MAbs in this panel were tested against a panel of apparently unrelated antigens. The results are shown in Figure 3. It was also asked whether or not thyroid hormones (T4 and T3) were capable of inhibiting the reactivity of these antibodies to Tg. The latter were included to test for the recognition of iodinated tyrosine residues that are unique to Tg. The results from these experiments (Fig. 3). clearly show three patterns of inhibition: those that appear to be uniquely specific for mTg and whose binding to Tg is not inhibited by other molecules; a second set of MAbs inhibited by both Tg and by thyroid hormones, but showing little or

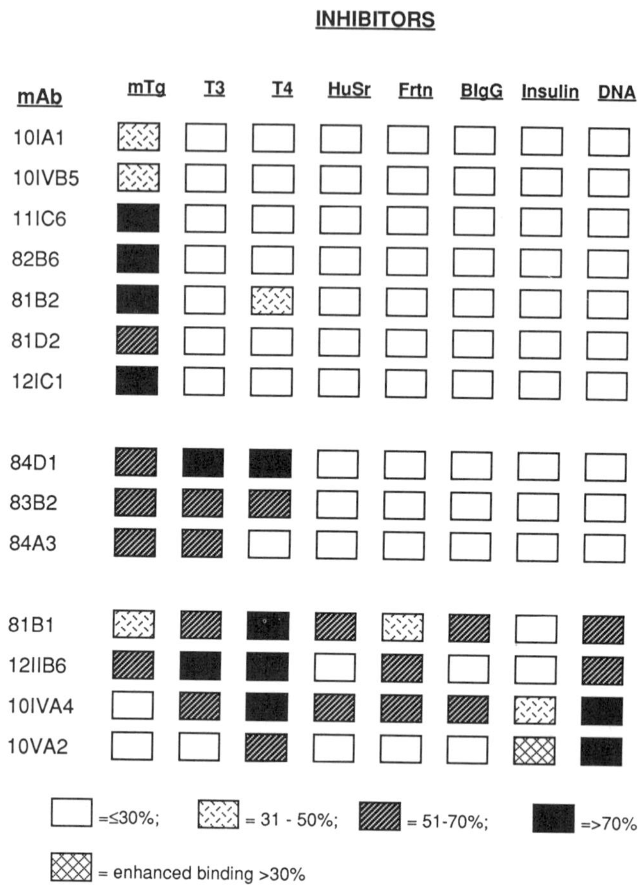

FIGURE 3 The inhibition of MAb binding to mTg by various competitors. MAbs were preincubated with the indicated inhibitor for 2 hr before addition of MAb to an ELISA assay. The inhibition of binding was taken as the percent reduction in OD as compared to MAb in absence of inhibitor. Inhibition by 1 mg/ml, except mTg (1.5 mg/ml) and human Igm serum (1-4 dilution). mTg, mouse Tg; HuSr, human IgM serum; Frtn, ferritin; BIgG, bovine immunoglobulin G.

no inhibition by unrelated compound; and a third group of antibodies inhibited by a variety of related and unrelated competitors including T3 and/or T4.

While these MAbs were fitted into the seven different reactivity patterns, shown in Figure 2, the antibodies within a reactivity group likely recognize different epitopes (Fig. 4). This is evident if one examines the microspecificity of these antibodies. For instance, while 84A3 appears to fit into reactivity pattern V, it also is inhibited by T3, whereas the other members of reactivity group VII do not.

Likewise, the antibodies in reactivity groups I thorugh IV also show similar heterogeneity in their binding; for instance, 10IA1 binds to mouse and rat Tg, but is not inhibited by T3 and T4. 10IVB5 recognizes mouse and rat and to some extent guinea pig, whereas 11IC6, group III, is mouse specific. 11IC6 and 84D1 show some similarity in that they belong to reactivity group III. However, they clearly show specificity differences, 11IC6 being mouse specific, whereas 84D1 reacts to various Tgs in addition to T3 and T4. We conclude that there are a large number of epitopes on the Tg molecule, but these epitopes may be confined to particular regions of the molecule.

The presence of anti-T3 and anti-T4 antibodies is not uncommon in the serum of autoimmune thyroiditis patients, as will be described later (56). Interestingly, we find here antibodies that show specificity for T3 alone and antibodies that recognize both T3 and T4. While 83B2 is inhibited by T3 and T4 and 84A3 by T3, both are specific for mTg. They are not then anti-T3/T4 Abs but seem to recognize T3/T4 in the context of the backbone structure of the mTg molecule.

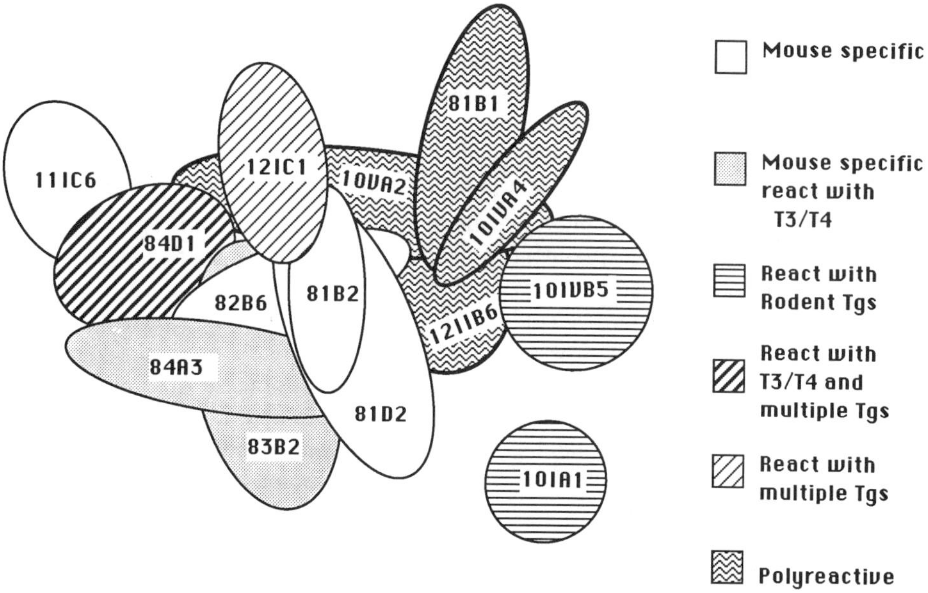

FIGURE 4 Inhibition of 12IIB6 and 12IC1 by various competitors (see Fig. 3). The concentration dependency of inhibition is shown for two IgG2a antibodies.

84D1 is also inhibited by T3 and T4. It, however, shows specificity for several Tgs but not necessarily all. This raises the possibility that this Ab is recognizing T3 and T4 structure in the context of an epitope conserved between species. As it is known that iodination of tyrosines occurs at several rather conserved locations throughout the Tg molecule, some of this heterogeneity may relate to the specific site at which these antibodies bind. Another possibility is that when condensation of iodotyrosines occurs there is a conformational change in the protein molecule and that some of these antibodies are recognizing this conformational change. While conformational changes are important in the binding of some anti-T4 antibodies (55), whether changes resulting from hormonogenesis play a role in autoimmune disease has yet to be examined. Dietary iodine, which presumably affects iodination levels, has been shown to be a predisposing factor for increased thyroiditis in the OS chicken (which is genetically predisposed to autoimmune thyroiditis), in the mouse EAT model, and in man (61–63).

The antibodies of group VII, 81B1, 10IVA4, and 12IIB6 are polyreactive. However, while they show reactivity to several compounds, each of these antibodies differs somewhat with respect to which inhibitors compete for binding to mTg or the concentration dependency of inhibition. It appears that some antibodies bind better to the other compounds than to mTg. 10VA2, for example, appears to be an anti-DNA Ab having lower affinity for mTg. The binding of DNA-reactive MAbs to MTg in these assays cannot, however, be explained by DNA contaminating the mTg preparation, for serum from an old MRL+/+ mouse known to have both anti ds- and ssDNA Ab activity failed to bind mouse Tg in an ELISA. Therefore, a determinant shared by DNA and Tg would appear to be a true target of the Ab.

The binding of the antibodies in group VII shows several interesting features. They are all inhibited by T3 and T4. In some cases, for instance, inhibition of 10VA2 by insulin, the inhibitor actually increased the binding to mTg. This inhibition was seen in all experiments using these MAbs. Inhibition by the various substances usually failed to follow normal concentration-dependent kinetics. In some cases inhibition was seen only at low inhibitor concentration. 12IIB6 is an IgG2a Ab which also demonstrates some degree of polyreactivity, while 12IC1, also an IgG2a, is mouse specific. The inhibition curves of these Abs are shown in Figure 5. We noted that the polyreactive antibodies appear to have a much higher background level of inhibition, that is, somewhere between 20 and 30% even in the low range of inhibitor. In some cases inhibition is better at low concentrations of inhibitor.

The basis of these inhibition patterns is unclear. It may be argued that the binding of these antibodies to Tg is nonspecific. We do not believe this is the case, as it is clear that these antibodies are capable of inhibiting the binding between themselves; that is, they belong to reactivity group VII, but they do not inhibit the binding of any of the other MAbs in the study. Therefore, they must be recognizing a unique site on the Tg molecule. Posttranslational modification of Tg may play a role in the binding of these antibodies. Glycosylated as well as phosphorylated regions of Tg may explain cross-reactivity to other proteins which share similar glycosylation or phosphorylation sites, and possibly to the reactivity

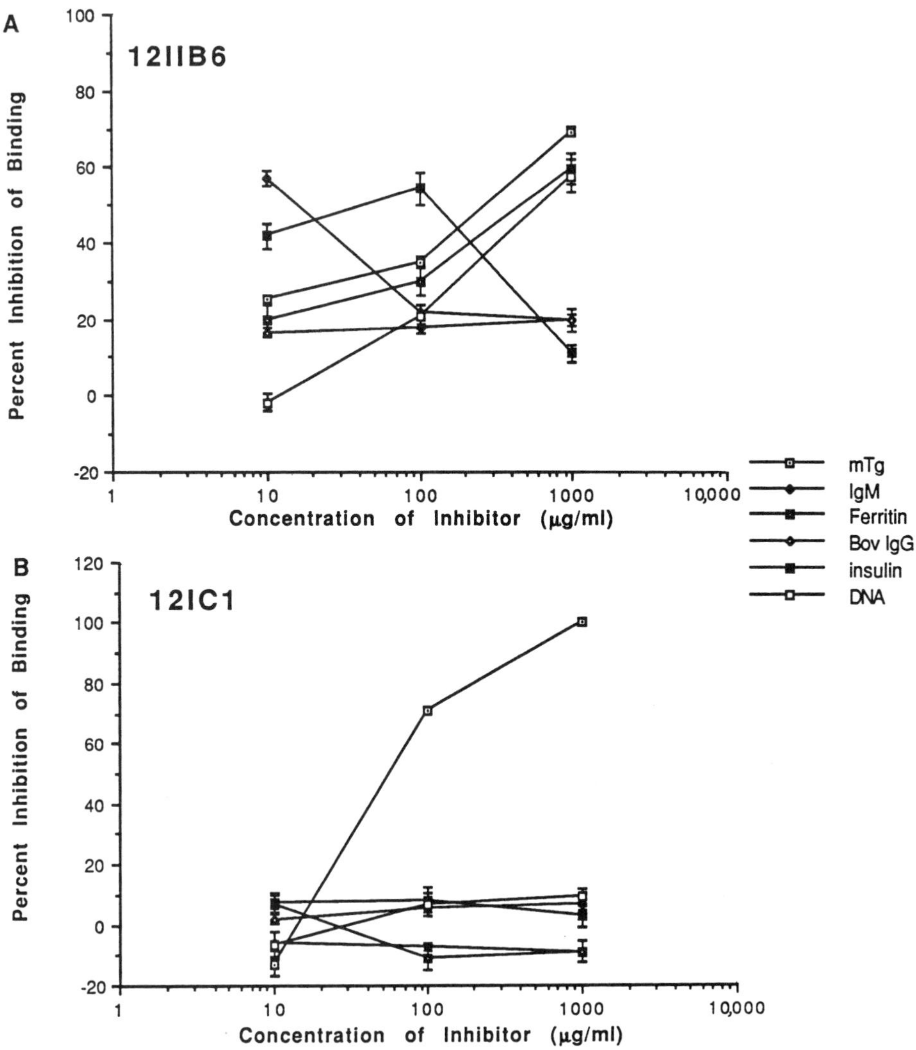

FIGURE 5 Summary of specificity and reactivity data. This Venn diagram summarizes the specificity and reactivity data from Figures 1, 2, and 3.

of many of these antibodies to phosphodeoxyribose backbone of DNA. These antibodies resemble the polyreactive MAbs occurring in autoimmune disease in mouse and human studied by others (64,65) and may represent "natural" antibodies selected by the B-cell repertoire on the basis of their reaction with Tg (66).

At the molecular level, Tg shows several types of repetitive domains. For instance, bovine Tg includes 10 repetitions of a 60-amino-acid motif. Peptides of various lengths are inserted within this repetitive unit. Small repetitions are also found in the central and carboxyl-terminal portion of the molecule. Similar repetitions were found for huTg. We have produced cyanogen bromide (CnBr) fragments of mTg and have studied this panel of MAbs for their binding to these fragments. As shown in Figure 6, when CnBr peptide fragments were sized on Sephadex 100, several peaks were obtained. Several of these fractions were tested for their ability to be bound by these MAbs. Three monoclonals were able to bind these fragments: 81B1, 10VA2 and 12IC1. Interestingly, two of these belong to the polyreactive group VII, whereas 12IC1 belongs to reactivity group VI.

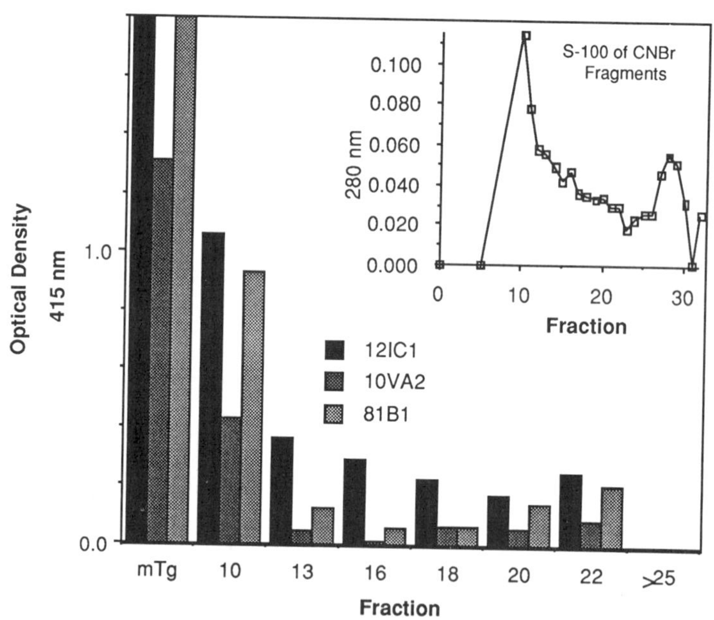

FIGURE 6 Binding of three MAbs to cyanogen bromide fragments of mTg. Reduced and alkylated MTg was cleaved using cyanogen bromide. Fragments were resolubilized using 3 M guanidine. The fragments were then separated on a Sephadex S-100 column (insert). Fractions were used to coat ELISA plates and the ability of the panel of MAbs to bind was assessed. Only three MAbs bound these fragments.

12IC1 shows reactivity to various Tgs, but no reactivity to T3 or T4, suggesting that it recognizes a backbone fragment of Tg. Interestingly, these antibodies were able to bind all six CnBr-Tg fragments tested, as shown in Figure 6. These results suggest that there is at least one repetitive epitope recognized by this panel of antibodies. However, as 12IC1 does not bind T3/T4 and fails to react with porcine Tg, 12IC1 is likely to be recognizing a second epitope common to many but not all Tgs. As these fragments are likely to be denatured after reduction and alkylation, the antibodies probably recognize the primary structure of the molecule and not conformational determinants.

B. Analysis of Immunoglobulin Gene Segment Usage in EAT

To further dissect the degree of heterogeneity of Tg autoantibodies induced in mice by immunization with mTg, immunoglobulin gene usage was assessed using hybridization or cDNA sequencing. Several of the antibodies in our panel have been completely or partially sequenced (67). Several V, (D), and J gene segments were used by the heavy and light chains of these antibodies. A summary of these results is given in Table 1. In this panel we found that four V_H subfamilies were used by these antibodies. This included six from J558, one from J606, one from 7183, and two from QPC52 subfamilies. The diversity shown at the nucleotide level indicates the Abs were encoded by different gene segments, even though they are of the same V-region family. This was true even within the J558 family, which is the most highly represented. The only exceptions were in the Vk21 subfamily from which two MAbs, 84A3 and 11IC6, appeared to use the same BALB/c Vk21E1.5 germline gene segment and 81D2 and 82B6, which appeared to use the same Vk9 gene segment. The first two antibodies were cloned from different mice and from different fusions. They also use different V_H subfamilies. These two antibodies are identical for the portion of the nucleotide sequence obtained except a three-base deletion in 11IC6 at the VJ-joining region. Both antibodies share a substitution at the second base of codon 91, which is different from that reported for Vk21E1.5. This may reflect an allelic difference between BALB/c and CBA/J. Three other substitutions at codons 21, 51, and 56 are also found in the 11IC6 in the region in which no sequence data were obtained for 84A3. The fine specificity of these Abs is also quite different (Fig. 3).

81D2 and 82B6 both appear to share the same Vk9 and Jk1 gene segments based on partial sequence data. They do differ at the V-J junction at which codon 95 has been deleted in 81D2. This difference suggests that they are different clones using the same gene segments.

One Ab, 10VA2, was found to use the EA6.0 germline gene segment, the prototype of the Vk1A subgroup (68). This germline gene is identical to that found in the MRL-DNA10 Ab kappa chain. This anti-DNA Ab arose spontaneously

TABLE 1 Summary of Heavy- and Light-Chain Gene Segment Use and Antibody Specificity

			Gene segments[b]				
			Heavy			Light	
MAb	Ig class	Reactivity group[a]	V_H	D	J_H	V_κ	J_κ
10IA1	μ,κ	I	7183[c]				
10IVB5	μ,κ	II					
11IC6	μ,κ	III	J606	SP2	2	21	2
84D1	μ,κ	III,IV	Q52[c]				
83B2	μ,κ	IV,V				8	1
81D2	μ,κ	V	J558[c]			9	1
82B6a[d]	μ,κ	V	Q52	SP2.7a	2	19	4
82B6b[d]						9	1
81B2	μ,κ	V					
84A3	μ,κ	V	J558[c]			21	1
12ICI	δ2a,κ	VI	J558	SP2.5	4	29	1
10VA2	μ,κ	VI,VII	J558	SP2.7a	3	1	1
12IIB6	δ2a,κ	VII	J558	SP2.5	4	4	1
81B1	μ,κ	VII	J558[c]	SP2.5	3	4	

[a]Defined in Fig. 2.
[b]Assignments are based on homology to V_H or V_κ families and D, J_H, and J_κ germline gene segments identified in the BALB/c strain.
[c]Determined by hybridization to RNA (100).
[d]Produces two productive kappa chains.

from the autoimmune MRL mouse. The anti-DNA reactivity of this kappa chain may explain the high degree of specificity of 10VA2 for DNA. What role the base substitutions in the heavy chain may play in binding Tg is not known.

The possible role that somatic mutation plays in the generation of autoantibodies has been an area of considerable study in recent years. In this panel we found mutations in 12IC1 at coding 9 of the JH gene and a 5th codon of J_K. Since no homology with known sequences was found in any of the V gene segments except 10VA2, the level of change due to somatic mutational processes cannot be assessed. While these data would be consistent with somatic mutation occurring in autoantibodies, the importance of these changes in the specificity of these Abs or the autoimmune process is not known.

The role of the natural Ab pool in the production of mTg-specific antibodies is not clear. It does appear from our data that these antibodies recognize a specific determinant or region on Tg, as they are cross-inhibitory and fail to inhibit the binding of the other antibodies in the panel. Yet to be determined is whether their binding is mediated through their antigen-binding site or via other regions of the Ab molecule.

Overall, the nucleotide and amino acid sequence data indicate that the Ab repertoire to mTg is derived from many different V-region families even when the MAbs fall in the same reactivity group. This diversity is further supported by the specificity analysis showing that these antibodies likely recognize many different epitopes. However, there appear to be immunodominant regions of the Tg molecule, as shown by their clustering to seven reactivity groups and a predominance of Abs within reactivity group V.

IV. STUDIES OF HUMAN AUTOIMMUNE THYROIDITIS

A. Genetics of Autoimmune Thyroid Disease

Evidence indicates that the development of autoimmune thyroid disease in humans represents the conjunction of several independent genetic and environmental events. Animal models of thyroid autoimmunity have given some insight into the types of genetic and environmental factors that can predispose to autoimmunity. This knowledge has been of use in approaching the study of human thyroid disease.

One consideration in human disease concerns the types of genetic traits that influence autoimmune thyroid disease. These traits may include one or more immunoregulatory genes, abnormality in maturation of the thymus, and disturbance in the structure or function of the thyroid gland. Individuals who inherit several defects are the ones most likely to develop autoimmune disease. The intervention of developmental and environmental factors may further favor the development of disease. Such factors as sex hormones, thyroid infection, or nutrition may contribute. Along these lines, it is important to point out that severe thyroiditis can be induced in genetically "resistant" mice if given a sufficiently strong antigenic stimulus, such as Tg combined with Freund's complete adjuvant. This picture seems to fit rather closely the clinical concept of an autoimmune diathesis. In families predisposed to the development of autoimmunity, different autoimmune diseases can develop in various members of the same family. These differences may be due in part to differing environmental influences in members of these families as well as differences in genetic constitution, including genetically predisposed abnormalities of various target organs.

B. Fine Specificities of Tg Autoantibodies

Since Tg autoantibodies were found in the serum of almost all patients with autoimmune thyroid disease (3) as well as in individuals having no clinical thyroid disease (69–73), it was hypothesized that certain Tg epitopes are relevant to the pathogenesis of autoimmune thyroid disease, while other epitopes are irrelevant.

A precise characterization of the epitopes and autoantibodies observed in autoimmune thyroid disease would be useful for understanding its pathogenesis.

Previous efforts to characterize the fine specificities and other qualities of anti-Tg antibodies have been hampered by the difficulties inherent in working with heterogeneous antisera from patients or experimental animals. Quantitative precipitation, used to estimate the number of combining sites on huTg recognized by autoantisera from CLT patients and from rabbits immunized with huTg, revealed that the molar ratios calculated for Ab to antigen were between 2:1 and 6:1 for thyroiditis antibodies, contrasting with approximately 40:1 for sera from rabbits immunized with huTg, as mentioned previously (51,57). These were the first indications that the response to Tg in patients with autoantibodies was limited to certain determinants. They suggested that only restricted parts of the molecule provide antigenic stimuli during autoimmunization. Rose and Stylos (74–76) studied the nature of hetero- and autoantisera directed against huTg by splitting the native Tg molecule enzymatically and analyzing the patterns of immunoreactivity of the fragments with various antisera. However, these studies shed little light on the fine specificities of the autoantibodies due to the limited reactivity of antibodies with protein fragments. Other investigators have performed similar studies in order to identify the immunogenic sites on Tg (77,78), but detailed immunochemical analysis has proven difficult.

Hybridoma technology is uniquely suited for use in detailed study of antigenic determinants. Preliminary investigations using anti-Tg MAbs prepared in mice supported the hypothesis that there are qualitative differences between the epitope specificities of anti-Tg antibodies of thyroiditis patients and those found in normal individuals.

Ruf et al. (52) described six distinct reactivity groups using their panel of murine MAbs to huTg. None of the epitopes identified by their 10 monoclonals seemed to contain carbohydrate moieties, tyrosines, iodotyrosines, or iodothyronines. Anti-Tg antibodies purified from the pooled sera of 48 patients with Graves' disease reacted with only one of the six clusters. They suggested that the antigenic determinants on Tg are not randomly distributed over the entire molecule, but are clustered in limited "autoantigenic regions." Furthermore, they concluded that, of the six antigenic regions described in their paper, only one is involved in autoimmune Ab production in Graves' disease. The same group of researchers also used these 10 monoclonals in competition studies with antibodies from a patient with Hashimoto's thyroiditis and from a patient with Graves' disease (79). Their results showed that the spectrum of antibodies in these patients did not differ from that found in a normal individual who also had Ab, although there were greatly increased concentrations of antibodies in the Graves' and Hashimoto's patients which were restricted to a few of the epitopes defined by the monoclonals. They hypothesized that immunoregulation failed in autoimmune thyroid diseases with respect to only selected epitopes on the Tg molecule.

Other recent information has been presented in studies comparing differences in the immune response to thyroid antigens between healthy individuals and those with disease. The results also support the concept that there is a qualitative difference in the immune response between these two groups. Piechaczyk et al. (58) compared the domains on the Tg molecule recognized by autoantibodies in sera from thyroiditis patients with those from healthy individuals. They obtained 15 MAbs, which they determined reacted to six different domains on the Tg molecule (80). With the limited number of domains they could distinguish, they found that sera from patients reacted mainly to one particular domain, while Tg autoantibodies from healthy individuals bound to other regions in a less restricted fashion. Delineation of the fine specificities of Tg autoantibodies is therefore a logical first step in the process to distinguish people with a genetic predisposition for development of disease.

C. Molecular Topography of huTg

Through the use of several hybridomas with different epitope specificities, we have been able to map the spatial relationships of many antigenic determinants and, to some extent, their chemical nature. Information concerning the evolutionary conservation of epitopes in other species was obtained by testing the reactivity of the MAbs with Tg from several other mammalian species (Fig. 7). Most MAbs (16/20) recognized a restricted number of different Tg indicating they see epitopes which are not widely shared among mammalian species, and even though no effort was made to select for MAbs which recognized uniquely human epitopes, 12 of 20 MAbs reacted only with huTg. Of the four MAbs that recognized epitopes widely shared among many mammalian species, three could be inhibited by T4 and T3. These three were the only MAbs that bound to Tg from all species tested. This finding suggests that Tg may vary considerably in its antigenic properties from one species to another, while the thyroxine itself, and perhaps the hormonogenic regions from which they arise, are at least partially conserved.

To further define the topographical relationship between the epitopes recognized, reciprocal Ab inhibition assays were performed as in the mouse EAT model. When the ability of one MAb to inhibit the binding of a second was tested, we distinguished 12 reactivity groups based mainly on the ability of one Ab to strongly inhibit another (Fig. 8). To present a better sense of the topograhical interaction between the Abs, a Venn diagram was created representing the ability of one Ab to interact with another (Fig. 9).

The pattern of shared determinant reactivities presented in Figures 8 and 9 indicates that there are topologically continuous antigenic regions in the native huTg molecule. These overlapping determinant clusters have been distinguished as "immunodominant," since 8 of the 20 MAbs in the panel define sites in these clusters,

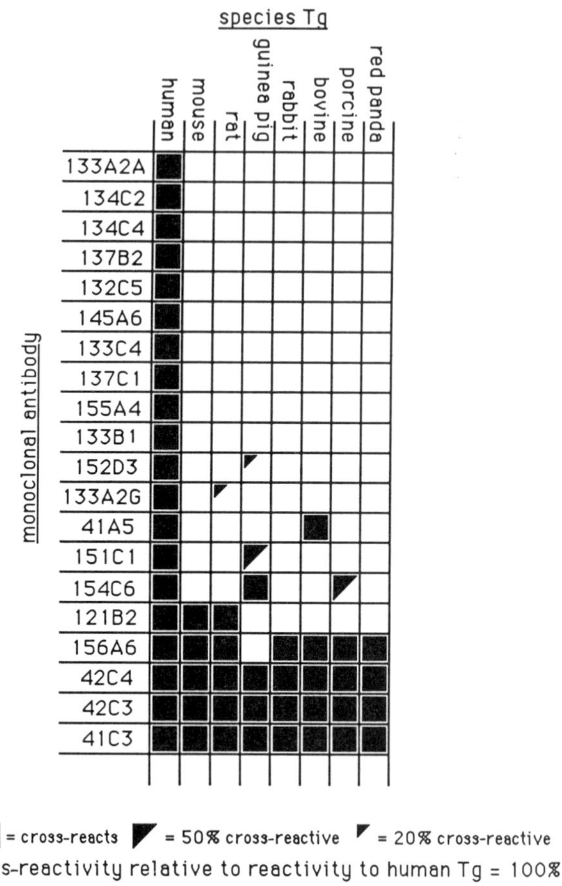

FIGURE 7 Thyroglobulin specificity of mouse anti-huTg MAbs. The MAbs containing culture supernatants were tested for binding to Tgs from the indicated sources in an ELISA assay. Relative binding to the species of Tg indicated is indicated.

reactivity groups 1–3. All of the MAbs in the immunodominant clusters react with huTg, and not with Tg from seven other species (Fig. 7).

Topologically interrelated epitopes are revealed by the high number of one-way inhibitions exhibited by a few MAbs. The best example is 133A2G, which was inhibited by 12 MAbs while it only inhibited 3 MAbs. The possible reasons for partial and one-way inhibitions have been discussed elsewhere (55). Therefore, we conclude that many of these Abs react with determinants present as a continuum over regions of the Tg molecule.

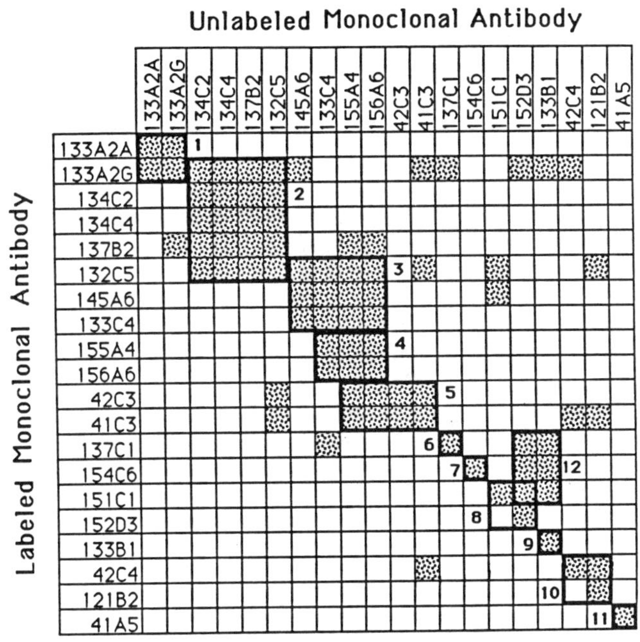

FIGURE 8 Reciprocal inhibition of the binding of mouse MAbs anti-huTg MAb to huTg. Labeled MAbs were tested for their ability to be inhibited from binding huTg by unlabeled MAbs. The ability of MAbs to inhibit one another is represented in this diagram. Based upon the clustering of interacting Abs, 12 reactivity groups were assigned, as indicated by the boxes.

Periodate oxidation followed by cyanoborohydride results in the formation of covalent bonds between the aldehydes and amino groups. This procedure can affect carbohydrate moieties on the Tg molecule by cross-linking them mainly to lysines and glutamines in the polypeptide portion of the molecule. The MAbs that have diminished or have lost their ability to bind Tg oxidized and reduced (ox/red) by this method may be reacting via a carbohydrate moiety or carbohydrate-dependent epitopes, or via epitopes dependent upon or near one or more of the cross-linked amino acids. We found that eight MAbs in our panel lost their ability to bind ox/red huTg, and three were found to be partially inhibited (Fig. 10). The Abs that were inhibited belonged to reactivity groups 3, 8, 9, 11, and one in group 4 (Fig. 8). While this does not prove that they are reactive with the carbohydrate chains of Tg, minimally it can be argued that the epitopes they recognized lie near a glycosylation site on the protein.

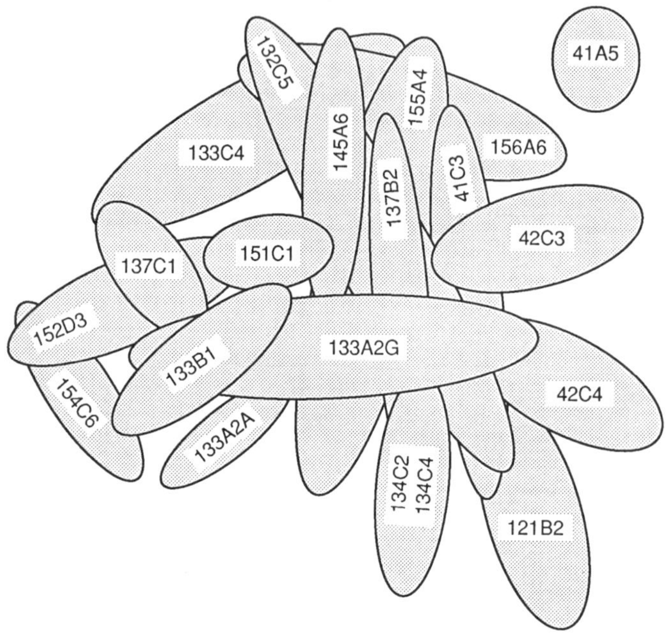

FIGURE 9 Topographical interpretation of the epitopic distribution of huTg antigenic determinant. This Venn diagram is a representation of the data from Figure 8.

Two MAbs reacted significantly better to oxidized/reduced huTg. They were also the only IgM antibodies in the panel (41C3 and 42C4 in Fig. 9). These IgM MAbs may represent "natural" autoantibodies from the normal Ab repertoire of the immunized mouse. Natural autoantibodies are likely to be of low affinity and cross-reactive, qualities both of these MAbs exhibit. Natural autoantibodies may react better with a distinctly foreign, denatured antigen than to a native one. This observation has been made by other investigators when looking at the reactivity of MAbs to denatured versus native antigens (81). The increased reactivity of these two Abs to ox/red huTg, in essence a denatured Tg, would be consistent with these observations.

Of the four MAbs which recognized epitopes widely shared among many mammalian species, three could be inhibited by T4 and T3 (Fig. 11). These three were the only MAbs which bound to Tg from all species tested. This finding suggests that Tg may vary considerably in its antigenic properties from one species to another; however, the hormonogenic regions may be more highly conserved, though not identical.

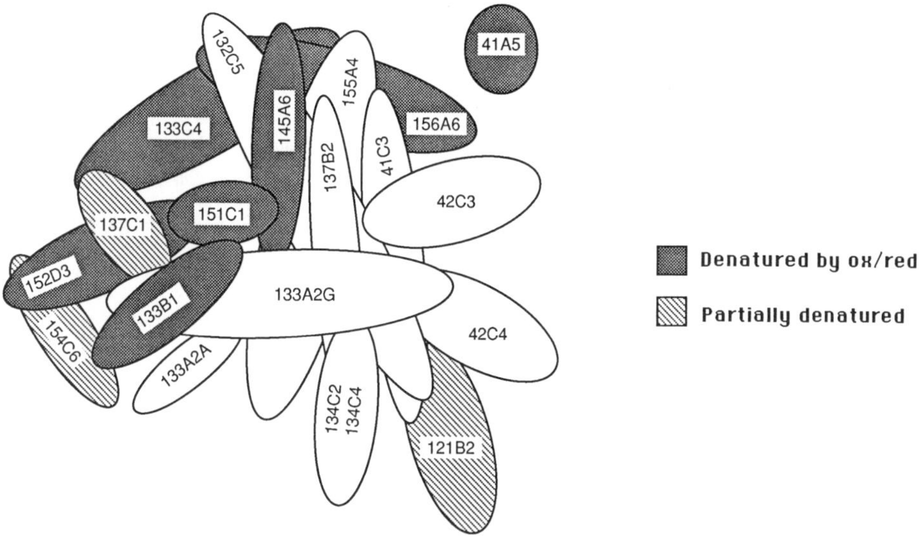

FIGURE 10 Inhibition of MAb binding by periodate treatment of huTg. HuTg was oxidized with periodate, then reduced with cyanoborohydride. The ability of the MAbs to bind this modified huTg was tested. MAbs which were completely or partially inhibited from binding are indicated in this Venn diagram.

Evidence that the regions neighboring the thyroxines are not identical comes from the reactivity patterns of two MAbs. One MAb (133B1), which bound only huTg, was inhibited by T4 but not by T3. The other MAb (41A5), which bound human and bovine Tg only, was inhibited by both T4 and T3. Since neither of these MAbs was able to bind Tg from other species, either the thyroxines are not part of the antigenic epitopes or the thyroxines are recognized in the context of residues unique to human and bovine Tgs. Interestingly, these two MAbs were incapable of binding oxidized/reduced huTg, unlike the other three MAbs, which were inhibited by T4 and T3, suggesting that carbohydrates may be part of the antigenic epitopes recognized by these two MAbs.

When the different reactivities of the MAbs are taken together (see Figs. 7–11), we felt we could discern 19 different determinants. The only two MAbs that apparently shared the same epitope specificity were 134C2 and 134C4. Each of the other epitopes defined by these MAbs could be distinguished from the others in the panel by one or more of the above-described criteria.

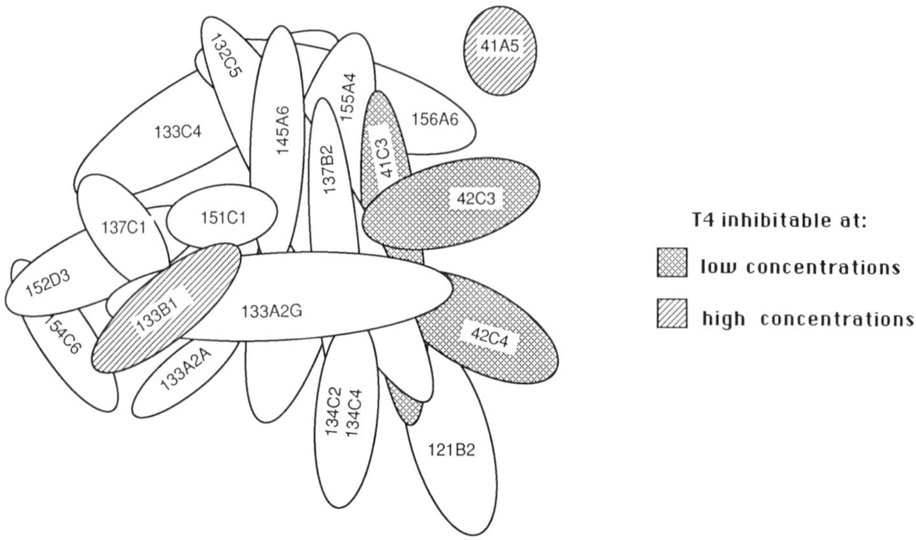

FIGURE 11 Inhibition of MAb binding by thyroid hormones. The ability of T4 and T3 hormones to inhibit the binding of mouse anti-huTg MAb to huTg was tested in an ELISA assay similar to that in Figure 3. Those MAbs that were inhibited at low and high concentrations of hormone are indicated in the Venn diagram.

D. Determinants on huTg Recognized by Autoantibodies

This section describes the use of the large, well-characterized panel of MAbs described to analyze the reactivity of human Abs to huTg (55). Previous investigations have studied randomly obtained populations of adult patients and normals (52,58,59,79,80,82–84). Presented are the results of inhibition studies comprised of sera from adult and juvenile individuals. In order to simplify the data, the results are presented for three categories of individuals. The first group is adult and juvenile CLT patients. The second is seronegative individuals, whether from the proband's family or from nondiseased normal families. The last group is seropositive individuals including individuals with possible subclinical disease.

Patient sera were tested in competitive inhibition ELISAs, which has been described by us in detail elsewhere (85). We have shown that the methods used to carry out the competitive inhibition assays are reliable even when dealing with Abs of dramatically different affinities. Therefore, we feel the technique is well suited for the analysis of the fine specificities of antibodies in complex mixtures, such as serum, where antibodies with multiple different affinities may be present.

Briefly, if a human serum, at a 1:100 dilution, inhibited a MAb 25% or more, as compared to baseline negative competition controls, then the human serum was considered to have autoantibodies that shared topographically related determinant specificity with that MAb. The value of 25% was selected as the one that gave the best discrimination between adult CLT positive and negative control groups. Although somewhat arbitrary, the 25% value is based on results of competitive inhibition ELISAs of the negative control serum versus each MAb. The average percent inhibition values plus two standard deviations (N = 28) obtained for each MAb inhibited by the negative control serum at a 1:100 dilution ranged from 6.8% for MAb 156A6 to 21.1% for 42C3. Thus, 25% is above the greatest of the average negative control values. The greatest of these values was selected as a conservative criterion of inhibition for all MAbs versus human sera.

Autoantibodies from adult CLT patients demonstrated predominant inhibition of the MAbs to 10 of the 19 determinants on huTg defined by the panel of mouse Abs (Fig. 12). All 10 of these determinants were restricted to huTg (Fig. 7), and none contained T4 or T3 residues (Fig. 11) (55). Eight of these 10 determinants are part of the three overlapping reactivity groups of determinant clusters on huTg that we have previously designated an "immunodominant region" on the basis of the large number of murine MAbs directed towards this region of the huTg molecule (55). Our results indicate, then, that the same region appears

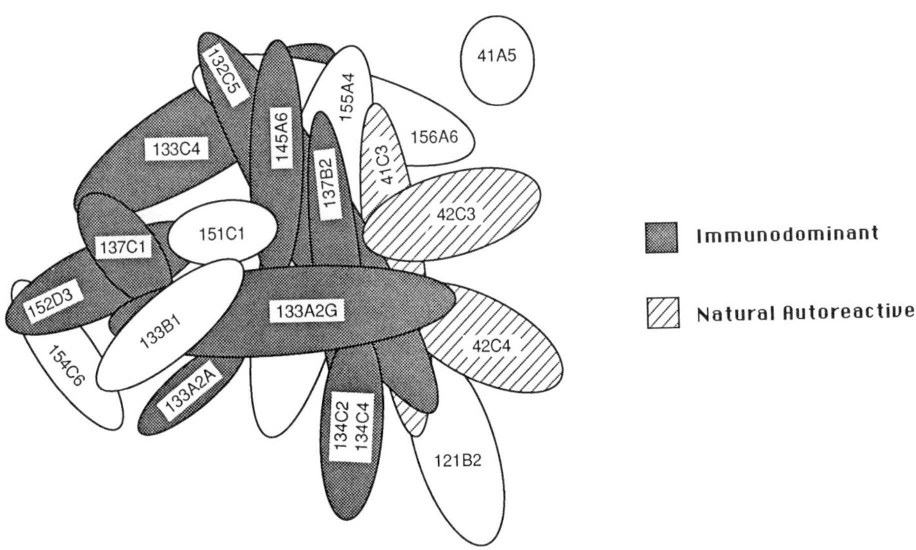

FIGURE 12 Immunodominant regions of HuTg. Based upon the relatively large number of MAbs recognizing these regions, they were designated as immunodominant (see Fig. 8).

to be immunodominant in CLT since 14 of 14 adult patients (100%) had autoantibodies to this region. The serum autoantibodies from 19 juveniles with clinical evidence of CLT reacted predominantly with the same 10 determinants as did the adults with disease. Among juvenile CLT probands, 53% had autoantibodies that recognized at least one of these 10 determinants. Eighty percent of CLT patients, adult and juvenile, that were able to inhibit one or more MAbs recognized determinants in this immunodominant region.

The pattern of determinant reactivities among these unrelated adult CLT patients was remarkably consistent. Out of 280 possible inhibitions (14 patients × 20 MAbs), 131 were found. Of these, 105 inhibitions were of these 10 MAbs. Although the pattern shown by the juvenile probands was more heterogeneous than that seen in the adult CLT patients, 60% of inhibitions (31/50) among juvenile CLT patients were of MAbs defining the 10 principal determinants. As a group, then, 75% (136 of 181) of the total inhibitions by sera from these patients were of these 10 MAbs. The average number of inhibitions of the immunodominant region per reactive juvenile individual was about 2 and, for adults, about 7.

It is important to note that the adult CLT patients also recognize determinants strongly inhibited by T4 and T3 (41C3, 42C3, and 42C4). We have defined Abs to these determinants previously as being naturally autoreactive because of their polyreactivity to all Tgs, their affinity, and most are IgM Abs (55). Six of 14 CLT adults had levels of Tg antibodies sufficient to inhibit these three MAbs. Of the 131 inhibitions shown by these patients, 9 were to this region with an average of about 1 inhibition per each patient. The juvenile patients showed 13 of 50 inhibitions. Together, 60% of patients reacted to these regions of Tg, representing 12% of the inhibitions. As will be seen, this is about the same incidence as in normal individuals (Table 2).

The pattern of determinant recognition among nondiseased control subjects was striking in that very few MAbs were inhibited. The sera from the nondiseased adult control individuals did not inhibit any particular determinant cluster, in contrast to sera from the adult CLT patients, who recognized the same determinants consistently. Only 2 out of 15 normal adults showed reactivity to the immunodominant region, each showing only 1 inhibition of this region. Of 15 unaffected, seronegative juveniles, 9 were able to inhibit 1 or more of the MAbs. Five of these individuals were able to inhibit 1 or more of the immunodominant determinants. In all, only 29% of unaffected, seronegative individuals could inhibit the immunodominant determinants. Out of the 480 possible inhibitions by the 24 reactive individuals, only 34 were found. Seven of these recognized the immunodominant determinants. The average number of inhibitions directed towards the immunodominant region in this population was less than 1 per reactive individual (Table 2).

Between the extremes of the diseased and the normal individual lie individuals who are seropositive (i.e., significant titer) for Tg autoantibodies and individuals

TABLE 2 Ability of Different Populations to Inhibit MAb Binding

Population[a]	No. patients[b] inhibiting MAb	Region inhibited[c] Immunodominant		Natural Ab		Other	
		% Pt[d]	% Inh[e]	% Pt	% Inh	% Pt	% Inh
CLT $n = 33$	30	80	75	60	12	40	13
Seropositive $n = 28$	10	60	63	60	33	10	4
Seronegative $n = 58$	24	29	21	54	70	8	9

[a]Patient populations were divided into CLT = adult and juvenile patients with overt thyroiditis, Seropositive = clinically unaffected and subclinical individuals with significant Tg Ab titer, Seronegative = Probands' family members and normal controls' family members who had no significant Tg Ab titer. n = number of individuals in category tested.
[b]Number of individuals in category capable of inhibiting one or more MAb.
[c]Regions which are defined as immunodominant, to which natural Abs react, and other regions.
[d]Percent of individuals, showing inhibition of MAb, capable of inhibiting MAbs defining this region.
[e]Percent of total inhibitions seen that are of MAb to this region.

who have apparent subclinical disease. Seven siblings of the juveniles with CLT were found in retrospect to have biochemical evidence of hypothyroidism, manifested as abnormally high levels of TSH in their blood. Six of these seven individuals had autoantibodies to Tg, and one had no detectable autoantibodies to Tg. Only three of the seven subclinically affected subjects inhibited the binding of MAbs to Tg. Interestingly, one of the three repeatedly had no detectable autoantibody to Tg by ELISAs or HAs. This individual inhibited only the one MAb defining one of the natural autoantibody determinants. The other two siblings with subclinical disease had autoantibodies to Tg that recognized determinants in the immunodominant region (as defined by the panel of MAbs). Unfortunately, the limited number of cases of subclinical disease and the small numbers of MAbs inhibited by them make interpretation of these results difficult, however, the tendency in seropositive individuals is toward a greater reactivity with the immunodominant region.

It had been shown previously that unaffected siblings of juveniles with CLT had a higher incidence of Tg autoantibodies than did children in unaffected control families (86). This finding was confirmed in the present study. Twenty-three of 37(62%) unaffected siblings of juvenile CLT patients were seropositive, whereas only 8 of 21 (38%) children from control families had autoantibodies to Tg.

The Tg antibodies from seropositive individuals including those above with subclinical disease showed a somewhat intermediate level of reactivity to the 10 principal immunodominant determinants. Six of 10, or 60% of seropositive individuals (unaffected and subclinical seropositive individuals), showed reactivity to the immunodominant region, with 17 of 27 inhibitions to this region. These seropositive individuals also had autoantibodies that reacted with T4- or T3-containing determinants. Sixty percent of reactive individuals inhibited MAbs to this region (Table 2). Nine of 27, or 33% of the inhibitions by antibodies from seropositive normal siblings were directed to T4- or T3-containing determinants.

Seronegative individuals showed a greater tendency to react preferentially with the T4- and T3-containing determinants. Seventy percent of inhibitions of seronegative individuals were with MAbs that defined the T3- or T4-containing determinants. This contrasts with the CLT patients themselves, whose sera recognized T4- or T3-containing determinants in only 12% of the inhibitions. As shown in Table 2, the relative number of inhibitions to the natural Ab sites decreases in the disease state. This likely reflects the change in the immune system during the disease process, where its concern for new, immunodominant epitope becomes its major focus. This is especially evident when the number of diseased and nondiseased individuals are compared in their inhibition of individual MAbs (Fig. 13). Clearly, the immune response in the nondiseased state is primarily toward the natural Ab regions, whereas in the disease state this natural Ab response does not change, but the immune system focuses upon the immunodominant region of Tg and other, apparently weaker determinants.

We feel these data support the view that the autoimmune response becomes more polyclonal as the titer rises encompassing a broader spectrum of determinants. The mature autoimmune response in adults with CLT is highly oligoclonal. In juvenile patients, however, the expansion of this clonality is limited (85). The immune response selects during this maturational process, species-restricted epitopes found in what appears to be a immunodominant region of the molecule. A major question yet to be resolved is whether the juvenile patient's repertoire will expand into that of the adult as that individual matures.

V. DISCUSSION

We have examined in depth three different immune responses to Tg. The mouse anti-mTg response is an example of an induced autoimmune response. The mouse anti-huTg response represents the response of an animal to a foreign antigen. Finally our analysis of the thyroiditis patient is an example of an autoimmune response in spontaneous disease. What is striking to us is the similarity of these responses. In all three, we have identified immunodominant domains on Tg to which a disproportionate number of Abs are directed. These domains appear to be phylogenetically unique since they are not shared by other species. We believe, then, that the Tg molecule is not highly conserved immunologically among species. The lack of reactivity to conserved epitopes outside of those recognized by the

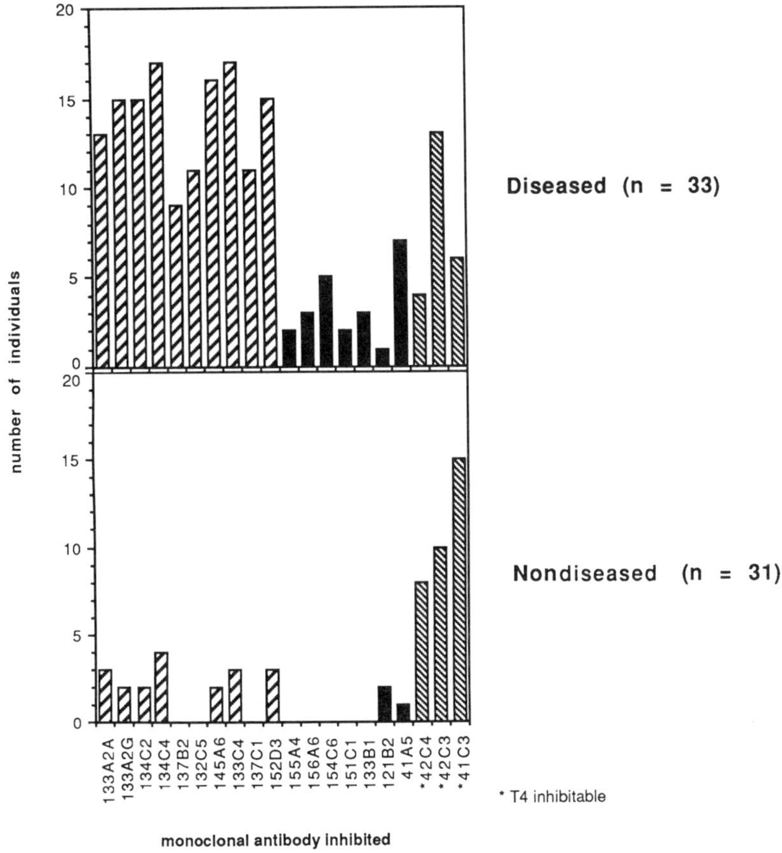

FIGURE 13 Frequency of specific Tg determinants in diseased and nondiseased individuals. The sera from patients with autoimmune thyroiditis inhibited MAbs that bind the immunodominant region (left 10 MAbs). The sera from both diseased and nondiseased individuals recognize the T3/T4 inhibitable natural Ab determinants (right 3 MAbs). Minor determinants of Tg are also recognized (middle 7 MAbs).

natural Ab pool may be a reflection of this. The finding of only 80% sequence homology between human and bovine Tgs also would support this. In the mouse, it appears that even the sequences around the hormonogenic sites are sufficiently different that T3/T4 reactive Abs are restricted by the backbone structure in these regions.

The remainder of the response to Tg is directed either to epitopes that are shared, and mainly identified by the natural Ab pool, or phylogenetically conserved regions of the molecule. The latter, in both the mouse/mouse and mouse/human response, appears to be a relatively minor proportion of the response, as judged by the small number of such Abs found in our mAb panels.

In both the mouse and human antisera, the natural Abs recognize a distinct epitope removed from the immunodominant region. These epitopes appear to be shared among species and likely represent a repetitive epitope as many of these Abs can react with multiple fragments of Tg (Fig. 6) (52,87). As all of our natural Abs are inhibited by thyroid hormone, it would be safe to infer they are recognizing the iodiotyrosine residues on the molecule. However, the polyreactive Abs from the mouse EAT model can react with several other molecules which are not known to be iodinated. One must then question what the Abs are recognizing. We believe because these Ab do not inhibit a large number of other MAbs in the panel, but do cross-inhibit one another, that they do recognize a distinct determinant. The fact that this occurs on CnBr fragments, DNA, insulin, etc. and is inhibitable by thyroid hormones is perplexing. One possibility is that it is seeing a carbohydrate moiety as suggested by the loss of reactivity of these Abs upon ox/red of Tg with periodate. Phosphorylation sites are another possibility especially in the case of anti-DNA reactivity. At present, however, the exact nature of this epitope is unknown.

We return to the question of why the hormonogenic portion of the molecule appears to be the site to which natural Abs are directed. There are several possible explanations for this predilection. First, the hormone-containing fragments are the portions of Tg most frequently in direct contact with the immune system since they are released into the bloodstream. The proteolytic breakdown of Tg into T4 and T3 may also allow the release of associated polypeptide fragments containing T4 or T3. The data indicate that determinant reactivities of the natural autoantibodies may be directed to T4- or T3-containing epitopes, including their immediate neighbors from the Tg molecule. This first explanation suggests that autoimmunization plays a part in the generation of natural autoantibodies. The second explanation grows directly from the issue of autoimmunization. Autoimmunization may occur throughout life, and some theories suggest that it has occurred throughout evolution. Natural autoreactive antibodies, especially those directed against commonly circulating autoantigens, may be necessary for "housekeeping," that is, the transportation and elimination of autoantigens, including products of dead or injured tissues. This could account for observations of the many naturally occurring autoreactive antibodies in normal humans and animals (discussed in Ref. 88). One would expect that if natural autoreactive antibodies are used for housekeeping, it would impose evolutionary pressure in favor of the selection of autoantibodies to the most conserved determinants on the autoantigens. The preference for conserved determinants was indeed observed in the present study.

While there is a unique, immunodominant domain on Tg to which the immune system is attracted, this is not a single epitope. In the mouse/mouse, mouse/human, and human/human (85) situations, the Abs to this region show heterogeneity. In the mouse/mouse response, differences in their ability to be inhibited by other MAbs in the panel and by thyroid hormones, and their immunoglobulin V gene usage, all suggest the Abs are seeing different but likely sterically close epitopes. Similarly, in the mouse/human response, the reciprocal inhibition studies between the Abs (Fig. 8) suggest these Abs also differ in the exact determinant to which they react. Likewise, in the human autoimmune situation, some patients are capable of inhibiting some, but not all members of the MAb panel that define the immunodominant region (85), indicating these sera are reacting with different epitopes within this region.

It is also clear from the results that the panel of MAbs does not completely describe the entire human Tg autoantibody repertoire. There were many patients and normal individuals with titers to Tg whose sera failed to inhibit our panel of MAbs. Clearly, there are autoantigenic determinants on the huTg molecule that are not recognized by any of the MAbs in this panel. The relative role of these in the progression of the disease is presently unknown. While the immunodominant domain we have described appears to be a good indicator of disease, especially in adult CLT patients (85), the high incidence of these antibodies in seropositive individuals, some of whom may never develop thyroiditis, suggests Abs to this region will not necessarily be predictive of disease. Clearly, increasing the size of the MAb pool will allow the detection of new determinants, some possibly being of use in defining individuals at greatest risk for developing full-blown disease.

Genetically, the MHC and immunoglobulin loci may be of importance in directing the Ab response to Tg. The restriction of reactivities to particular autoantigenic determinants may result from particular immune response genes. Class II gene products play an important role in the selection of antigens for presentation to T cells. Those individuals with class II haplotypes capable of presenting thyroid antigens would logically be more predisposed to the development of thyroid autoimmunity and autoimmune thyroid disease. This would account for relationships between HLA-DR types and autoimmune thyroid diseases that have been described by others (89–91). The T-cell help derived from the presentation of self antigens would also likely induce cytotoxic T cells. The involvement of cell-mediated immunity (CMI) in the pathogenesis of thyroiditis is undoubtedly important based on our studies of experimental thyroiditis in mice (92,93). Whether the same immunodominant region is also involved in T-cell responses is presently under investigation.

The data were also examined for evidence of common determinant recognition among members of the same families. Since the propensity to develop autoantibodies to Tg was apparently inherited by the juveniles with CLT and their siblings from their parents (86,94), similar determinant recognition patterns might be predicted. No such pattern of inheritance of autoantibody fine specificity could be discerned. Therefore, the inherited tendency toward thyroid autoimmunity appears to be not primarily due to the inheritance of autoantibody specificities. Likewise, there were no correlations of HLA-A or -B haplotypes with particular specificities of autoantibody. Data about HLA-DR haplotypes are not available at this time.

Our studies in the mouse have not indicated a restricted immunoglobulin gene usage by these autoreactive Abs. The heavy- and light-chain usage of these is derived from several V_H and V_K gene segments using several D and J regions. The size of V gene pool is unknown. The fact that we found two V gene segments repeated (Table 1) in this small sampling may argue that some preference for particular V gene segments may occur. However, at this point, we believe the potential pool is large. We have estimated the frequency of mTg-reactive Abs in mouse at about 1/2500 LPS-responsive B cells (99). The natural Ab pool, which also may have been detected, is also included in this figure. However, we have found that 75% of the clones detected in these limiting dilution assays show no detectable reactivity to huTg. We would suggest from this that the majority of mTg-reactive B cells we detected do not belong to the natural Ab pool. Therefore, the potential number of V genes used in the Tg autoantibody response could be large.

One surprising feature about the MAb panels generated is their lack of cross-species reactivity. It can be shown that sera from animals immunized with heterologous Tg do in fact cross-react with autologous Tg (92,95–97). An explanation for this discrepancy is not totally obvious. One could clearly argue that these cross-reactive Abs belong totally to the natural Ab pool and that immunization, especially with adjuvant, may drive these Abs to be expressed at high levels. The high frequency of heterologous Tg-reactive hybridomas detected by LPS stimulation (98) may be a reflection of this natural Ab pool. The lack of these Abs in the MAb panels may reflect some type of selective process either in terms of B cells that can lead to stable, productive hybridomas, or by the screening process. The latter we do not feel is likely the case, as ELISA assays can detect Abs with low affinities. The isolation of 10VA2 in the mouse/mouse response supports this possibility. This Ab is clearly an anti-DNA Ab with some affinity for mTg. We are presently attempting to generate cross-reactive hybridomas in these systems to examine their specificities in greater detail.

We argue that these cross-reactive Abs are not important in the autoimmune response. This inference comes from our studies of human patients. The autoantibody responses to autologous Tg in humans with CLT are largely, but not completely, restricted to a few determinants on the huTg molecule. These determinants were found only on huTg, indicating that the autoimmune response to Tg in CLT patients is principally directed toward the more recently evolved portions of the molecule. Even though the titers of autoantibodies were different in different patients, the patterns of determinant reactivities were remarkably consistent. The pattern of autoantigenic determinants recognized by sera from subjects without detectable thyroid disease was clearly different from that seen with thyroiditis patients. The nondiseased subjects recognized a higher proportion of determinants that contained T4 or T3, i.e., a natural Ab pool. Natural autoantibodies in individuals without any clinical or biochemical evidence of thyroid disease are generally of low titer and have low affinity. This is reflected in the low-level responses and small numbers of determinant specificities in the normal control families.

A comparison of the adult CLT patients with the juvenile sufferers indicates differences between the immunological responses of these two groups. Adult disease is characterized by high titers of autoantibody to Tg and by a high proportion of antibodies directed to the 10 principal immunodominant determinants. Juveniles with CLT, with few exceptions, tend to have lower autoantibody titers to Tg and fewer reactivities to the 10 principal determinants. It is not clear if these differences reflect the same disease being influenced by the maturational state of the individual, or whether there may exist two forms of disease with different genetic factors and etiological events influencing the onset of disease. The difference between adults and juveniles suggests that the fine specificities of autoantibodies reflect the pathological processes in the thyroid. The autoimmune response becomes more polyclonal as the titer rises, encompassing a broader spectrum of determinants. The mature autoimmune response in adults with CLT is polyclonal. In juvenile patients, however, the expansion of this clonally is limited (85).

Some event, as yet unknown, causes the natural low level of autoimmunity to increase above normal. This increase could probably be detected as an increase in autoantibody titer and in the number of determinants recognized, and may be reflected in the autoantibody status of individuals tested before the onset of thyroiditis. As the pathological processes proceed, there is an increase in the quantity of thyroid autoantibodies, but the determinant specificities of the early autoantibodies are restricted to a very few sites on the Tg molecule, as seen in the subclinical cases of juvenile CLT. These individuals are euthyroid, but already have biochemical indicators of injury to the thyroid gland by the immune system. The inflammatory response grows, and more thyroid gland is destroyed, releasing thyroid autoantigens into the general circulation at a higher rate, and increasing the probability that concentrations of macromolecular autoantigens will reach thresholds necessary for activation of more lymphocytes with higher affinities and different specificities. The juveniles with CLT may be a reflection of this early stage in the disease. The ongoing inflammatory process recruits greater numbers of lymphocytes, which, in turn, increase the overall diversity of the autoantibody response. In later stages of autoimmunity, B cells within the thyroid gland itself could be important antigen-presenting cells for the continued development of disease (62).

Autoantibodies may contribute to the disruption of the gland, freeing more antigen into the circulation, and thus completing the positive feedback loop. The practical limit of such a vicious cycle of autoimmunization would be saturation of every possible determinant on the autoantigens or the total destruction of the gland. However, the immune response is not random, and autoantibody specificity is controlled in such a way that certain determinants are preferred. Predominant specificities would shift toward species-specific determinant reactivities in addition to natural autoreactivity to conserved epitopes. The result of this scenario, carried to its logical conclusion, would be saturation of nearly every immunodominant determinant on the Tg molecule, subject to the built-in restrictions of clonal selection. This situation describes very well the Ab status of the adults with long-standing CLT where virtually every immunodominant epitope is saturated.

REFERENCES

1. Witebsky, E., and Rose, N. R. 1956. Studies on organ specificity IV. Production of rabbit thyroid antibodies in the rabbit. *J. Immunol., 76*: 408–416.
2. Rose, N. R., and Witebsky, E. 1956. Studies on organ specificity. V: Changes in the thyroid glands of rabbit following active immunization with rabbit thyroid extracts. *J. Immunol., 76*: 417–427.
3. Roitt, I. M., Doniach, D., Campbell, P. N., and Hudson, R. V. 1956. V: Autoantibodies in Hashimoto's disease. *Lancet, 2*: 820–821.
4. Van Herle, A. J., Vassart, G., and Dumont, J. E. 1979. Control of thyroglobulin synthesis and secretion. I. *N. Engl. J. Med., 301*: 239–249.
5. Van Herle, A. J., Vassart, G., and Dumont, J. E. 1979. Control of thyroglobulin synthesis and secretion. II. *N. Engl. J. Med., 301*: 307–314.
6. Vassart, G., Refetoff, S., Brocas, H., Dinsart, C., and Dumont, J. E. 1975. Translation of thyroglobulin 33S messenger RNA as a means of determining thyroglobulin quaternary structure. *Proc. Natl. Acad. Sci. USA, 72*: 3839–3843.
7. Vassart, G., Verstreken, L., and Dinsart, C. 1977. Molecular weight of thyroglobulin 33 S messenger RNA as deterined by polyacrylamide gel electrophoresis in the presence of formamide. *FEBS Lett., 79*: 15–18.
8. Vassart, G., and Brocas, H. 1980. Restriction mapping of synthetic thyroglobulin structural gene as a means of investigating thyroglobulin structure. *Biochim. Biophys. Acta, 610*: 189–194.
9. Chebath, J., Chabaud, O., Berge Lefranc, J. L., Cartouzou, G., and Lissitzky, S. 1977. Molecular weight of the thyroglobulin messenger RNA of sheep thyroid gland. *Biochem. Biophys. Res. Commun., 79*: 267–273.
10. Chebath, J., Chabaud, O., Becarevic, A., Cartouzou, G., and Lissitzky, S. 1977. Thyroglobulin messenger ribonucleic acid translation in vitro. *Eur. J. Biochem., 77*: 243–252.
11. Berge Lefranc, J. L., Cartouzou, G., Malthiery, Y., Perrin, F., Jarry, B., and

Lissitzky, S. 1981. Cloning of our DNA fragments complementary to human thyroglobulin messenger RNA. *Eur. J. Biochem.*, *120*: 1–7.

12. van Ommen, G. J., Arnberg, A. C., Baas, F., Brocas, H., Sterk, A., Tegelaers, W. H., Vassart, G., and de Vijlder, J. J. 1983. The human thyroglobulin gene contains two 15-17 kb introns near its 3′-end. *Nucleic Acids Res.*, *11*: 2273-2285.
13. Targovnik, H. M., Pohl, V., Christophe, D., Cabrer, B., Brocas, H., and Vassart, G. 1984. Structural organization of the 5′ region of the human thyroglobulin gene. *Eur. J. Biochem.*, *141*: 271–277.
14. Baas, F., van Ommen, G. J., Bikker, H., Arnberg, A. C., de Vijlder, J. J. 1986. The human thyroglobulin gene is over 300 kb long and contains introns of up to 64 kb. *Nucleic Acids Res.*, *14*: 5171–5186.
15. van Ommen, G. B. J., Baas, B., Arnberg, A. C., Pearson, P. L., and de Vijlder, J. J. M. 1984. Chromosome mapping and polymorphism study of the human thyroglobulin gene. *Cytogenet. Cell Genet.*, *37*: 562.
16. Perry, P., and Wolff, S. 1974. New Giemsa method for the differential straining of sister chromatids. *Nature, 251*: 156–158.
17. Baas, F., Bikker, H., Geurts van Kessel, A., Melsert, R., Pearson, P. L., de Vijlder, J. J., and van Ommen, G. J. 1985. The human thyroglobulin gene: A polymorphic marker localized distral to C-MYC on chromosome 8 band q24. *Hum. Genet.*, *69*: 138–143.
18. Vassart, G., Brocas, H., Cabrer, B., Christophe, D., de Martynoff, G., Leriche, A., Mercken, L., Parma, J., Pohl, V., Targovnik, H., and Van Heuverswyn, B. 1985. Structure and expression of the thyroglobulin gene. In *Thyroglobulin—The Prothyroid Hormone* (M. C. Eggo and G. N. Burrow, eds.). Raven Press, New York, pp. 55–68.
19. Taylor, B. A., and Rowe, L. 1987. The congenital goiter mutation is linked to the thyroglobulin gene in mouse. *Proc. Natl. Acad. Sci., USA, 84*: 1986–1990.
20. Malthiery, Y., and Lissitzky, S. 1987. Primary structure of human thyroglobulin deduced from the sequence of its 8448-base complementary DNA. *Eur. J. Biochem.*, *165*: 491–498.
21. Mercken, L., Simons, M. J., Swillens, S., Massaer, M., and Vassart, G. 1985. Primary structure of bovine thyroglobulin deduced from the sequence of its 8,431-base complementary DNA. *Nature, 316*: 647–651.
22. Durand, J., Malthiery, Y., Chabaud, O., and Lissitzky, S. 1987. C-terminal extremity of ovine thyroglobulin shows strong interspecies homologies. *C R Soc. Biol.* (Paris), *181*: 258-266.
23. Di Lauro, R., Obici, S., Condliffe, D., Ursini, V. M., Musti, A., Moscatelli, C., and Avvedimento, V. E. 1985. The sequence of 967 amino acids at the carboxy-end of rat thyroglobulin. Location and surroundings of two thyroxine-forming sites. *Eur. J. Biochem.*, *148*: 7–11.
24. Schumacher, M., Camp, S., Maulet, Y., Newton, M., MacPhee Quigley, K., Taylor, S. S., Friedman, T., and Taylor, P. 1986. Primary structure of Torpedo californica acetylcholinesterase deduced from its cDNA sequence. *Nature, 319*: 407–409.
25. Koch, N., Lauer, W., Habicht, J., and Dobberstein, B. 1987. Primary structure of the gene for the murine Ia antigen-associated invariant chains (Ii). An

alternatively spliced exon encodes a cysteine-rich domain highly homologous to a repetitive sequence of thyroglobulin. *EMBO J.*, *6*: 1677–1683.
26. Kohno, Y., Naito, N., Hiyama, Y., Shimojo, N., Suzuki, N., Tarutani, O., Niimi, H., Nakajima, H., and Hosoya, T. 1988. Thyroglobulin and thyroid peroxidase share common epitopes recognized by autoantibodies in patients with chronic autoimmune thyroiditis. *J. Clin. Endocrinol. Metab.*, *67*: 899–907.
27. McLachlan, S. M., and Rapoport, B. 1989. Evidence for a potential common T-cell epitope between human thyroid peroxidase and human thyroglobulin with implications for the pathogenesis of autoimmune thyroid disease. *Autoimmunity*, *5*: 101–106.
28. Spiro, M. J. 1977. Presence of a glucuronic acid-containing carbohydrate unit in human thyroglobulin. *J. Biol. Chem.*, *252*: 5424–5430.
29. Herzog, V. 1986. Secretion of sulfated thyroglobulin. *Eur. J. Cell Biol.*, *39*: 399–409.
30. Eggo, M. C., Drucker, D., Cheifetz, F., and Burrow, G. N. 1983. Posttranslational modification of prothyroid hormone. *Can. J. Biochem. Cell. Biol.*, *61*: 662–669.
31. Spiro, M. J., and Gorski, K. M. 1986. Studies on the posttranslational migration and processing of thyroglobulin: use of inhibitors and evaluation of the role of phosphorylation. *Endocrinology*, *119*: 1146–1158.
32. Consiglio, E., Acquaviva, A. M., Formisano, S., Liguoro, D., Gallo, A., Vittorio, T., Santisteban, P., De Luca, M., Shifrin, S., Yeh, H. J., and Kohn, L. D. 1987. Characterization of phosphate residues on thyroglobulin. *J. Biol. Chem.*, *262*: 10304–10314.
33. Yamaoto, K., Tsuji, T., Tarutani, O., and Osawa, T. 1985. Phosphorylated high mannose-type and hybrid-type oligosaccharide chains of human thyroglobulin isolated from malignant thyroid tissue. *Biochim. Biophys. Acta*, *838*: 84–91.
34. Herzog, V., Neumuller, W., and Holzmann, B. 1987. Thyroglobulin, the major and obligatory exportable protein of thyroid follicle cells, carries the lysosomal recognition marker mannose-6-phosphate. *EMBO J.* *6*: 555–560.
35. Czarnocka, B., Ruf, J., Ferrand, M., Carayon, P., and Lissitzky, S. 1985. Purification of the human thyroid peroxidase and its identification as the microsomal antigen involved in autoimmune thyroid diseases. *FEBS Lett.*, *190*: 147–152.
36. Kimura, S., Kotani, T., McBride, O. W., Umeki, K., Hirai, K., and Ohtaki, S. 1987. Human thyroid peroxidase: complete cDNA and protein sequence, chromosome mapping, and identification of two alternately spliced mRNAs. *Proc. Natl. Acad. Sci. USA*, *84*: 5555–5559.
37. Magnusson, R. P., Chazenbalk, G. D., Gestautas, J., Seto, P., Filetti, S., Degroot, L. J., and Rapoport, B. 1987. Molecular cloning of the complementary deoxyribonucleic acid for human thyroid peroxidase. *Mol. Endocrinol.*, *1*: 856–861.
38. Ui, N., Tarutani, O., Kondo, Y., and Tamura, H. 1961. Chromatographic fractionation of hog thyroglobulin. *Nature*, *191*: 1199–1201.
39. Salvatore, G., Salvatore, M., Cahnmann, H. J., and Robbins, J. 1964. Separation of thyroidal iodoproteins and purification of thyroglobulin by gel filtration and density gradient centrifugation. *J. Biol. Chem.*, *239*: 3267–3274.
40. Bouchilloux, S., Rolland, R., Torresani, J., Roques, M., and Lissitzky, S. 1964. Microheterogeneite de la thyroglobulin purification par chromatographie sur diethylaminoethyl cellulose et interpretation. *Biochim. Biophys. Acta*, *93*: 15–30.

41. Lissitzky, S. 1984. Thyroglobulin entering into molecular biology. *J. Endocrinol. Invest.*, *7*: 65–76.
42. Vassart, G., and Dumont, J. E. 1973. Identification of polysomes synthesizing thyroglobulin. *Eur. J. Biochem.*, *32*: 322–330.
43. Palmiter, R. D. 1974. Magnesium precipitation of ribonucleoprotein complexes. Expedient techniques for the isolation of undergraded polysomes and messenger ribonucleic acid. *Biochemistry, 13*: 3606-3615.
44. Di Lauro, R., Obici, S., Acquaviva, A. M., and Alvino, C. G. 1982. Construction of recombinant plasmids containing rat thyroglobulin mRNA sequences. *Gene, 19*: 117–125.
45. Marriq, C., Arnaud, C., Rolland, M., Lissitzky, S. 1980. An approach to the structure of thyroglobulin. Hormone-forming sequences in porcine thyroglobulin. *Eur. J. Biochem.*, *111*: 33–47.
46. Marriq, C., Rolland, M., and Lissitzky, S. 1982. Structure-function relationship in thyroglobulin: Amino acid sequence of two different thyroxine-containing peptides from porcine thyroglobulin. *EMBO J.*, *1*: 397–401.
47. Marriq, C., Rolland, M., and Lissitzky, S. 1983. Amino acid sequence of the unique 3,5,3′-triiodothyronine-containing sequence from porcine thyroglobulin. *Biochem. Biophys. Res. Common.*, *112*: 206–213.
48. Lejeune, P. J., Marriq, C., Rolland, M., and Lissitzky, S. 1983. In vitro and in vivo iodination of human thyroglobulin in relation to hormone release. *FEBS Lett.*, *156*: 77–82.
49. Lamas, L., and Taurog, A. 1977. The importance of thyroglobulin structure in thyroid peroxidase-catalyzed conversion of diiodotyrosine to thyroxine. *Endocrinology, 100*: 1129–1136.
50. Maurizis, J. C., Marriq, C., Michelot, J., Rolland, M., and Lissitzky, S. 1979. Thyroid peroxidase-induced thyroid hormone synthesis in relation to thyroglobulin structure. *FEBS Lett.*, *102*: 82–86.
51. Roitt, I. M., Campbell, P. N.,and Doniach, D. 1958. The nature of the thyroid autoantibodies present in patients with Hashimoto's thyroiditis (lymphadenoid goitre). *Biochem. J.*, *69*: 248–256.
52. Ruf, J., Carayon, P., Sarles-Philip, N. Kourilsky, F., and Lissitzky, S. 1983. Specificity of monoclonal antibodies against human thyroglobulin; comparison with autoimmune antibodies. *EMBO J.*, *2*: 1821–1826.
53. Rose, N. R., Accavitti, M., Pydnyn, E. F., Leon, M. A., and Brown, R. K. 1982. The use of hybridoma antibodies to probe the antigenic determinants of thyroglobulin. *Adv. Exp. Med. Biol.*, *150*: 23–35.
54. Kondo, E., and Kondo, Y. 1984. Monoclonal antibodies to hog thyroglobulin recognizing disulfide-dependent conformational structures. *Mol. Immunol.*, *21*: 581–588.
55. Bresler, H. S., Burek, C. L., and Rose, N. R. 1990. Autoantigenic determinants on human thyroglobulin: I. Determinant specificities of murine monoclonal antibodies. *Clin. Immunol. Immunopathol.*, *54*: 64–75.
56. Himsworth, R. L., Byfield, P. G. H., and Copping, S. 1983. Studies on the antigenicity of human thyroglobulin. *Life Sci.*, *32*: 119–125.

57. Shulman, S., and Witebsky, E. 1960. Studies on organ specificity IX. Biophysical and immunochemical studies on human thyroid autoantibody. *J. Immunol., 85*: 559–567.
58. Piechaczyk, M., Bouanani, M., Salhi, S. L., Baldet, L., Bastide, M., Pau, B., and Bastide, J-M. 1987. Antigenic domains on the human thyroglobulin molecule recognized by autoantibodies in patients' sera and by natural autoantibodies isolated from the sera of healthy subjects. *Clin. Immunol. Immunopathol., 45*: 114–121.
59. Kotani, T., Maeda, M., Ohtaki, S., Kobayashi, S., and Okuyama, H. 1985. Analyses of the specificity of mouse monoclonal antibodies to syngeneic and allogeneic thyroglobulins. *Clin. Immunol. Immunopathol., 34*: 147–157.
60. Esquivel, P. S., Rose, N. R., and Kong, Y. C. 1977. Induction of autoimmunity in good and poor responder mice with mouse thyroglobulin and lipopolysaccharide. *J. Exp. Med., 145*: 1250–1263.
61. Bagchi, N., Brown, T. R., Urdanivia, E., and Sundick, R. S. 1985. Induction of autoimmune thyroiditis in chickens by dietary iodine. *Science, 230*: 325–327.
62. Champion, B., Hutchings, P., Rayner, D., Page, K., Byfield, P., Chan, J., Roitt, I., and Cooke, A. 1987. Autoantigenicity of murine thyroglobulin. In *Thyroid Autoimmunity* (A. Pinchera, S. H. Ingbar, J. M. McKenzie, and G. F. Fenzi, eds.). Plenum Press, New York, pp. 181–187.
63. Tajiri, J., Higashi, K., Morita, M., Umeda, T., and Sato, T. 1986. Studies of hypothyroidism in patients with high iodine intake. *J. Clin. Endocrinol. Metab., 63*: 412–417.
64. Casali, P., Prabhakar, B. S., and Notkins, A. L. 1988. Characterization of multireactive autoantibodies and identification of Leu-1 + B lymphocytes as cells making antibodies binding multiple self and exogenous molecules. *Int. Rev. Immunol., 3*: 17–45.
65. Rose, N. R., Accavitti, M., Pydyn, E. F., Leon, M. A., and Brown, R. K. 1982. The use of hybridoma antibodies to probe the antigenic determinants of thyroglobulin. In *Immunobiology of Proteins and Peptides-II* (M. Z. Atassi, ed.). Plenum Publishing Corporation, New York, pp. 23–35.
66. Guilbert, B., Dighiero, G., and Avrameas, S. 1982. Naturally occurring antibodies against nine common antigens in human sera. I. Detection, isolation and characterization. *J. Immunol., 128*: 2779–2787.
67. Gleason, S. L., Gearhart, P., Rose, N. R., and Kuppers, R. C. 1990. Autoantibodies to thyroglobulin are encoded by diverse V-gene segments and recognize restricted epitopes. *J. Immunol., 145*: 1768–1775.
68. Heinrich, G., Traunecker, A., and Tonegawa, S. 1984. Somatic mutation creates diversity in the major group of mouse immunoglobulin k light chain. *J. Exp. Med., 159*: 417–435.
69. Khangure, M. S., Dingle, P. R., Stephenson, J., Bird, T., Hall, R., and Evered, D. C. 1977. A long-term follow up of patients with autoimmune thyroid disease. *Clin. Endocrinol.* (Oxf), *6*: 41–48.
70. Aho, K., Gordin, A., Sievers, K., and Takala, J. 1983. Thyroid autoimmunity in siblings: a population study. *Acta Endocrinol.* [Suppl] (Copenh), *251*: 11–15.
71. Bigazzi, P. E., and Rose, N. R. 1985. Autoimmune thyroid disease. In *The*

Autoimmune Diseases (N. R. Rose and I. R. MacKay, eds.). Academic Press, Inc., New York, pp. 161–199.

72. Mori, T., and Kriss, J. P. 1971. Measurements by competitive binding radioassay of serum anti-microsomal and anti-thyroglobulin antibodies in Graves' disease and other thyroid disorders. *J. Clin. Endocrinol. Metab.*, *33*: 688–698.
73. Scherbaum, W. A., Stockle, G., Wichmann, J., and Berg, P. A. 1982. Immunological and clinical characterization of patients with untreated euthyroid and hypothyroid autoimmune thyroiditis. Antibody spectrum, response to TRH and clinical study. *Acta Endocrinol.* (Cophen), *100*: 373–381.
74. Rose, N. R.,and Stylos, W. A. 1969. Splitting of human thyroglobulin. I. Reduction and alkylation. *Clin. Exp. Immunol.*, *5*: 129–140.
75. Stylos, W. A., and Rose, N. R. 1969. Splitting of human thyroglobulin. II. Enzymatic digestion. *Clin. Exp. Immunol.*, *5*: 285–297.
76. Stylos, W. A., and Rose, N. R. 1977. Splitting of human thyroglobulin. IV. The antigenicity of the pepsin-derived fragments. *Clin. Exp. Immunol.*, *27*: 245–253.
77. Metzger, H., Sharp, G. C., and Edelhoch, H. 1962. The properties of thyroglobulin VII. The immunologic activity of thyroglobulin fragments. *Biochemistry*, *1*: 205–214.
78. Mates, G. P., and Shulman, S. 1968. Studies on thyroid proteins. IV. Haemagglutinating activity of molecular fragments of human thyroid proteins. *Immunology*, *14*: 89–98.
79. Ruf, J., Carayon, P., and Lissitzky, S. 1985. Various expressions of a unique anti-human thyroglobulin antibody repertoire in normal state and autoimmune disease. *Eur. J. Immunol.*, *15*: 268–272.
80. Piechaczyk, M., Chardes, T., Cot, M-C., Pau, B., and Bastide, J-M. 1985. Production and characterization of monoclonal antibodies against human thyroglobulin. *Hybridoma*, *4*: 361–367.
81. Figuet, B., Djavadi Ohaniance, L., and Goldberg, M. E. 1984. Some monoclonal antibodies raised with a native protein bind preferentially to the denatured antigen. *Mol. Immunol.*, *21*: 673–677.
82. Kurata, A., Ohta, K., Mine, M., Fukuda, T., Ikari, N., Kanazawa, H., Matsunaga, M., Izumi, M., and Nagataki, S. 1984. Monoclonal antihuman thyroglobulin antibodies. *J. Clin. Endocrinol. Metab.*, *59*: 573–579.
83. Bellet, D., Schlumberger, M., Bidart, J. M. Assicot, M., Caillou, B., Motte, P., Vignal, A., and Bohuon, C. 1983. Production and *in vitro* utilization of monoclonal antibodies to human thyroglobulin. *J. Clin. Endocrinol. Metab.*, *56*: 530–533.
84. Chan, C. T. J., Byfield, P. G. H., Himsworth, R. L., and Shepherd, P. 1987. Human autoantibodies to thyroglobulin are directed towards a restricted number of human specific epitopes. *Clin. Exp. Immunol.*, *69*: 516–523.
85. Bresler, H. S., Burek, C. L., Hoffman, W. H., and Rose, N. R. Autoantigenic Determinants on Human Thyroglobulin: II. Determinants recognized by autoantibodies from patients with chronic autoimmune thyroiditis compared to autoantibodies from healthy subjects. *Clin. Immunol. Immunopathol.*, *54*: 76–86.
86. Burek, C. L., Hoffman, W. H., and Rose, N. R. 1982. The presence of thyroid autoantibodies in children and adolescents with autoimmune thyroid disease and in their siblings and parents. *Clin. Immunol. Immunopathol.*, *25*: 395–404.

87. de Baets, M. H., Theunissen, R., Kok, K., de Vijlder, J. J. M., and van Breda Vriesman, P. J. C. 1987. Monoclonal antibodies to human thyroglobulin as probes for thyroglobulin structure. *Endocrinology, 120*: 1104–1111.
88. Dighiero, G., Lymberi, P., Guilbert, B., Ternynck, T., and Avrameas, S. 1986. Natural autoantibodies constitute a substantial part of normal circulating immunoglobulins. In *Autoimmunity: Experimental and Clinical Aspects* (R. S. Schwartz and N. R. Rose, eds.). The New York Academy of Sciences, New York, pp. 135–145.
89. Farid, N. R., Sampson, L., Noel, E. P., Barnard, J. M., Mandeville, R., Larsen, B., Marshall, W. H., and Carter, N. D. 1979. A study of human leukocyte D locus related antigens in Graves' disease. *J. Clin. Invest., 63*: 108–113.
90. Weissel, M., Hofer, R., Zasmeta, H., and Mayr, W. R. 1980. HLA-DR and Hashimoto's thyroiditis. *Tissue Antigens, 16*: 256–257.
91. Farid, N. R., Sampson, L., Moens, H., and Barnard, J. M. 1981. The association of goitrous autoimmune thyroidits with HLA-DR5. *Tissue Antigens, 17*: 265–268.
92. Simon, L. L., Justen, J. M., Giraldo, A. A., Krco, C. J.,and Kong, Y. C. 1986. Activation of cytotoxic T cells and effector cells in experimental autoimmune thyroiditis by shared determinants of mouse and human thyroglobulins. *Clin. Immunol. Immunopathol., 39*: 345–356.
93. Kuppers, R. C., Neu, N., and Rose, N. R. 1988. Animal models of autoimmune thyroid disease. In *Immunogenetics of Endocrine Disorders* (N. R. Fand, ed.). Alan R. Liss, Inc., New York, pp. 111–131.
94. Burek, C. L., Rose, N. R., Najar, G. M., Gimelfarb, A., Zmijewski, C. M., Polesky, H. F., and Hoffman, W. H. 1984. Autoimmune thyroid disease. In *Clinical Immunology,* Volume 1—*Immunogenetics* (C. David and G. S. Panayi, eds.). Butterworth & Co., Ltd., Kent, pp. 207–233.
95. Rose, N. R., Twarog, F. J., and Crowle, A. J. 1971. Murine thyroiditis: importance of adjuvant and mouse strain for the induction of thyroid lesions. *J. Immunol., 106*: 698–704.
96. Clagett, J. A., and Weigle, W. O. 1974. Roles of T and B lymphocytes in the termination of unresponsiveness to autologous thyroglobulin in mice. *J. Exp. Med., 139*: 643–660.
97. Romball, C. G., and Weigle, W. O. 1983. T and B cell reactivity in experimental autoimmune thyroiditis. *Life Sci., 32*: 127–138.
98. Souroujon, M., White-Scharf, M. E., Andre-Schwartz, J., Gefter, M., and Schwartz, R. S. 1988. Preferential autoantibody reactivity of the preimmune B cell repertoire in normal mice. *J. Immunol., 140*: 4173–4179.
99. Kuppers, R. C. 1991. The fequency of LPS-responsive B cells to autologous and heterologous thyroglobulin. *Cell. Immunol., 132*: 94–101.
100. Monestier, M., Manheimer-Lory, A., Bellon, B., Painter, C., Dang, H., Talal, N., Zanetti, M., Schwartz, R., Pisetsky, D., Kuppers, R., Rose, N., Brochier, J., Klareskog, L., Holmdahl, R., Erlanger, B., Alt, F., and Bona, C. 1986. Shared idiotopes and restricted immunoglobulin variable region heavy chain genes characterize murine autoantibodies of various specificities. *J. Clin. Invest., 78*: 753–759.

15

Chronic Infections and Autoimmunity

M. Abu-Shakra
Soroka Medical Center, Beer-Sheva, Israel

Y. Shoenfeld
Sheba Medical Center, Tel-Hashomer, Israel

I. INTRODUCTION

The term "autoimmune" is applied to a wide spectrum of diseases in which the immune system damages otherwise normal components of the individual. One of the hallmarks of autoimmune disorders is the presence of autoantibodies and/or self-reacting cells. However, the occurrence of these autoantibodies or cells is not sufficient to induce autoimmune diseases. Furthermore, their presence even in high titers is not necessarily associated with apparent disease. For example, high concentrations of autoantibodies can be measured in healthy family members of patients with autoimmune diseases (1–3) as well as in patients with monoclonal gammopathies (4–6) who have no clinical manifestations of autoimmunity. Similarly, potentially virulent autoimmune T cells have been isolated from lymphoid tissues of seemingly healthy experimental animals (7–9).

Therefore, it is clear that besides the presence of self-recognizing cells or autoantibodies, other factors are necessary. Among those factors are immune defects (complement component deficiencies, suppressor T-cell defects), hormonal constellation (high estrogen levels), genetic background (HLA DR2, DR3, or DR4 or Gm allotypes), and environmental elements (10–13).

The appearance of a trigger mechanism in an individual with the "proper" immunologic, genetic, and hormonal background may lead to the development of an overt autoimmune disease. Such a trigger mechanism may be a common and ubiquitous one. The environmental factors may act as a trigger mechanism. The major environmental agents include the sun (14) (which may alter an autoantigen by UV radiation), drugs (15), and infections (16).

The association between infectious agents and autoimmune disorders was reported with acute infections as well as with infections with a chronic course. Observations that link acute infections and autoimmune phenomena include the temporal relationship between a specific infection and the appearance of disease, for example, the appearance of rheumatic fever following streptococcal infection (17) and the onset of diabetes mellitus type I following mumps or coxsackievirus infection (18,19). Infectious agents were also found to be related to the etiology of chronic rheumatic disease, including reactive arthritis (Reiter's disease, psoriatic arthritis, and the arthritis associated with inflammatory bowel disease), ankylosing spondylitis, Lyme disease, and rheumatoid arthritis. This issue has recently been reviewed (16,20). Furthermore, there are many viral, bacterial, and parasitic infections which are frequently associated with the appearance of autoantibodies in the host (16). Autoantibodies including rheumatoid factor, anti-DNA, anticardiolipin, and anti–red blood cells were detected in the sera of healthy animals immunized with viral or bacterial products (21), as well as by the incubation of normal peripheral blood lymphocytes with bacterial components such as lipopolysaccharide (22–24).

Recently, Shoenfeld and Cohen (16) reviewed the association between acute infectious diseases and autoimmunity. In this chapter we will review the evidence implicating certain chronic infectious agents as triggering events in the breakdown of tolerance and the appearance of autoimmune diseases. We will discuss mainly the association between autoimmunity and tuberculosis, syphilis, AIDS, malaria, *Leishmania*, and schistosomiasis.

II. MYCOBACTERIAL AUTOANTIBODIES AND AUTOIMMUNITY

The most pathogenic bacteria of the genous mycobacterium are *Mycobacterium tuberculosis* and *M. leprae*, which induce tuberculosis and leprosy, respectively. Tuberculosis is a chronic infection characterized by the formation of granulomas in infected tissues. The usual site of disease is the lungs, but other organs may be involved. On the other hand, leprosy is a chronic granulomatous infection which attacks superficial tissues, especially the skin and peripheral nerves.

Several autoantibodies were detected in the sera of patients with *M. tuberculosis* and *M. leprae* infections. Among these antibodies one can find antinuclear factor (25), rheumatoid factor (26,27), anticardiolipin, anti-DNA (25–27), and antibodies against synthetic polynucleotides (27). The diversity of autoantibodies in the sera of patients infected with mycobacteria is not limited to nuclear components, extending to erythrocytes (28), thyroglobulin (29), and spermatozoa (30). Table 1 shows the incidence of autoantibodies in the sera of patients with tuberculosis.

Monoclonal anti-Tb antibodies were found to bind to ssDNA, as well as to other polynucleotides (31). The binding of the anti-TB antibodies to ssDNA could be inhibited by prior incubation of these monoclonal antibodies with ssDNA and various polynucleotides. It was also found that hybridoma-derived monoclonal anti-DNA antibodies from humans and mice with SLE reacted with three mycobacterial cell wall glycolipids shared by all mycobacteria. These autoantibodies and the monoclonal anti-TB antibodies competed with each other on their binding to ssDNA, and several of the anti-TB antibodies carried a common anti-DNA idiotype (16/6 Id) (31). This idiotype appears to be important clinically. Its titer correlates with disease activity in patients with SLE (32), and recently we induced an SLE-like syndrome by serial injections of this idiotype in murine strains that are not susceptible to spontaneous autoimmune diseases (33,34).

Further studies show that 60% of sera of patients with active tuberculosis had increased levels of the 16/6 Id compared to only 1 out of 28 matched controls (27).

Recently, we found a high incidence (22%) of anti-TB glycolipids antibodies in sera of patients with monoclonal gammopathies (35), some of which show anti-DNA and other antinuclear antigens activities. This is an additional evidence for the mycobacterial-nuclear antigens cross-reactivity, which may suggest a possible role of infection in autoimmune conditions.

The reactivity of sera from some patients with SLE to three glycolipids derived from *M. bovis* membranes was comparable to the response seen with the sera of patients with active tuberculosis. However, a subset of patients was found to have extremely low levels, even below those recorded in a group of normal healthy controls. This group of patients had cerebritis (36). All these findings lead to a suggestive antigenic mimicry existing between mycobacterial and cerebral glycolipids (37), and these data are supported by a recent study demonstrating the binding of mouse monoclonal anti-*M. tuberculosis* antibodies to brain, reacting as antineuronal antibodies and by the ability of mycobacterial glycolipids to inhibit the reaction between brain tissue and antineuronal antibodies derived from sera of patients with SLE and cerebritis (38).

These studies emphasize the pathogenic role of cross-reactive antimycobacterial antibodies and antineuronal antibodies in SLE, especially among patients with an associated neuropsychiatric disease (37). These autoantibodies may penetrate the central nervous system via a "leaky" blood-brain barrier damaged by a vasculitic process entailing a cytopathic effect on brain tissue.

Another association between autoimmunity and tuberculosis was detected by studying the immunoglobulin structure. An essential feature of IgG is the conserved N-glycosylation site in their CH_2 domains at position ASn297. The oligosaccharide units attached at this site interact with each other and help to

TABLE 1 Autoantibodies Detected in the Sera of Patients with Mycobacterial Infection

Autoantibody	Incidence	Ref.
Antinuclear factor	46%	25
Rheumatoid factor	10–40%	25–27
Anticardiolipin	5–10%	25–27
Anti-ssDNA	30%	27
Anti-DNA idiotype (16/6) Id	60%	27
Anti-RBC	rare	28
Antithyroglobulin	rare	29
Antispermatozoa	rare	30

maintain the structural relationship between the heavy chains. It was found (39) that the IgG from patients with rheumatoid arthritis (RA) had an increased number of oligosaccharide moieties whose outer arms lack galactose and terminate in N-acetylglucosamine residue. This truncation exposes portions of IgG Fc usually concealed by the overlying oligosaccharides. The truncated oligosaccharides may also make the IgG "sticky" through a lectin-like effect.

In studies of over 30 different autoimmune and infectious diseases, only patients with tuberculosis (TB) and Crohn's disease have an identical defect (40). Enzymatic studies have revealed that various lymphocytes subpopulations in patients with RA and Crohn's disease have significant abnormalities of the enzyme galactosyltransferase, compared with healthy normal controls. In RA patients, enzyme activity was significantly reduced in B cells but normal in T cells. In contrast, in the patients with TB and Crohn's disease, enzyme activity was impaired in both T and B cells (41).

Cellular studies revealed that a T-cell clone specific for *M. tuberculosis* which was arthritogenic, recognized antigens present in human synovial fluid, chondrocyte culture medium, and proteoglycans purified from cartilage (42). The clinical importance of molecular mimicry between myobacteria and self antigen was highlighted by the report that patients treated with BCG immunotherapy developed severe arthritis (43). In animals it was found that some rat strains developed an autoimmune-like arthritis after immunization with *M. tuberculosis* (44), and the arthritis can be transferred to unimmunized rats by T-cell clones from immunized rats or by T-cell clones such as the A2 clone. A subclone of this, A2B, responded to both *M. tuberculosis* and to the core protein part of a proteoglycan antigen in cartilage. Another clone, A2C, did not induce arthritis, but was protective and seemed to act as suppressor-inducer of T cells. Both the A2B and A2C clones recognized the 65 kD antigen from *M. bovis* BCG, which is a heat shock protein (HSP).

The HSP related to homologous proteins in higher eukaryotes as well as in bacteria (45). Self-epitopes present in stress proteins could be necessary by-products of their phylogenetic conservation. Antigens cross-reactivity with the 65 kD *M. bovis* BCG protein are present in some mycobacteria (44), and this antigen is also related to another antigen shared by more than 50 different bacterial species including Klebsiella, Shigella, Salmonella, Yersinia, and Campylobacter, all suspected of being involved in human arthritis (44–46).

Human studies showed that peripheral blood T lymphocytes from patients with RA bind to purified protein derivative (PPD), although they responded poorly to other mitogens such as phytohaemagglutinin and pokeweed mitogen (47). Holoshitz et al. (48) found that sera of patients with rheumatoid arthritis react with an acetone-precipitable fraction of *M. tuberculosis*, which cross-reacts with human cartilage. RA patients had more pronounced T-cell responses to the antigen than patients with degenerative joint diseases or healthy controls.

Waxman (49) found that tuberculin test responsiveness was decreased in rheumatoid arthritis patients. Bahar et al. (50) reported that responses to four new tuberculins—tuberculin, leprosin A, scrofalin, and vaccine—were found to be significantly reduced in 46 patients with RA in comparison with a control group. Except for tuberculin itself, the same was found in 111 patients with tuberculosis. This similarity suggests that similar regulatory mechanisms may control the responses to tuberculins in RA and tuberculosis (51). HLA studies showed that rheumatoid patients with the HLA-DR4 haplotype, which is known to be associated with RA, had significantly greater responses to all four reagents than did non-DR4 patients.

Ottenhoff (51) found that HLA-DR4 was associated with high responsiveness to tuberculin tests in patients with leprosy, similar to HLA-DR4 positive RA patients. Bahar et al. (50) postulated that the immunopathology of RA is similar to that of mycobacterial infection, and a contact with environmental mycobacteria may regulate a tissue-damaging immune response directed at antigenic determinants common to joint tissue and mycobacteria.

To summarize, mycobacterial infection induces with autoimmune disorders through antigeninc similarity between the host antigens and mycobacteria. However, although autoimmune phenomena are frequent in mycobacterial infection, only in those patients with the "proper" immunogenetic background (e.g., HLA-DR4) will autoimmune disease ensue after the infection.

III. SYPHILIS AND AUTOIMMUNITY

Syphilis is a chronic systemic infection caused by *Treponema pallidum* and characterized by a primary lesion associated with regional lymphadenopathy followed by a secondary bacteremic stage associated with generalized mucocutaneous lesions and generalized lymphadenopathy and, in about one third of untreated cases, a tertiary stage characterized by progressive destructive mucocutaneous, musculoskeletal, parenchymal lesions, or central nervous system disease.

A role of circulating immune complexes (CICs) in the pathogenesis of secondary syphilis has been postulated both in human diseases (52) and in animal models (53). CICs were detected in the sera of patients with syphilis (54) as well as in sera of rabbits with experimental secondary syphilis (53,55). These complexes have been implicated in the pathogenesis of the glomerulonephritis that may complicate human secondary syphilis (56). Jorizzo et al. (57) studied nine subjects with active secondary syphilis. All patients tested had CICs on Clq or Raji cell assay. *Treponema pallidum*-specific antigens were detected in CICs. Biopsy of early cutaneous lesions revealed immunoreactants (IgG,C3) in three of nine subjects and treponemal antigens in six of eight subjects. *T. pallidum* antigens and IgG have been demonstrated in glomeruli in the rare glomerulonephritis that accompanies secondary syphilis (56,57). In addition, the histopathologic findings of leukocytoclastic vasculitis in the early lesions of secondary syphilis (58) and the decreased complement levels (CH_{50}, C3) (59) all support a CICs-mediated pathogenesis for lesions in human secondary syphilis.

On the other hand, the importance of endogenous antigens, such as those that develop as part of an autoimmune response in SLE (60), made it difficult to discount the possibility that CICs in syphilis represent only a by-product of the infection. Infection-induced tissue destruction may give rise to altered host antigens that in turn could invoke autoimmune phenomena (61).

Isolation of CICs from reactive sera by polyethylene glycol precipitation followed by anti-Clq affinity chromatography, and immunoblot assays revealed that beside IgG, C3, Clq, and treponemal antigens, fibronectin, fibronectin-binding protein, fibronectin degradation products, and antifibronectin autoantibodies were consistently present in most of the complexes (62–64).

Fibronectin, a molecule capable of interacting with many cell types, has binding sites for collagen, heparin, fibrin, and several microorganisms, including treponema antigens (64). It also has a possible opsonic role in promoting phagocytosis (65).

Antifibronectin antibodies were detected in the CICs and sera of patients with secondary syphilis (66). The mechanism(s) of the production of these autoantibodies could be related to (1) conformational changes that occur as a result of binding to treponemas, or (2) primary complexes treponema–antitreponemal antibody and the complement component Clq may bind fibronectin in such a way that hidden epitopes on the molecule are subjected to antigen processing and, in turn, lead to the formation of "secondary" complexes composed of fibronectin degradation products and antifibronectin autoantibodies (64,67).

In humans, the role of these CICs in processing tissue damage is not well defined. However, animal studies (68,69) demonstrated damage to glomerular basement membranes after immunization with denatured fibronectin. These findings suggest that the relation between the nephrotic syndrome in secondary syphilis and CICs is less than casual, and additional work is needed to clarify this issue.

Besides the presence of antifibronectin antibodies, several autoantibodies have been detected in the sera of patients with syphilis. In addition to anticardiolipin autoantibodies (70), antibodies have been demonstrated to laminin and collagen (66), IgG (rheumatoid factor) (71), and muscle creatine kinase (72). Table 2 shows the autoantibodies reported in the sera of patients with syphilis.

The mechanism of anticreatine kinase (anti-CK) autoimmune response is not known. It is possible that CK, like cardiolipin, is released from affected mitochrondia of mammalian cells (72). The release of normally sequestered host enzyme may give rise to the formation of autoantibodies. Alternatively, *T. pallidum* may act as an adjuvant or carrier in sensitization against the creatine-kinase (72). The significance of these autoantibodies in the clinical manifestations of syphilis is not clear. However, a number of observations of human syphilis suggest that autoimmune reactions may participate in the development of pathogenic lesions. It was found that early dermal lesions are paralleled by the appearance of anticardiolipin antibodies and the titer of these autoantibodies decreases with the resolution of the skin rashes (73). These observations suggest that syphilitic dermal lesions may result from autoimmune reactions to host antigens. However, *T. pallidum*-mediated toxicity (74) caused by endotoxin-like activity cannot be excluded.

Anticardiolipin antibodies were reported in several autoimmune diseases. However, antiphospholipid antibodies from patients with syphilis bind cardiolipin but exhibit little cross-reactivity with negatively charged phospholipids. On the other hand, antibodies to phospholipids from patients with autoimmune disorders exhibited little or no binding to the VDRL antigen, but cross-reacted with both cardiolipin and negatively charged phospholipids (76).

The role of autoimmune response in the immunity-inducing process in syphilis is a challenge for further investigation.

TABLE 2 Autoantibodies Detected in the Sera of Patients with Syphilis

Autoantibody	Ref.
Anticardiolipin	70
Rheumatoid factor	71
Anti–creatine kinase	72
Antifribronectin	62–64
Antilaminin	66
Anticollagen	66
Antilymphocytic	75

IV. AIDS AND AUTOIMMUNITY

The acquired immunodeficiency syndrome (AIDS) is a consequence of infection with the human immunodeficiency virus (HIV). Patients diagnosed with AIDS exhibit qualitative and quantitative defects in helper T lymphocytes, causing impaired cell-mediated immunity. The spectrum of the clinical manifestations of this syndrome includes opportunistic infections (*Pneumocystis carinii* pneumonia, *Mycobacterium avium*, and cytomegalovirus infection), Kaposi's sarcoma, lymphoid neoplasms, neuropsychiatric disease, and other disorders (77).

The pathogenesis of acquired immunodeficiency syndrome (AIDS) is not well known despite intensive research in recent years. Ziegler and Stites (78) proposed the hypothesis that human immunodeficiency virus triggers an autoimmune response of the immune system, a "host vs. host" reaction, and that AIDS is an autoimmune disease directed at the immune system. They based their hypothesis on the assumption that HIV binds to CD4 molecules of helper T lymphocytes and imitates the class II MHC antigen, which is the normal ligand for this receptor. As a result of this binding, the normal immune response to the HIV would then recognize and cross-react to "self," i.e., class II–bearing cells. An anti-idiotypic response to the CD4 antigen ensues, with consequent disruption of communication between CD4 lymphocytes and antigen-processing cells. This hypothesis was supported by clinical and serologic findings. Patients with AIDS can present clinical manifestations of autoimmune diseases including fever, rash, lymphadenopathy, renal dysfunction, and neurologic disorders (77,78). Furthermore, several hematologic abnormalities widely recognized in AIDS patients (79) currently appear to be autoimmune in nature.

Several autoantibodies were reported in AIDS, including anti-RBC (80), antineutrophil (81), antiplatelet (82), and antilymphocyte (83). These autoantibodies were found to bind to the target cells and induce anemia, neutropenia, thrombocytopenia, and lymphopenia, respectively. Table 3 shows the autoantibodies reported in the sera of patients with AIDS.

Indirect support for this hypothesis is obtained upon comparison of SLE and AIDS (84). Both diseases exhibit normal B cell numbers with polyclonal B-cell activation, manifested by hypergammaglobulinemia, presence of ANA, rheumatoid factor, anti-idiotypic antibodies (85), and CICs with IgG, IgA, and IgM (87–89). The CICs have also been implicated in the clinical manifestations of immune thrombocytopenic purpura (ITP) and hemolytic anemia, which are frequently observed in SLE and AIDS (81,90). Impaired T-cell activity, as indicated by delayed hypersensitivity skin test anergy (87,91) and reduced T-cell proliferative response to mitogens (91), was also detected in both diseases. However, in AIDS there is a reduction in T-helper cells, while T-suppressor cells are functionally normal, as opposed to their decreased number and function in some patients with active SLE (91).

TABLE 3 Autoantibodies in the Sera of Patients with AIDS

Autoantibody	Ref.
Antinuclear antibody	85
Rheumatoid factor	85
Antiplatelets	82
Anti–red blood cells	80
Antilymphocytes	83
Antineutrophils	81
Antisperm	86

Two additional findings draw the parallel between AIDS and SLE even closer and further substantiate the claim that AIDS is an autoimmune disease. The first is the presence of natural autoantibodies (92) and the second is a high incidence of SLE patients found to harbor antibodies to HIV and HTLV-I (93), implicating a viral etiology of SLE.

Finally, AIDS patients are characterized by their ability to produce acid-labile alpha-interferon (94). The only other disease states associated with this interferon are autoimmune diseases, including rheumatoid arthritis, vasculitis, and SLE (95,96). The role of the interferon is not clear; it may be associated with the above-mentioned impaired lymphocyte function (97) and the high levels of beta-2-microglobulin in serum from patients with AIDS and SLE (98).

Table 4 summarizes the common immunologic features in AIDS and SLE. However, all of these evidences are merely "circumstantial" and far from conclusive, certainly regarding the clinical and serological aspects of the disease. While HIV infection has been associated with each of the clinical manifestations of AIDS (95), an immunologic mechanism has been implicated as well, and the evidence remains insufficient to claim autoimmune pathogenesis.

The mechanism(s) of B-cell activation and hyperglobulinemia in AIDS could be explained by (102):

1. Known polyclonal activator (PBA) such as cytomegalovirus or Epstein-Barr virus.
2. HIV itself could act as a PBA without infecting B cells.
3. T cells from HIV subjects may be acting as PBA.
4. The HIV-related decline in T-cell number and/or function may also lead to loss of regulatory T-cell function, allowing B-cell hyperactivity to go unleashed.

However, the pronounced humoral and cellular dysfunction may be explained by alternative immunologic mechanisms of autoantibody production, via the web of connections between idiotypes, anti-idiotypes, and normal cellular components.

TABLE 4 Common Immunologic Features in AIDS and SLE

Immunologic feature	Ref.
B-cell activation	85
Increased immune complexes	89
Increased levels of beta-2-microglobulin	98
Acid-labile α-interferon production	94
Decreased lymphokine production (IL_1, IL_2)	99
Decreased natural killer cell activity	99,100
Lymphopenia	88,100
Lymphocytotoxic antibodies	
Decreased response to mitogens	91
Skin test anergy	87,91
Natural autoantibody production	101

Anti-idiotype antibodies, inherent components of immunoregulatory network, may arise following viral infection and may cross-react with self-antigens, resulting in autoimmunity (10).

V. MALARIA AND AUTOIMMUNITY

Malaria is a protozoan disease transmitted to humans by the bite of *Anopheles* mosquitoes. It is characterized by fever, rigors, splenomegaly, anemia, and chronic relapsing course. The humoral response to malaria in humans is characterized by high serum levels of IgG and IgM antibodies (103). Only a small proportion of these antibodies has antimalaria antigen activity, the remainder showing anti-IgG (rheumatoid factor) (104), antinuclear (105), anti-ssDNA, anti-smooth muscle, anti-Sm/RNP (106), anti-parietal cells (107), antilymphocytic (108) and anti-RBC antibodies (109).

Adu et al. (110) found that healthy Ghanaians living in a holoendemic malarious area had a higher incidence of antinuclear antibodies (ANA) and a higher mean titer of anti-ssDNA autoantibodies than healthy Caucasians who had not been exposed to malaria. Similar findings of high incidence of ANA were reported in the sera of apparently healthy individuals living in malarious areas of Nigeria, Uganda, and Liberia (111), but not in Thai residents (106).

A significant correlation was found between the detection of these autoantibodies and the presence of high titers of antimalaria antibodies, suggesting that the development of ANA was related to malaria infection. However, the persistence of these autoantibodies did not correlate with the parasitemia once the initial infection was established and treated (112).

The precise mechanism(s) leading to development of autoantibodies in malaria is not known. Possible explanations include:

1. Cross-reactivity between the foreign antigens and host proteins (113).
2. Polyclonal B-cell activation by malarial mitogens (114,115), possibly through a T-cell factor (116); the production of high levels of IgM antibody directed to nonparasite antigens during malaria infection support his hypothesis. Culture supernatants from infected human RBC transformed lymphocytes not only from individuals immune to malaria, but also from individuals not previously exposed to malaria (117).
3. Antigenic variation on the surface of parasites (118). It has been found that several antigens of *Plasmodium falciparum* contain repeats with related sequences (119), and that these repeats play an important role of "baffling" the host immune response and lead to an increase in the number of somatic mutants with autoreactivity.

The clinical significance of the autoantibodies in malaria is not known. There are no reports of autoimmune disease development secondary to malaria infection. One of the common renal findings in falciparum malaria in man is immune complex glomerulonephritis (120); however, it is not clear if there is any role for the autoantibodies in the pathogenesis of the glomerulonephritis. The role of these autoantibodies in patients with malaria in relation to the development of sequelae remains questionable. There is clearly a need for additional studies on the nature of the antibodies and the mechanism leading to their production.

VI. *LEISHMANIA* AND AUTOIMMUNITY

Leishmania are obligate intracellular protozoa that reside within mononuclear phagocytes of their host. Depending on the *Leishmania* species, the infected host develops localized or disseminated disease. The first form of leishmaniasis is characterized by cutaneous and mucocutaneous lesions, which are caused in the old world by *L. tropica*, *L. major*, *L. aethiopica*, and in the new world by *L. mexicana* and *L. braziliensis* (121).

Visceral leishmaniasis, or kala azar, is caused primarily by *L. donovani*. This form of leishmaniasis is characterized by the production of high titers of nonspecific immunoglobulins and, to a lesser extent, by specific antibodies against the parasite (122). On the other hand, in the first form of leishmaniasis, antibodies specific to the parasite are demonstrable, whereas the serum immunoglobulin levels are normal (123).

Like in malaria infection, several autoantibodies were detected in the sera of patients with leishmaniasis including anti-IgG (rheumatoid factor) (124–125), antitubulin, antiactin (126), anti-DNA, anti-Sm/RNP, anti-SSA/SSB, and anti-smooth muscle (127–128). These autoantibodies were found in visceral as well as in mucocutaneous leishmaniasis.

Recently, we examined the sera of 29 patients with visceral leishmaniasis and 14 patients with cutaneous leishmaniasis for autoantibody activity against a panel of nine nuclear antigens, employing an enzyme-linked immunosorbent assay (ELISA). Anti-SM, RNP, SS-A, and SS-B antibodies were present in high titers in 83, 86, 36, and 73% of the patients with visceral leishmaniasis and in 7, 14, 25, and 25% of the patients with the cutaneous form. The binding of visceral leishmaniasis serum antibodies to ribonucleoproteins was inhibited by prior incubation of serum with either leishmanial membrane antigens from four different species of leishmania or intact cells of *L. donovani* (127).

The presence of autoantibodies in the sera of patients with leishmaniasis could be related to polyclonal B-cell activation (128), release of sequestered antigens when surrounding host tissue and cells are damaged (128), and cross-reactivity between parasite and host antigens (127). All of these mechanisms will be discussed in detail later in this chapter.

Circulating immune complexes have also been identified in patients with leishmaniasis (128–129). A close correlation was found between CICs and anti-IgG antibodies in mucocutaneous leishmaniasis, suggesting that part of detected CICs could be formed by IgG and anti-IgG antibodies (130). Desjeux et al. (130) found that subjects with the cutaneous form or only one mucocutaneous lesion presented mean levels of CICs similar to control groups. This finding suggests an association between the development of severe mucocutaneous lesions and the appearance of CICs.

In visceral leishmaniasis CICs may participate in the pathogenesis of the disease. Patients with this form of leishmaniasis present symptoms similar to those observed in serum sickness (131). Glomerular lesions with deposition of immunoglobulin and C components in glomeruli have been demonstrated (132). The CICs may play a role in the pathogenesis of anemia in American visceral leishmaniasis (133).

The mechanisms involved in the generation of CICs during visceral leishmaniasis are not well understood. The reaction of circulating parasites with their corresponding antibodies could be involved in the formation of CICs (134). However, parasite antigens were not found in CICs purified from the serum of patients with visceral leishmaniasis (135). On the other hand, CICs may also be formed by a reaction between autoantibodies and autoantigens, such as a reaction between immunoglobulin and rheumatoid factor (136) or interaction between auto anti-idiotypic antibodies and idiotypic determinants of immunoglobulin, such reaction having been demonstrated in murine African trypanosomiasis (137).

VII. SCHISTOSOMIASIS AND AUTOIMMUNITY

There are three major schistosome species that infect humans. The clinical manifestations of *Schistosomia mansoni* and *S. japonicum* are hepatic, while

S. haematobium adults are found mostly in the venules of the urinary tract and cause disease primarily of the ureters and the bladder.

The pathologic hallmark of schistosomal infection is a granulomatous inflammation surrounding the helminth eggs. However, like malaria and leishmaniasis, glomerulonephritis associated with immune complex deposition, consisting of immunoglobulin, complement components and parasite antigens, has been documented in patients with schistosomiasis (138–139). Immune complexes were found in renal tissue as well as in the circulation (140,141). Deposition of CICs is believed to account for the most common immunopathologic mechanism of glomerulonephritis (142), although complexes were only detected in 64% of patients with schistosomiasis and renal disease. The absence of CICs might indicate that (1) the level of pathogenic IC were below the level of sensitivity of the assays; (2) the level of CIC may fluctuate based on the titer of antibodies and amount of antigens in the serum; and (3) formation of IC in situ in the renal glomeruli (143).

The presence of autoantibodies has been reported during schistosoma infections in man and in experimental models. Anti-DNA, rheumatoid factor, antisperm, antilymphocyte, and anticollagen antibodies were detected in schistosomiasis (143–146).

Recently, Thomas et al. (147) found high levels of anti-DNA idiotype (16/6 Id), as well as anticardiolipin antibodies in the sera of patients with schistosomiasis and filariasis. They also found a positive correlation between the 16/6 Id level and anticardiolipin antibodies, suggesting that the 16/6 Id contained lipid-binding antibodies.

Possible explanations for the presence of these autoantibodies in schistosomiasis include polyclonal B-cell activation, molecular mimicry between host and parasite proteins, and antigenic variation on the surface of parasites (144).

The role of rheumatoid factor in schistosomiasis is not clear. The presence of this factor may represent nonspecific polyclonal activation of B cells (144). However, RF may participate in monoclonal phagocytic clearance of CICs by increasing the size of the complexes and possibly avoiding deposition in the glomerular basement membrane (148). RF production might thus represent a protective mechanism in patients with schistosomiasis.

Autoimmune mechanisms may play a role in the pathogenesis of the visceral fibrosis in schistosomiasis. In *Schistosoma mansoni*-infected mice, autoantibodies and T-cell responsiveness to collagen have been reported (146). These autoantibodies were also found in some patients with connective tissue disorders, including rheumatoid arthritis (149), scleroderma (150), idiopathic pulmonary fibrosis (151), and relapsing polychondritis (152). T-cell responses to collagen in connective tissue diseases might play a role in inducing chronic inflammatory and fibrosis formation. On the other hand, mice immunized with collagen developed arthritis (153), which provides some support for the hypothesis that anticollagen responses may be pathogenic.

It is possible that collagen-responding T cells in *Schistosoma mansoni*-infected mice release lymphokines which might recruit inflammatory cells and stimulate fibroblasts to migrate and synthesize collagen (154). These cells might be important primarily in hepatic fibrogenesis in humans.

VIII. MECHANISMS FOR MICROBE-INDUCED AUTOIMMUNITY

Microbes may induce autoimmune phenomena by several mechanisms including molecular mimicry, production of autoantibodies, polyclonal activation of B cells, altered self antigens, and others. The ways whereby microbes can induce autoreactivity are summarized in Table 5 and are discussed in this section.

IX. MOLECULAR MIMICRY BETWEEN MICROBIAL AND HOST ANTIGENS

This theory is based on antigenic similarity between antigens of host tissues and infectious agents (16). In these cases, the antimicrobial response may cross-react with molecules that have similar antigenic determinants. The molecular mimicry of microbial epitopes to cellular proteins may be responsible for the large variety of autoantibodies produced after microbial infection (16).

Antigenic cross-reactivity between host and microbes is supported by the following studies:

Monoclonal anti-DNA antibodies derived from SLE patients bound to mycobacteria and the binding was inhibited by DNA (31).

Inhibition of binding of anti-Sm/RNP and anti-SS-B to their autoantigens by four different *Leishmania* species, implying that Sm, RNP, and SS-B share epitopes with common leishmanial antigens (127).

Jahnke et al. (155) showed amino acid homologies between several animal viruses and myelin basic protein, a protein whose encephalitogenic site of 10 amino acids induces experimental allergic encephalomyelitis.

Additional support for the molecular mimicry theory has been summarized by Shoenfeld and Cohen (16).

X. MODIFICATION OF SOMATIC HOST CELL

Infection of cells may induce alteration of host antigens secondary to the release of microbial products or as a result of the accompanying inflammatory reaction by one of the following mechanisms (156):

1. Release of sequestered antigens when surrounding host tissue and cells are damaged. The newly exposed antigens are recognized as foreign by the host.
2. Alterations of host cell proteins which are no longer recognized as "self."

TABLE 5 Mechanisms for Microbe-Induced Autoimmunity

Molecular mimicry
Modified self antigens
Release of sequestered antigens
Alteration of host cell proteins
Incorporation of microbial antigens into host cells
Polyclonal activation of B cells
Abnormal expression of immunoregulatory molecules
Idiotypic network

For example, lysosomal enzymes released from polymorphonuclear cells could alter host globulins and thus induce antigammaglobulin antibodies (rheumatoid factor) (157).

3. Incorporation of viral antigens into host cells. For example, viral genetic material may be incorporated into the nucleus of megakaryocyte encoding viral antigens which appear on platelets. Circulating antibodies are generated against platelets bearing viral antigens (158).

XI. POLYCLONAL B-CELL ACTIVATION

The presence of autoantibodies in the sera of patients with chronic infection could be related to polyclonal B-cell activation. During polyclonal activation, all B-cell clones are expanded, including clones producing natural autoantibodies which are present at low levels under normal conditions (127). These result in hypergammaglobulinemia and high titers of autoantibodies. It was found that parasite-derived antigens from *Leishmania*, malaria, and *Schistosoma* parasites are mitogenic and trigger the production of immunoglobulin with autoantibody activity (127).

Polyclonal activation of B cells has also been proposed as the mechanism responsible for the presence of autoantibodies in the sera of patients with chronic viral and bacterial infections (16) besides parasitic infections.

The polyclonal activator could be certain bacterial polysaccharides or cell wall products such as endotoxin, or mycobacterial and parasitic fractions (159).

XII. ABNORMAL EXPRESSION OF IMMUNOREGULATORY MOLECULES

Microbial infections can induce abnormal expression of MHC class II antigens (160). During the inflammatory response, activated T cells secrete lymphokines such as gamma-interferon, which is the best known inducer of DR antigen. As a result, somatic cells are induced to express class II molecules, thus forming a cell capable of presentation of autoantigens to autoimmune T lymphocytes (161). Thus, the self-antigen per se is not altered by the infection; rather the self-antigen becomes immunogenic for T lymphocytes as a consequence of associated class II MHC molecules.

XIII. THE IDIOTYPIC NETWORK

Another theory which may explain the induction of autoimmunity entails the anti-idiotypic network. Jerne (162) postulated that any given individual possesses thousands of idiotypes reflecting the infinite conformational possibilities of foreign antigen structures. Each antigen induces a set of antibodies (idiotypes), which in turn induces a set of anti-idiotypes. Therefore, similar to the manner in which an antibody removes an antigen circulating in the bloodstream, an anti-idiotype may be triggered and terminate the production of another idiotype. If the idiotypes and antiidiotypes recognize each other's antigen-binding sites, the anti-idiotype may mimic the structure of the antigen, in which case both the antigen and anti-idiotype will have a structure that is complementary to the binding site of the idiotypic antibody.

The viral ligands have complementary shapes to the viral receptors on the host cells. Therefore, the host antiviral ligand antibodies might have the same shape as the host's own viral receptors, that is, the antibody might mimic the structure of a self-antigen. Hence, an anti-idiotype to such an idiotypic antibody will bind the host antigen that serves as the receptor for the virus (163).

Fields et al. (164) found that immunization with monoclonal antiviral ligand antibody induced anti-idiotypic antibodies that react with the viral receptor of the host cell.

It has been possible to induce anti-idiotypic antibodies to the insulin receptor by immunizing mice with insulin (165). In a similar way anti-idiotypic antibodies to acetylcholine receptor, TSH receptor, and beta-adrenergic receptors were produced by immunizing animals with acetylcholine, TSH, and ligands that fit the beta receptors, respectively (165–167). The clinical significance of these anti-idiotypic antibodies in the induction of autoimmune diseases was reviewed recently by Shoenfeld and Cohen (16).

The pathological effects of the antireceptor antibodies were found to be transient. By immunizing mice with insulin, the generation of anti-insulin receptor antibodies induced diabetes for only 1–2 weeks. Somehow, the immune system stopped producing the antireceptor antibodies, and the mice became resistant to repeated immunization with insulin.

This observation brings us back to the fact that although autoantibodies or autoreactive lymphocytes are necessary for the development of autoimmune diseases, their mere presence is not sufficient. Disease appears to involve a failure of the immune system to regulate the self-reacting lymphocytes allowing progression or exacerbation of their effects. What the regulatory factors are, how they work to prevent autoimmune diseases, and what causes their failure are question to which there are no certain answers at the present time.

XIV. THERAPEUTIC IMPLICATIONS

We will close this chapter by briefly considering specific therapy of autoimmune diseases. Since infectious agents were found to be related to the development of autoimmune diseases, one of the goals of therapy to induce immune tolerance to the self-antigen.

This preventive therapy could be achieved by vaccination against microbes. However, there are no effective vaccines against most of the etiologic agents of chronic infections. On the other hand, vaccination against tuberculosis by BCG immuization may be one of the trigger mechanisms for autoimmunity. A second approach of therapy is to immunize with nonpathogenic anti-idiotypic antibodies to antimicrobial agent antibodies, thus suppressing autoimmune idiotypic antibodies (168). Yet another approach is the use of T cells in therapy to exploit the ability of the immune system to respond to its own components. T lymphocytes may be used because, as helpers and suppressors, they are the primary regulatory components of the system. Moreover, the real damage in many autoimmune diseases seems to be produced by autoreactive T cells. Cohen et al. (169) have succeeded in vaccinating laboratory animals against a variety of experimental autoimmune diseases by inoculating the animals with autoimmune T lymphocytes. Results obtained by using this approach have been encouraging. It was also possible to induce remission of already established adjuvant arthritis with suitable T cells (170). Helper T lymphocytes line that recognize critical self antigens attenuated by irradiation, so that they can no longer cause disease, are inoculated into rats or mice. The recipients were found to acquire resistance to the specific autoimmune disease (171). For example, it was possible to vaccinate mice against autoimmune thyroiditis with T lymphocytes reactive to self thyroglobulin (8). Ben-Nun et al. (172) found that lines of T cells reactive to myelin basic protein could be used to vaccinate rats against experimental autoimmune encephalomyelitis induced by active immunization to that antigen. The antiself receptors of the T lymphocytes appear to function as immunogens and induce an immune response that suppresses the potential for autoimmune diseases of particular specificity (173).

Another way to induce suppression of autoreactive T cells was achieved by vaccination with the 65 kD mycobacterial heat shock protein (HSP). Van Eden et al. (174) demonstrated that pretreatment of rats with mycobacterial 65 kD HSP resulted in resistance to *Mycobacterium tuberculosis*-induced adjuvant arthritis.

It was also found that intraperitoneal administration of 65 kD HSP to rats protected against the streptococcal cell wall induced chronic erosive polyarythritis (175). In such protected rats, mycobacterial- and streptococcal-specific T cell responses were suppressed, as compared with responses in arthritis rats, raising the possibility that the 65 kD HSP possesses a specific T-cell immunosuppressive activity.

XV. SUMMARY

The studies summarized in this chapter indicate that chronic bacterial, viral, and parasitic infections can serve as a trigger factor of autoimmune reactivity according to various mechanisms. The relationship between microbes and autoimmunity could be manifested by the presence of autoantibodies, autoimmune complexes, or T cells with autoactivity. The presence of autoimmune phenomena in chronic infections could be related to polyclonal B-cell activation, molecular mimicry between microbial and host antigens, altered self, abnormal expression of immunoregulatory molecules, and the anti-idiotypic network.

In most cases, the appearance of self-reactivity in the sera of patients with chronic infections is not associated with clinical manifestations. These findings suggest that autoimmune disease is the result of a combination of factors including immunologic, genetic, hormonal, and environmental. Infectious agents have a role in the breakdown of tolerance and the appearance of autoreactivity. However, only patients with the proper immunogenetic and hormonal background may develop clinical manifestations of autoimmune disease.

In spite of the extensive knowledge that has accumulated, the specific relationship between infections and autoimmunity is still obscure. Clearly, additional studies are required to clarify the relevance of microbes to the pathogenesis of autoimmune diseases.

REFERENCES

1. Lipman, S. M., Arnett, F. C., Conley, C. L., Ness, P. M., Meyers, D. A., and Blas, W. B. 1982. Genetic factors predisposing to autoimmune diseases: autoimmune hemolytic anemia, chronic thrombocytopenic purpura and systemic lupus erythematosus. *Am. J. Med.*, *73*: 827–840.
2. Isenberg, D. A., Shoenfeld, Y., Walaport, M., Mackworth-Young, C., Dudeney, C., Toddopokpopet, A., Brill, S., Weinberger, A., and Pinkhas, J. 1985. Detection of cross reactive anti-DNA antibody idiotypes in the serum of systemic lupus erythematosus patients and their relatives. *Arthritis Rheum.*, *28*: 999–1007.
3. Seligman, M., and Buet, J. C. 1977. Antibody activity of human myeloma globulins. *Sem. Hematol.*, *10*: 163–177.
4. Shoenfeld, Y., Segol, G., Segol, O., Klajman, A., Stollar, B. D., and Isenberg, D. A. 1987. Detection of antibodies to total histones and their subfractions in systemic lupus erythematosus patients and their asymptomatic relatives. *Arthiritis Rheum.*, *30*: 169–175.
5. Shoenfeld, Y., El-Roeiy, A., Ben-Yehuda, D., and Pick, A. P. 1987. Detection of

anti-histone activity in sera of patients with monoclonal gammopathies. *Clin. Immunol. Immunopathol.*, *42*: 250–258.

6. Abu Shakra, M., Krupp, M., Argov, S., Buskila, D., Slor, H., and Shoenfeld, Y. 1989. The detection of anti-Sm-RNP activity in sera of patients with monoclonal gammopathies. *Clin. Exp. Immunol.*, *75*: 349–353.
7. Ben-Nun, A., and Cohen, I. R. 1981. The rapid isolation of clonal antigen-specific T lymphocyte line capable of mediating autoimmune encephalomyelitis. *Eur. J. Immunol.*, *11*: 195–199.
8. Maron, R., Zerubavel, R., Friedman, A., and Cohen, I. R. 1983. T Lymphocyte line specific for thyroglobulin produces or vaccinates against autoimmune thyroiditis in mice. *J. Immunol.*, *1312*: 2316–2322.
9. Naparstek, Y., Holoshitz, J., Eisenstein, S., Reshef, T., Rappaport, S., Chemke, J., Ben-Nun, A., and Cohen, I. R. 1982. Effector T lymphocyte line cells migrate to the thymus and persist there. *Nature, 300*: 262–264.
10. Shoenfeld, Y., and Schwartz, R. S. 1984. Immunologic and genetic factors in autoimmune diseases. *New Engl. J. Med.*, *311*: 1019–1029.
11. Shoenfeld, Y., and Isenberg, D. A. 1989. *The Mosaic of Autoimmunity*. Elsevier, Amsterdam, pp. 1–540.
12. Shoenfeld, Y., and Isenberg, D. A. 1989. The mosaic of autoimmunity. *Immunol. Today, 10*: 123–126.
13. Abu-Shakra, M., and Shoenfeld, Y. 1989. The Gm allotypes and autoimmune diseases. *Immunol. Res.*, *8*: 281–291.
14. Salama, A., and Mueller-Eckhardt, C., 1987. On the mechanisms of sensitization and attachment of antibodies to RBC in drug-induced immune hemolytic anemia. *Blood, 69*: 1006–1010.
15. Dawkins, R. L., Garlepp, M. J., and McDonald, B. L. 1981. Myasthenia gravis and D-penicillamine. *J. Rheumatol.*, *7*: 169–172.
16. Shoenfeld, Y., and Cohen, I. R. 1987. Infection and autoimmunity. In *The Antigens*. Vol. 7 (M. Sela, ed.). Academic Press, San Diego, pp. 307–325.
17. Zabriskie, J. B. 1982. Rheumatic fever; a streptococcal-induced autoimmune disease. *Pediatr. Ann.*, *11*: 383–396.
18. King, M. L., Bidwell, D., Voller, A., Bryant, J., and Banatvala, J. E. 1983. Coxsackie-B virus specific IgM responses in children with insulin-dependent (type 1) diabetes mellitus. *Lancet, 1*: 1397–1399.
19. Christiansen, M. L., Pachman, L. M., Maryjowski, M. C., and Friedman, J. M. 1983. Antibody to coxsackie-B virus increased incidence in sera from children with recently diagnosed juvenile dermatomyositis, *Arthritis Rheum.*, *26* (Suppl): S26.
20. Sagg, M. S., and Bennett, J. C. 1987. The infectious etiology of chronic rheumatic diseases. *Sem. Arthiritis Rheum.*, *17*: 1–23.
21. Dziarski, R. 1982. Preferential induction of autoantibody secretion in polyclonal activation by peptidoglycan and lipopolysaccharide I. In vitro studies. *J. Immunol.*, *128*: 1018–1025.
22. Dziarski, R. 1982. Preferential induction of autoantibody secretion in polyclonal activation by peptidoglycan and lipopolysaccharide II. In vivo studies. *J. Immunol.*, *128*: 1026–1030.

23. El-Roiey, A., Sela, O., Isenberg, D. A., Feldman, R., Colaco, B. C., Kennedy, R. C., and Shoenfeld, Y. 1987. The sera of patients with klebsiella infection contain a common anti-DNA idiotype (16/6 Id) and anti-polynucleotide activity. *Clin. Exp. Immunol., 67*: 507–515.
24. El-Roiey, A., Gross, W. L., Leundemann, J., Isenberg, D. A., and Shoenfeld, Y. 1986. Preferential secretion of a common anti-DNA idiotype (16/6 Id) and antipolynucleotide antibodies by normal mononuclear cells following stimulation with klebsiella pneumoniae. *Immunol. Lett., 12*: 313–317.
25. Lindqvist, K. L., Coleman, R. E., and Osterland, C. K. 1970. Autoantibodies in chronic pulmonary tuberculosis. *J. Chron. Dis., 22*: 717–725.
26. Singer, J. M., Plotz, C. M., Peralta, F. M., and Lyons, H. C. 1972. The presence of anti-gamma globulin factors in sera of patients with active pulmonary tuberculosis. *Ann. Intern. Med., 56*: 545–552.
27. Sela, O., El-Roeiy, A., Isenberg, D. A., Kennedy, R. C., Colaco, C. B., Pinkhas, J., and Shoenfeld, Y. 1987. A common anti-DNA idiotype in sera of patients with active pulmonary tuberculosis. *Arthritis Rheum., 30*: 50–56.
28. Murray, H. W. 1978. Transient autoimmune hemolytic anemia and pulmonary tuberculosis. *New Engl. J. Med., 299*: 488.
29. Bonomo, L., Dammacco, F., and Pinto, L. 1963. Thyroglobulin antibodies in leprosy. *Lancet, 2*: 807–809.
30. Gupta, S. C., Chabra, B., and Mehrotra, T. N. 1982. A study of antispermatozal antibodies in leprosy. *Int. J. Lepr., 50*: 43–46.
31. Shoenfeld, Y., Vilner, Y., Coates, A. R. M., Joyce, R., Lavie, G., Shaul, D., and Pinkhas, J. 1986. Monoclonal anti-tuberculosis antibodies react with DNA and monoclonal anti-DNA autoantibodies react with mycobacterium tuberculosis. *Clin. Exp. Immunol., 66*: 255–261.
32. Isenberg, D. A., Shoenfeld, Y., Madaio, M. P., Rauch, J., Reichlin, M., Stollar, B. D., and Schwartz, R. S. 1984. Anti-DNA antibody idiotypes in systemic lupus erythematosus. *Lancet, ii*: 417–422.
33. Mendlovic, S., Brocke, S., Shoenfeld, Y., Ben-Bassat, M., Meshorer, A., Bakimer, R., and Mozes, E. 1988. Induction of a systemic lupus erythematosus-like syndrome in mice by a common human anti-DNA idiotype. *Proc. Natl. Acad. Sci. USA, 85*: 2226–2264.
34. Abu Shakra, M., and Shoenfeld, Y. 1990. The human anti-DNA idiotype (16/6 Id) pathogenic role in autoimmunity. *Human Ant. Hybridomas, 1*: 10–14.
35. Buskila, D., Abu-Shakra, M., Amital-Teplizki, H., Coates, A. R. M., Krupp, M., Sukenik, S., and Shoenfeld, Y. 1989. Serum monoclonal antibodies from patients with multiple myeloma react with mycobacterial phosphoinositides and nuclear antigens. *Clin. Exp. Immunol., 76*: 378–383.
36. Teplizki, H., Buskila, D., Argov, S., Isenberg, D. A., Coates, A. R. M., Sukenik, S., and Shoenfeld, Y. 1987. Low serum anti-mycobacterial glycolipid antibody titers in sera of patients with systemic lupus erythematosus associated with central nervous system involvement. *J. Rheumatol., 14*: 507–511.
37. Shoenfeld, Y., and Isenberg, D. A. 1988. Mycobacteria and autoimmunity. *Immunol., Today, 9*: 178–181.

38. Avinoach, I., Teplizki, H., Kuperman, O., Coates, A. R. M., Sukenik, S., and Shoenfeld, Y. 1990. Characteristics of antineuronal antibodies in SLE patients with and without central nervous system involvement: The role of mycobacterial cross-reacting antigens. *Isr. J. Med. Sci.*, *26*: 367–373.
39. Parekh, R. B., Dwek, R. A., Sutton, B. J., Fernandes, L., Leung, A., Stanworth, D., and Rademacher, T. 1985. Association of rheumatoid arthritis and primary osteoarthritis with changes in the glycosylation pattern of total serum IgG. *Nature*, *316*: 452–457.
40. Parekh, R. B., Isenberg, D. A., and Rook, G. 1989. A comparative analysis of disease associated changes in the galactosylation of serum IgG. *J. Autoimmunity*, *2*: 101–114.
41. Axford, J., MacKenzie, L., Lydyard, P. M., Hay, F. C., Isenberg, D. A., and Roitt, I. M. 1987. Reduced B-cell galactosyltransferase activity in rheumatoid arthritis. *Lancet*, *2*: 1486–1488.
42. Van Eden, W., Holoshitz, J., and Nevo, A. 1985. Arthritis induced by a T lymphocyte clone that responds to mycobacterium tuberculosis and to cartilage proteoglycans. *Natl. Acad. Sci.*, *82*: 5117-5120.
43. Torisu, M., Miyahara, T., and Shinohara, N. 1983. A new side effect of BCG immunotherapy—BCG induced arthritis in man. *Cancer Immunol. Immunother.*, *5*: 77–83.
44. Holoshitz, J., Matitiau, A., and Cohen, I. R. 1984. Arthritis induced in rats by cloned T lymphocytes responsive to mycobacteria, but not to collagen type II. *J. Clin. Invest.*, *73*: 211-215.
45. Minota, S., Cameron, B., Welch, W. J., and Winfield, J. B. 1988. Autoantibodies to the constitutive 73-KD member of the hsp 7 family of heat shock proteins in systemic lupus erythematosus. *J. Exp. Med.*, *168*: 1475–1480.
46. Meeting Report: International meeting on the association between rheumatoid arthritis and mycobacterial infection. *Autoimmunity*, *2*: 73–76 (1988).
47. Abrahamsen, T. G., Froland, S. S., and Natvig, J. B. 1978. In vitro mitogen stimulation of synovial fluid lymphocytes from rheumatoid arthritis and juvenile rheumatoid arthritis patients: Dissociation between the response to antigens and polyclonal mitogens, *Scand. J. Immunol.*, *7*: 81–90.
48. Holoshitz, J., Drucker, I., Yaretzky, A., Van Eden, W., Klajman, A., Frenkel, A., and Cohen, I. R. 1986. T lymphocytes of rheumatoid arthritis patients show augmented reactivity to a fraction of mycobacteria cross-reactive with cartilage. *Lancet*, *2*: 305–309.
49. Waxman, J., Lockshin, M. D., Schnapp, J. J., and Doneson, I. N. 1973. Cellular immunity in rheumatic disease, 1. Rheumatoid arthritis. *Arthritis Rheum.*, *16*: 499–506.
50. Bahr, G. M., Sattar, M. A., Stanford, J. L., Shaaban, M. A., Shimali, A. I., Chugh, T. D., Rook, G. A., and Behbenhani, K. 1989. HLA-DR and tuberculin tests in rheumatoid arthritis and tuberculosis. *Ann. Rheum. Dis.*, *48*: 63–68.
51. Ottenhoff, T. H., Torres, P., and Terencio. J. 1986. Evidence for an HLA-DR4 associated immune response gene for M. tuberculosis. A clue to the pathogenesis of rheumatoid arthritis. *Lancet*, *2*: 310–313.
52. Solling, J., Solling, K., Jakobsen, K. U., and Form. E. 1978. Circulating immune complexes in syphilis. *Acta Derm. Venereol.*, *58*: 263–267.

53. Baughn, R. E., Adams, C. B., and Musher, D. M. 1982. Immune complexes in experimental syphilis: A methodologic evaluation. *Sex Transm. Dis.*, *9*: 170–177.
54. Woznicko-Orlowska, G., and Milgrom, F. 1981. Immune complexes in syphilis sera. *J. Immunol.*, *127*: 1048–1051.
55. Baughn, R. E., Tung, K. S. K., and Musher, D. M. 1980. Detection of circulating immune complexes in the sera of rabbits with experimental syphilis; possible role in immunoregulation. *Infect. Immun.*, *29*: 575–582.
56. Gamble, C. N., and Reardan, J. B. 1975. Immunopathogenesis of syphilitic glomerulonephritis. *New Engl. J. Med.*, *292*: 449–454.
57. Jorizzo, J. L., McNeely, M. C., Baughn, R. E., Solomon, A. R., Cavallo, T., and Smith, E. B. 1986. Role of circulating immune complexes in human secondary syphilis. *J. Infect. Dis.*, *153*: 1014–1022.
58. McNeely, M. C., Jorizzo, J. L., Solomon, A. R., Smith, E. B., Cavallo, T., and Sanchez, R. 1986. Cutaneous secondary syphilis: preliminary immunohistopathologic support for immune complexes lesion pathogenesis. *J. Am. Acad. Dermatol.*, *14*: 564–571.
59. Baughn, R. E., McNeely, M. C., Jorizzo, J. L., and Musher, D. M. 1986. Characterization of the antigenic determinants and host components in immune complexes from patients with secondary syphilis. *J. Immunol.*, *136*: 1406–1414.
60. Gilliand, B., and Mannik, M. 1987. Immune complex disease. In *Harrison's Principles of Internal Medicine* (R. G. Petersdorf, R. D. Adams, J. K. Isselbacher, J. D. Wilson, eds.). McGraw-Hill, New York, pp. 1414–1418.
61. Baughn, R. E., Wicher, V., Jakubowski, A., and Wicher, K. 1987. Humoral response in Treponema-pallidum infected guinea pigs: Circulating immune complexes and autoimmune responses. *J. Immunol.*, *138*: 4435–4440.
62. Baughn, R. E., and Musher, D. M. 1983. Isolation and preliminary characterization of circulating immune complexes from rabbits with experimental syphilis. *Infect. Immun.*, *42*: 585–593.
63. Baughn, R. E., Adams, C. B., and Musher, D. M. 1983. Circulating immune complexes in experimental syphilis: identification of treponemal antigens and specific antibodies to treponemal antigens in isolated complexes. *Infect. Immun.*, *42*: 585–593.
64. Baughn, R. E. 1987. Role of fibronectin in the pathogenesis of syphilis. *Rev. Infect. Dis.*, *984*: S372–S385.
65. Proctor, R. A., Mosher, D. F., and Olbrantz, P. J. 1981. Fibronectin binding to staphylococcus aureus. *J. Biol. Chem.*, *35*: 29–54.
66. Fitzgerald, T. J., Repesh, L. A., Blanco, D. R., and Miller, J. N. 1984. Attachment of *Treponema pallidum* to fibronectin, laminin, collagen IV, and blockage of attachment by immune rabbit IgG. *Br. J. Vener. Dis.*, *60*: 357–363.
67. Fitzgerald, T. J., and Repesh, L. A. 1985. Interaction of fibronectin with *Treponema pallidum*. *Geniotourin. Med.*, *61*: 147–155.
68. Murphy-Ullrich, J. E., Oberley, T. D., and Mosher, D. F. 1982. Glomerular and vascular injury in mice following immunization with heterologous and autologous fibronectin. *Virchows Arch.*, *39*: 305–321.
69. Murphy-Ullrich, J. E., Oberley, T. D., and Mosher, D. F. 1984. Detection of autoantibodies and glomerular injury in rabbits immunized with denatured human fibronectin monomer. *Am. J. Pathol.*, *117*: 1–11.

70. Kumar, V., Klingman, J. D., and Wicher, K. 1977. Host response to Treponema pallidum infection: Quantitative changes of lipids in rabbit organs. *Int. Arch. Appl. Immunol., 55*: 476–480.
71. Mustakallio, K. K., Lassus, A., and Wager, O. 1967. Autoimmune phenomena in syphilitic infections: Rheumatoid factor and cryoglobulins in different stages of syphilis. *Int. Arch. Allergy Appl. Immunol., 31*: 417–426.
72. Strugneel, R. A., Williams, W. F., Raines, G., Pedersen, J. S., Drummond, L. P., Toh, B. H., and Faine, S. 1986. Autoantibodies to creatinine kinase in rabbits infected with Treponema pallidum. *J. Immunol., 136*: 667–671.
73. O'Neill, P. 1976. A new look at the serology of treponemal disease. *Br. J. Vener. Dis., 52*: 296–299.
74. Fitzgerald, T. J., Repesh, L. A., and Oakes, S. G. 1982. Morphology destruction of cultured cells by the attachment of *Treponema pallidum. Br. J. Vener. Dis., 58*: 1–11.
75. De Jong, N. H., Koehorst, J. A., van der Sluis, J. J. 1980. Autolymphocytotoxins in syphilis. *Br. J. Vener. Dis., 56*: 297–301.
76. Harris, E. N., Charavi, A., Wasley, G., and Hughes, G. 1987. Use of an ELISA and of inhibition studies to distinguish between antibodies to cardiolipin from patients with syphilis or autoimmune disorders. *J. Inf. Dis., 157*: 23–31.
77. Fauci, A. S. 1988. The human immunodeficiency virus: infectivity and mechanisms of pathogenesis. *Science, 239*: 617–622.
78. Ziegler, J. L., and Stites, D. P. 1986. Hypothesis: AIDS is an autoimmune disease directed at the immune system and triggered by a lymphotropic retrovirus. *Clin. Immunol. Immunopathol., 41*: 305–313.
79. Spivak, J. L., Bender, B. S., and Quinn, T. C. 1984. Hematologic abnormalities in the acquired immune deficiency syndrome. *Am. J. Med., 77*: 224–228.
80. Gupta, S., and Licorish, K. 1984. The Coombs' test and the acquired immunodeficiency syndrome. *Ann. Intern. Med., 100*: 462.
81. Murphy, M. F., Metcalfe, P., Waters, A. H., Linch, D. C., Cheigsong-Popov, R., Carne, C., and Weller, I. V. D. 1985. Immune neutropenia in homosexual men. *Lancet, 1*: 217–218.
82. Walsh, C. M., Nardi, M. A., and Karpatkin, S. 1984. On the mechanism of thrombocytopenia purpura in sexually active homosexual men. *N. Engl. J. Med., 311*: 635–639.
83. Dorsett, B., Cronin, W., Chuma, W., and Ioachim, H. L. 1985. Antilymphocyte antibodies in patients with the acquired immune deficiency syndrome. *Am. J. Med., 78*: 621–626.
84. Malatzky-Goshen, E., and Shoenfeld, Y. 1989. AIDS and autoimmunity. *Autoimmunity, 3*: 201–212.
85. Zolla-Pazner, S. 1984. Serology. In *Basics on AIDS: A Guide to Clinician's Laboratory Studies in AIDS* (Melbye, M., P. Ebbeson, R. J. Bigger, eds.). Munksgard, Copenhagen, pp. 151–172.
86. Adam, L. E., Donovan-Brand, R., Friedman-Kien, A., El Ramahi, K., and Hess, E. V. 1988. Sperm and seminal plasma antibodies in AIDS and other associated syndromes. *Clin. Immunol. Immunopathol., 46*: 442–449.
87. Seligman, M., Chess, L., Fahey, J. L., Fauci, A. S., Lachmann, P. J., L'Age-Stehr,

J., Ngu, J., Pinching, A. J., Rosen, F. S., and Spira, T. J. 1984. AIDS—an immunologic reevaluation. *N. Engl. J. Med., 311*: 1286-1292.

88. Delfraissy, J. F., Segond, P., Selanaud, F., Wallon, C., Massisa, P., and Dormont, J. 1982. Depressed primary in vitro antibody response in untreated systemic lupus erythematosus. T helper cell defect and lack of defective suppressor cell function. *Clin. Exp. Immunol., 48*: 513-518.
89. McDougal, J. S., Hubbard, M., and Nickelson, J. K. 1985. Immune complexes in the acquired immunodeficiency syndrome (AIDS): relationship to disease manifestation, risk group and immunologic defect. *J. Clin. Immunol., 5*: 130-138.
90. Toy, P. T., Reid, M. E., and Burns, M. 1985. Positive direct antiglobulin test associated with hyperglobulinemia in acquired immuno-deficiency syndrome (AIDS). *Am. J. Hematol., 19*: 145-150.
91. Gottleib, M. S., Groopman, J. E., Weinstein, W. H., Fahey, J. L., and Detels, R. 1983. The acquired immunodeficiency syndrome (UCLA Conference). *Ann. Int. Med., 99*: 208-220.
92. Matsiota, P., Chamaret, S., Montagnier, L., and Avrameas. S. 1987. Detection of natural autoantibodies in the serum of anti-HIV-positive individuals. *Ann. Inst. Pasteur. Immunol., 138*: 223-233.
93. Olsen, R. G., Tarr, M. J., Mathes, L. E., Whisler, R., du Plessis, D., Schultz, E. J., and Blakeslee, J. R. 1987. Serological and virological evidence of human T-lymphotropic virus in systemic lupus erythematosus. *Med. Microbiol. Immunol., 176*: 53-64.
94. DeStefanou, E., Friedman, R. M., Friedman-Kien, A. E., Goedert, J. J., Henriksen, D., Preble, G. T., Sonnabend, J. A., and Vilcek, J. 1982. Acid labile human leukocyte interferon in homosexual men with Kaposi's sarcoma and lymphadenopathy. *J. Inf. Dis., 146*: 451-459.
95. Preble, D. T., Black, R. J., Friedman, R. M., Klippel, J. H., and Vilcek, J. 1982. Systemic lupus erythematosus: Presence in human serum of an unusual acid-labile leukocyte interferon. *Science, 216*: 429-431.
96. Arvin, A. M., and Miller, J. J. 1985. Acid labile alpha-interferon in the sera and synovial fluids from patients with juvenile arthritis. *Arthritis Rheum., 27*: 582-585.
97. Sonnefield, G. 1980. Modulation of immunity by interferon. In *Lymphokine Reports*, Vol. 1 (Pick, E. E.,ed.). Academic Press, New York, p. 113.
98. Evrin, P. E., and Storm, T. 1984. Beta-2-microglobulin and its binding activity in serum from patients with SLE. *Ann. Rheum. Dis., 42*: 267-274.
99. Rook, A. H., Masur, H., Lane, H. C., Fredrick, W., Fausi, A. S., and Quinnan, G. V. 1983. Interleukin-2 enhances the depressed natural killer and cytotoxic activities of lymphocytes from patients with the acquired immunodeficiency syndrome. *J. Clin. Invest., 72*: 398-403.
100. Fauci, A. S. 1984. Immunologic abnormalities in the AIDS. *Clin. Res., 32*: 491-499.
101. Lane, H. C., Masui, H., Edgar, L. C., Rook, A. H., and Fauci, A. S. 1983. Abnormalities of B-cell activation and immunoregulation in patients with AIDS. *N. Engl. J. Med., 309*: 453-458.
102. Via, C. S., and Shearer, G. M. 1989. Autoimmunity and the acquired immune deficiency syndrome. *Autoimmunity, 1*: 753-756.

103. Rowe, D. S., McGregor, I. A., Smith, S. J., Hall, P., and Williams, K. 1968. Plasma immunoglobulin concentration in West African (Gambian) community and in a group of healthy British adults. *Clin. Exp. Immunol.*, *3*: 63–79.
104. Greenwood, B. M., Muller, A. S., and Valkenburg, H. A. 1971. Rheumatoid factor in Nigerian sera. *Clin. Exp. Immunol.*, *8*: 161–173.
105. Voller, A., O'Neill, P., and Humphrey, D. 1972. Serological studies in Tanzania. II. Antinuclear factor and malarial indices in population living at different altitudes. *J. Trop. Med. Hug.*, *75*: 136–139.
106. Boonpucknavig, S., and Ekapanyakuld, S. 1984. Autoantibodies in sera of Thai patients with *Plasmodium falciparum* infection. *Clin. Exp. Immunol.*, *58*: 77–82.
107. Sharper, A. G., Kaplan, M. H., Mody, N. J., and McIntyre, P. A. 1968. Malaria antibodies and autoantibodies to heart and other tissues in the immigrant and indigenous people of Uganda. *Lancet*, *1*: 1342–1343.
108. Wells, R. A., Pavanand, K., Zolyomi, S., Permpanich, B., and MacDermott, R. P. 1980. Anti-lymphocytotoxic antibodies in sera of Thai adults infected with plasmodium falciparum or plasmodium vivax. *Clin. Exp. Immunol.*, *39*: 663–667.
109. Rosenberg, E. B., Strickland, G. T., Sen-Lain, Y., and Whalen, G. E. 1973. IgM antibodies to red cells and autoimmune anemia in patients with malaria. *Am. J. Trop. Med. Hyg.*, *22*: 146–150.
110. Adu, D., Williams, D. G., Quakyi, I. A., Voller, A., Anim-Addo, Y., Bruce-Tagoe, A. A., Johnson, G. D., and Holborow, E. J. 1982. Anti-ssDNA and antinuclear antibodies in human malaria. *Clin. Exp. Immunol.*, *49*: 310–316.
111. Greenwood, B. M., Herrick, M. E., and Holborow, E. J. 1970. Speckled antinuclear factor in African sera. *Clin. Exp. Immunol.*, *7*: 75–83.
112. Phanuphak, P., Tirwatpong, S., Hanvanich, M., Panmuong, W., Moollar, P., Vejjajiva, S., Sitprija, V., Intaraprasert, R., and Phanthumkosol, D. 1983. Autoantibodies in falciparum malaria: A sequential study in 183 Thai patients. *Clin. Exp. Immunol.*, *53*: 627–633.
113. Koffler, D., Carr, R., Agnello, V., Thoburn, T., and Kunkel, H. G. 1971. Antibodies to polynucleotides in human sera: antigenic specificity and relation to disease. *J. Exp. Med.*, *134*: 294–312.
114. Rosenberg, Y. J. 1978. Autoimmune and polyclonal B-cell responses during malaria. *Nature*, *274*: 170–172.
115. Greenwood, B. M. 1974. Possible role of B-cell mitogen in hypergammaglobulinaemia in malaria and trypanosomiasis. *Lancet*, *1*: 435–436.
116. Poels, L. G., Van Niekerk, C. C., van der Sterrenreti, V., and Jerusalem, C. 1980. *Plasmodium berghei* T-cell dependent autoimmunity. *Exp. Parasitol.*, *49*: 97–105.
117. Greenwood, B. M., and Vick, R. M. 1975. Evidence for a malaria mitogen in human malaria. *Nature*, *257*: 592–594.
118. Hommei, M., David, P. H., and Oligin, L. D. 1983. Surface alterations of erythrocytes in *Plasmodium falciparum* malaria. Antigenic variation, antigenic diversity and the role of spleen. *J. Exp. Med.*, *157*: 1137–1148.
119. Anders, R. F., Shi, P. T., Scanion, D. B., Leach, S. J., Coppel, R. L., Brown, G. V., Stahl, H. D., and Kemp, D. J. 1986. Antigenic repeat structure in proteins of plasmodium falciparum. Synthetic peptides as antigen. Ciba Foundation Symposium, Wiley, Chichester, p. 164.

120. Boonpucknavig, V., Sitprija, V. 1979. Renal disease in acute Plasmodium falciparum infection in man. *Kidney Int.*, *16*: 44–52.
121. Marsden, P. D. 1984. Selective primary health care: Strategies for controls of disease in the developing world. XIV. Leishmaniasis. *Rev. Infect. Dis.*, *6*: 736–744.
122. Rezai, H. R., Ardehali, S. M., Amirhakimi, G., and Kharazmi, A. 1978. Immunological features of kala-azar. *Am. J. Trop. Hyg.*, *27*: 1079–1083.
123. Pearson, R. D. 1983. The immunobiology of leishmaniasis. *Rev. Infect. Dis.*, *5*: 907–927.
124. Carvalho, E. M., Andrews, B. S., Martinelli, R., Dutra, M., and Rocha, M. 1983. Circulating immune complexes and rheumatoid factor in schistosomiasis and visceral leishmaniasis. *Am. J. Trop. Med. Hyg.*, *32*: 61–68.
125. Desjeux, P., Santoro, F., Afchian, D., Lovens, M., and Capron, A. 1980. Circulating immune complexes and anti-IgG antibodies in mucocutaneous leishmaniasis. *Am. J. Trop. Med. Hyg.*, *29*: 195–198.
126. Howard, M. K., and Miles, M. A. 1986. Anti-tubulin antibodies in visceral leishmaniasis. *Trans. Roy. Soc. Trop. Med. Hyg.*, *80*: 493–494.
127. Argov, S., Jaffe, C. L., Krupp, M., Slor, H., and Shoenfeld, Y. 1989. Autoantibody production by patients infected with leishmania. *Clin. Exp. Immunol.*, *76*: 561–568.
128. Galvao-Crasto, B., Sa'Ferreira, J. A., Marzochi, K. F., Marzochi, M. C., Coutinho, S. G., and Lambert, P. H. 1984. Polyclonal B-cell activation, circulating immune complexes and autoimmunity in human American visceral leishmaniasis. *Clin. Exp. Immunol.*, *56*: 58–66.
129. Carvalho, E. M., Andrews, B. S., Martinelli, R., Dutra, M., and Rocha, H. 1983. Circulating immune complexes and rheumatoid factor in visceral leishmaniasis and schistosomiasis. *Am. J. Trop. Med. Hyg.*, *32*: 61–68.
130. Desjeux, P., Santoro, F., Afchin, D., Loyens, M., and Capron, A. 1980. Circulating immune complexes and anti-IgG antibodies in mucocutaneous leishmaniasis. *Am. J. Trop. Med. Hyg.*, *29*: 195–198.
131. Pugin, P., and Miescher, P. A. 1982. Le kala-azar. Etude clinique et physiopathologique a propos d'un noveau cas observ'e en Suisse. *Schweiz. Med. Wochenschr.*, *109*: 265–269.
132. Batto, T., Hoshino-Shimizu, S., Amato-Neto, V., Duarte, I. S., and Penna, D. O. 1975. Glomerular involvement in human kala-Azar. A light immunofluorescent and electron microscopic study based on kidney biopsies. *Am. J. Trop. Med. Hug.*, *24*: 9–16.
133. Carvalho, L. C., Badara, R., Carvalho, E. M., Lannes-Vieira, J., Vinhaes, L., Orge, G., and Marsochi, M. C. 1986. Nature and incidence of erythrocyte-bound IgG and some aspects of the physiopathogenesis of anaemia in American visceral leishmaniasis. *Clin. Exp. Immunol.*, *64*: 495–502.
134. Lambert, P. H., and Houba, V. 1974. Immune complexes in parasitic disease. *Prog. Immunol.*, *5*: 57–63.
135. Casali, P., and Lambert, P. H. 1979. Purification of soluble immune complexes from serum using polymethylmetacrilate beads coated with conglutinin of Clq. *Clin. Exp. Immunol.*, *37*: 295–309.

136. Ramso-Niembro, F., Fourinie, G., and Lambert, P. H. 1982. Induction of circulating immune complexes and their renal localization acute or chronic polyclonal B-cell activation in mice. *Kidney Int.*, *21*: S29–S38.
137. Rose, L., Goldman, M., and Lambert, P. H. 1982. Simultaneous induction of an idiotype corresponding anti-idiotypic antibodies, and immune complexes during African trypanosomiasis in mice. *J. Immunol.*, *128*: 79–85.
138. Takao, H. A., and Gould, D. B. 1975. Immune complex nephropathy in schistosomiasis. *Ann. Intern. Med.*, *83*: 148–154.
139. Hashino-Shimizu, S., de Brito, T., Kanamura, H., Canto, A. L., Silva, O. A., Campos, A. R., and Silva, L. C. 1976. Human schistosomiasis: *Schistosoma mansoni* antigen detection in renal glomeruli. *Trans. R. Soc. Trop. Med. Hyg.*, *70*: 492–496.
140. Lawley, T. J., Ottesen, E. A., Hiatt, R. A., and Gazze, L. A. 1979. Circulating immune complexes in acute schistosomiasis. *Clin. Exp. Immunol.*, *37*: 221–227.
141. Phillips, T. M., and Draper, C.C. 1975. Circulating immune complexes in schistosomiasis due to *Schistosoma mansoni*. *Br. Med. J.*, *2*: 476–477.
142. Border, W. A. 1979. Immune complex detection in glomerular diseases. *Nephron*, *24*: 105–113.
143. Carvalho, E. M., Andrews, B. S., Martinelli, R., Dutra, M., and Rocha, M. 1983. Circulating immune complexes and rheumatoid factor in schistosomiasis and visceral leishmaniasis. *Am. J. Trop. Med. Hyg.*, *32*: 61–68.
144. Fischer, E., Camus, D., Santoro, F., and Capron, A. 1981. *Schistosoma mansoni*: Autoantibodies and polyclonal B cell activation in infected mice. *Clin. Exp. Immunol.*, *46*: 89–97.
145. Al Abdel, H., El Atribi, A., Abdel Hafiz, A., and Aidaros, M. 1975. Azoospermia in bilharziasis and the presence of sperm antibodies. *J. Reprod. Fertil.*, *42*: 403–410.
146. Wyler, D. J., Lammie, P. J., Michael, A. I., Rosenwasser, L. J., and Phillips, S. M. 1987. *In vitro* and *in vivo* evidence that autoimmune reactivity to collagen develops spontaneously in schistosoma mansoni-infected mice. *Clin. Immunol. Immunopath.*, *44*: 140–148.
147. Thomas, M. A., Frampton, G., Isenberg, D. A., Shoenfeld, Y., Akin-sola, A., Ramsay, M., and Williams, D. G. 1989. A common anti-DNA antibody idiotype and anti-phospholipid antibodies in sera from patients with schistosomiasis and filariasis with and without nephritis. *Autoimmunity*, *2*: 803–812.
148. Carson, D. A., Bayer, A. S., Eisenberg, R. A., Lawrence, S., and Theofilopoulos, A. N. 1978. IgG rheumatoid factor in subacute bacterial endocarditis: Relationship to IgM rheumatoid factor and circulating immune complexes. *Clin. Exp. Immunol.*, *31*: 100–103.
149. Solinger, A. M., Bhatnagar, R. S., and Stobo, J. D. 1981. Cellular, molecular and genetic characteristics of T cell reactivity to collagen in man. *Proc. Natl. Acad. Sci.*, *78*: 3877–3881.
150. Stuart, J. M., Postethwaite, A. E., and Kang, A. H. 1976. Evidence for cell-mediated immunity to collagen in progressie systemic sclerosis. *J. Lab. Clin. Med.*, *88*: 601–607.

151. Kravis, T. C., Ahmed, A., Brown, T. E., Fulmer, J. D., and Crystal, R. E. 1976. Pathogenic mechanisms in pulmonary fibrosis: Collagen induced migration inhibition factor production and cytotoxicity mediated by lymphocytes. *J. Clin. Invest.*, *58*: 1223–1232.
152. Foidart, J. N., Shizeto, A., Martin, G. R., Zizic, T. M., Barnett, E. V., and Lawley, T. J. 1978. Antibody to type II collagen in relapsing polychrondritis. *N. Engl. J. Med.*, *299*: 1203–1207.
153. Stuart, J. M., Townes, A. S., and Kang, A. H. 1982. Nature and specificity of the immune response to collagen in type II collagen induced arthritis in mice. *J. Clin. Invest.*, *69*: 673–683.
154. Johnson, R. L., and Ziff, M. 1976. Lymphokine stimulation of collagen accumulation. *J. Clin. Invest.*, *58*: 240–252.
155. Jahnke, V., Fisher, E. F., and Alvoral, E. C. 1985. Sequence homology between certain viral proteins and proteins related to encephalomyelitis and neuritis. *Science*, *229*: 282–284.
156. Rager-Zisman, B. 1988. Virus-induced autoimmunity. *Isr. J. Med. Sci.*, *24*: 363–365.
157. Mahmoud, A. F., Kellermeyer, R. W., and Warren, S. 1974. Monospecific antigranulocyte sera against human neutrophils, eosinophils, basophils and myeloblasts. *Lancet*, *2*: 1163–1166.
158. Richard, H. A. 1983. Immune thrombocytopenias. *Hosp. Pract.*, *18*: 187–204.
159. Williams, R. C. 1978. In *Autoimmunity: Genetic, Immunologic, Virologic and Clinical Aspects* (N. Talal, ed.). Academic Press, New York, p. 457.
160. Bottazzo, G. F., Todd, I., Mirakian, R., Belfiore, A., and Pujol-Borrell, R. 1986. Organ specific autoimmunity: 1986 overview. *Immunol. Rev.*, *94*: 137–169.
161. Pober, J. S., Gimbrone, M. A., Cotran, R. S., Reiss, C. S., and Ault, K. A. 1983. Ia expression by vascular endothelium is inducible by activated T cells and by human gamma interferon. *J. Exp. Med.*, *157*: 1339–1353.
162. Jerne, N. K. 1974. Toward a network theory of the immune system. *Ann. Immunol.*, *125*: 373–377.
163. Plotz, P. H. 1982. Autoantibodies are anti-idiotype antibodies to antiviral antibodies. *Lancet*, *1*: 824–826.
164. Fields, N. B., and Green, M. I. 1982. Genetic and molecular mechanisms of viral pathogenesis: Implications for prevention and treatment. *Nature*, *300*: 19–23.
165. Wasserman, N. H., Penn, A. S., Freiruth, P. I., Treptow, N., and Erlanger, B. F. 1982. Anti-idiotypic route to anti-acetylcholine receptor antibodies and experimental myasthenia gravis. *Proc. Natl. Acad. Sci.*, *79*: 4810–4814.
166. Islam, M. N., Pepper, B. M., Brioner-Urinu, R., and Farid, N. R. 1983. Biological activity of anti-thyrotropin anti-idiotypic antibody. *Eur. J. Immunol.*, *13*: 57–63.
167. Strosberg, A. D., Couraud, P. O., and Schreiber, A. 1981. *Immunol. Today*, *2*: 75.
168. Kennedy, R. C., Eichberg, J. W., and Landford, R. 1987. Anti-idiotypic antibody vaccine for type B viral hepatitis in chimpanzees. *Science*, *232*: 220–223.
169. Cohen, I. R., Holoshitz, J., and van Eden, W. 1985. T lymphocytic clones illuminate pathogenesis and affect therapy of experimental arthritis. *Arthritis Rheum.*, *28*: 841–845.

170. Holoshitz, J., Naparstek, Y., and Ben-Nun, A. 1983. Line of T lymphocytes induce or vaccinate against autoimmune arthritis. *Sciences, 129*: 56–58.
171. Lider, O., Kavin, N., Shinitzky, M., and Cohen, I. R. 1987. Therapeutic vaccination against adjuvant arthritis using autoimmune T cells treated with hydrostatic pressure. *Proc. Natl. Acad. Sci., 84*: 4577–4580.
172. Ben-Nun, A., Wekerle, H., and Cohen, I. R. 1981. Vaccination against autoimmune encephalomyelitis with T lymphocyte line cell reactive against myelin basic protein. *Nature, 292*: 60–61.
173. Cohen, I. R., Ben-Nun, A., Holoshitz, J., Maron, R., and Zerubauel, R. 1983. Vaccination against autoimmune disease with lines of autoimmune T lymphocyte. *Immunol. Today, 4*: 227–230.
174. Van Eden, W., Thole, J. E., Van der Zee, R., Noordzig, A., Van Embolen, J. D., Hansen, E. J., and Cohen, I. R. 1988. Cloning of the mycobacterial epitope recognized by T lymphocytes in adjuvant arthritis. *Nature, 331*: 171–173.
175. Winfield, J. B. 1989. Stress proteins, arthritis and autoimmunity. *Arthritis Rheum., 32*: 1497–1504.

16

Chemical-Induced Autoimmunity

L. Pelletier, B. Bellon, H. Tournade, C. Dubey, J. C. Guery, A. Saoudi, F. Hirsch, and P. Druet
Hôpital Broussais, Paris, France

I. INTRODUCTION

Many drugs or toxins can induce immune manifestations and autoimmunity in susceptible individuals. Numerous compounds, particularly metals (nickel, chromium, mercurials, gold salts), are able to trigger either delayed-type hypersensitivity (DTH) skin reactions or autoimmune manifestations. A DTH reaction is the consequence of an immune reaction mediated by CD4+ T-helper cells specific for the toxin or an autoantigen modified by the toxin. Autoimmunity is an immune response (antibody or cell-mediated) towards an autoantigen. In humans, the role of environmental pollutants and of professional exposure is probably underestimated in immunologically mediated diseases. For example, mercury has been the major component of tooth-filling materials for the last past 150 years; it was considered as inert material. However, it has recently been shown that substantial quantities of Hg from amalgam appeared in various body tissues as early as 29 days after sheep had received occlusal amalgam fillings into 12 molar teeth (1).

It is often difficult to discriminate an immune response specific for any drug (or a metabolite) and a response against an autoantigen. Numerous drugs are associated with the occurrence of autoantibodies (Table 1) (2); however, the

TABLE 1 Autoantibodies Found in Several Drug-Induced Autoimmune Disorders

Drug	Autoantibody to:	Clinical features
Methyldopa, Procainamide, chlorpropamide	Red blood cells	Anemia
Carbamazepine, gold salts	Platelet	Thrombopenia
Lithium, anticonvulsant,	Thyroglobulin/microsomes	Thyroid dysfunction
D-Penicillamine	Intercellular substance of the skin	Pemphigus
D-Penicillamine	Acetylcholine receptor	Myasthenia gravis
Hydrocarbon solvents?	GBM	Glomerulopathy
Methicilline	TBM	Tubulointersitial nephritis
Halothane	Trifluoroacetylated carboxylesterase	Hepatitis
Tienilic acid	Cytochrome p-450	Hepatitis
Hydralazine, D-penicillamine, etc.[a]	Nuclear components	Lupus-like disease

GBM, glomerular basement membrane; TBM, tubular basement membrane.
[a]Antinuclear factors are found in most of the patients with drug-induced lupus-like diseases. The fine specificities of the autoantibodies and the main toxins responsible are considered in the text.

pathogenic role of these antibodies has been demonstrated in rare occasions (3). In addition, little attention has been paid to the role of cellular immune responses in drug-induced autoimmunity (4). These autoimmune manifestations are observed only in some individuals, and the role of genetic factors has been recently considered. The development of experimental models during the past few years has clarified the mechanisms at play in several situations.

In this chapter, we will consider some features of chemical-induced autoimmunity in humans. We will describe experimental models that will be useful to propose mechanisms of induction of autoimmunity. In the last part, we will discuss how a toxin may activate a cell.

II. CHEMICAL-INDUCED AUTOIMMUNITY IN HUMANS

Skin, kidney, liver, platelets, or red blood cells are preferential targets for toxin-induced immunologically mediated reactions (reviewed in Refs. 3,5–9). Clinical features of these manifestations are summarized in Table 2. Kidney will be chosen as an example of targeted organ (5,7,9). Depending upon the histologic lesions, several mechanisms have been proposed. D-Penicillamine and gold salts induced essentially membranous nephropathies (10–11) thought to be immune complex–mediated (9). Lithium salts induced preferentially a glomerulopathy with minimal

TABLE 2 Drug-Induced, Immunologically Mediated Clinical Manifestations

Organ	Clinical manifestations	Toxin
Skin	Rashes, prurit, eczema, urticaria	Gold, D-penicillamine, antibiotics
	Syndrome of Lyell	Sulfonamides
Liver	Acute or chronic hepatitis, Cirrhosis	Halothane, tienilic acid, alphamethyldopa, isoniazid, procainamide, gold
Kidney	Glomerular linear Ig deposits	D-penicillamine, solvents
	Immune complex–type glomerulonephritis	Mercurials, gold salts, drugs with SH groups
	Glomerular minimal changes	D-penicillamine, lithium
	Tubulointerstitial nephritis	NSAID, antibiotics (methicillin)
Platelets	Thrombopenia	Heparin, hypnotics, quinine, quinidine
		Methyldopa, rifampicin
Red blood cells	Hemolytic anemia	Methyldopa, penicillin and related, sulfonamides, levodopa, chlorpromazine, hydantoin, procainamide, rifampicin
Systemic disease	Lupus-like disease	Procainamide, hydralazine, isoniazid, D-penicillamine

glomerular changes presumably due to lymphokines produced by activated T cells (12). These lymphokines would modify the capillary permeability and trigger proteinuria in this way.

Some drugs or toxins are responsible for systemic autoimmunity (as reviewed in Refs. 2,6). Thus, hydralazine, D-penicillamine, procainamide, isoniazid, anticonvulsant drugs, silica, and polyvinyl chloride can trigger various autoimmune diseases such as a lupus-like syndrome, scleroderma, myasthenia, and pemphigus (Tables 1, 2). Most of the patients exhibit circulating antinuclear factors including antihistone antibodies and sometimes anti–native DNA antibodies. It is noteworthy that the same drug can induce either an organ-specific disease or systemic autoimmunity. Most of the time, one individual exhibits only one type of clinical manifestation. D-penicillamine can induce glomerulopathy or myasthenia or pemphigus or a lupus-like disease (reviewed in Refs. 6,7). Mercurials can induce a glomerulopathy (5) or can be responsible for a clinical illness mimicking Kawasaki's syndrome, characterized by fever, erythematous mucosa, enlargement of lymph nodes, and an increase of total serum IgE concentration (13).

Genetically determined differences play an important role in the development of drug-induced autoimmunity. Gold- and D-penicillamine–induced proteinuria are more frequent among poor sulfoxydators or DR-3 positive patients (14,15). Poor acetylators or DR-4 positive patients are more susceptible to hydralazine-induced lupus-like disease (16,17).

Numerous experimental models have been developed in an attempt to understand mechanisms of drug-induced immune disorders. Several will be described here.

III. EXPERIMENTAL MODELS

Interestingly, the same agent can induce DTH, organ-specific autoimmunity, or systemic disease. Thus mercurid chloride induces skin hypersensitivity in a strain of guinea pigs (18), a membranous nephropathy in some strains of rats (19,20), and a systemic disease in Brown-Norway (BN) rats (21–24). Similarly, D-penicillamine can induce a neuromuscular disease in guinea pigs (25) reminiscent of myasthenia gravis (26) and a lupus-like disease in BN rats (27–28). These examples show that it may be extremely difficult, and perhaps inappropriate, to differentiate toxin-induced DTH and autoimmunity. Mercury-induced autoimmune disease in the BN rat is one of the best studied models.

A. Effects of Mercuric Chloride in Rats

1. Mercury-Induced Autoimmunity in BN Rats

Nontoxic amounts of mercuric chloride (1mg/kg, s.c, three times a week) induce an autoimmune disease in BN rats (21–24). The main features of the disease are summarized in Table 3. In the second week after the first $HgCl_2$ injection, an enlargement of spleen and lymph nodes is found due to proliferation of both $CD4^+$ T-helper/inducer and B cells (23,29). Autoantibodies to anti–glomerular basement membrane (GBM), DNA, IgG, type II collagen, and thyroglobulin as well as antibodies specific for exogenous antigens (trinitrophenol hapten, sheep red blood cells, etc.) are detected from the end of the first week (23,24,30). The titers of all these antibodies peak at weeks 2–3 and then spontaneously decrease, although injections of $HgCl_2$ are continued (21–24). Serum immunoglobulin concentrations increase from week 1, peak at week 2, and then decrease; all the isotypes follow these kinetics, but the magnitude of enhancement is different: IgM, IgG, and IgA concentrations are increased twofold, threefold, and fivefold, respectively; IgE is mainly affected since it exhibits a 10^3-fold enhancement at the peak (23,29,31). Anti-GBM autoantibodies found deposited from day 7 in a linear pattern along the glomerular capillary wall are likely responsible for the proteinuria and the nephrotic syndrome observed in this model (21,22,24). Later on, a membranous glomerulopathy of unknown pathogenesis is observed

TABLE 3 Similarities Between $HgCl_2$-, Gold Salt-, and D-Penicillamine-Induced Autoimmunity

	$HgCl_2$	Gold	D-penicillamine
Lymphoproliferation ($CD4^+$/B cells)	+	+	+
Autoantibodies (anti-GBM, antinuclear)	+	+	+
Hyper Ig (IgE)	+	+	+
Anti-GBM-mediated glomerulopathy	+	+	+
Membranous glomerulopathy	+	+	−
Anti-class II T cells (1/frequency)	5000	50000	100000
Autoregulation of the disease	+	+	+
Genetic control	BN susc. LEW res.	BN susc. LEW res.	BN susc. LEW res.

GBM, glomerular basement membrane; susc., susceptible; res., resistant.
[a]The frequency of anti-class II T cells was determined by limiting dilution analysis of lymph node cells from diseased rats.

(22,24). BN rats injected with $HgCl_2$ also developed a mucositis and a Sjogren's syndrome (32). Mercuric chloride induces in BN rats a B-cell polyclonal activation. T cells are required for the mercury-induced disease to occur since (1) T-cell-depleted BN rats do not display the autoimmune disorders (33) and (2) T cells from diseased BN rats can transfer the disease in naive syngeneic recipients (34). Finally, autoregulation is another key feature of this disease. Although mercury injections are pursued for 2 months, autoimmune manifestations progressively resolved (21–24,29). Suppressor T cells (35) and/or anti-idiotypic antibodies (36) could participate in this regulatory phenomenon.

2. *Genetic Control*

The susceptibility to mercury-induced autoimmunity is genetically controlled, as shown in Table 4 (37). The strains tested bearing the RT1-1 haplotype are resistant in contrast to BN rats (RT1-n). The study of segregants between BN and Lewis (LEW) rats demonstrates that susceptibility is inherited as an autosomal and dominant trait and depends upon three to four genes, one of them being linked to the major histocompatibility complex (MHC) class II genes. Both MHC and non-MHC genes are required since BN.1L and LEW.1N rats are resistant while (BN.1L × LEW.1L) F_1 rats are susceptible. Other strains were tested and some develop an immune complex–type glomerulonephritis. For example, Weening et al. (19,20,38) showed that PVG/c rats (RT1-c) and DZB (RT1-u) rats develop an immune complex–type glomerulonephritis and antinuclear antibodies.

TABLE 4 Mercury-Induced Glomerulopathy in the Rat

Strain	RT-1 haplotype	Anti-GBM GN	ICGN
BN	n	+	+
LEW.1N	n	−	−
ACI.1N	n	−	−
LEW, F.344	l	−	−
BN.1L	l	−	−
AS, BS	l	−	−
BN.1L × LEW.1N	l/n	+	+
LOU, WAG	u	−	−
Wistar Furth	u	−	+
DZB	u	−	+
PVG/c, AUG	c	−	+
DA, AVN	a	−	+
BDV	d	−	+
BUF	b	−	+
OKA	k	−	+
AS 2	f	−	+

Anti-GBM GN, anti-glomerular basement membrane antibody-mediated glomerulonephritis; ICGN, immune complex-mediated glomerulonephritis.

B. Effects of Mercuric Chloride in Other Species

$HgCl_2$ induces in rabbits an autoimmune disease quite similar to the one observed in BN rats (39). The susceptibility of mice to mercury-induced autoimmunity was recently studied by several authors (40–44) (Table 5). As found in rats, susceptibility is genetically controlled. A lymphoproliferation, an increase in total serum IgG and IgE concentrations, circulating antinucleolar antibodies, and an immune complex–type glomerulonephritis were described in mice bearing the $H\text{-}2^s$ haplotype (A-SW, SJL, B10-S). In contrast, DBA/2 mice expressing the $H\text{-}2^d$ haplotype were completely resistant to induction of mercury-induced autoimmune disease.

C. D-Penicillamine and Gold Salt–Induced Autoimmunity in Rats

BN rats inoculated with D-penicillamine (27,28) and gold salts (45) display autoimmune disorders quite similar to the ones following $HgCl_2$ injections (Table 3). A cross-reactive idiotype detected in the three models suggests that the same B-cell clones are stimulated during this polyclonal B-cell activation (46). In $HgCl_2$-injected BN rats, autoimmune disorders are more intense than in gold salt– and D-penicillamine–treated BN rats. A nephrotic syndrome or a proteinuria are found in all the rats from the first group versus 50% in the second and none

TABLE 5 Genetic Control of Mercury-Induced Autoimmunity in Mice

Strain	Haplotype	Increase in total PFC	Serum hyper Ig	ANA (homogen/ nucleolar)	ICGN	Anti-TNP Abs
SJL	s	+[a]	M, G1, G2b[b]	+/+	+[c]	+
B10S	s	+[a]	?	+/+	+	?
A.SW	s	+[a]	M, G, E	+/+	+	?
C57BL/6J	b	−	E[d]	+/−	−	−
BALB/c	d	+	G1, G2a[b]	−/−	+[c]	−
DBA/2	d	−	−	−/−	−	?

ANA, antinuclear antibodies; ICGN, immune complex–type glomerulonephritis.
[a]Associated with a splenic cell hyperplasia. SJL, A.SW and B10S have nuclear antibodies specific for histones and fibrillarin.
[b]Serum IgE concentration was not determined.
[c]Antinuclear antibodies were eluted from kidneys of $HgCl_2$-injected SJL mice but not from those of $HgCl_2$-injected BALB/c mice.
[d]There was an increase in serum IgE concentration without modification of the other Ig classes.

in the third. Similarly, enhancement of serum IgE concentration is the highest in the first group (around 5 mg/ml), (31) and 5- and 10-fold lower in gold- and D-penicillamine–treated BN rats, respectively (28). The intensity of the disease is related to the frequency of anti–class II autoreactive T cells in the three models. These cells could be responsible for the induction of B-cell polyclonal activation as discussed below. The mechanisms of spontaneous regulation are $CD8^+$ T-cell independent (28,47) and probably partly common at least for $HgCl_2$ and D-penicillamine models. Wistar rats injected with D-penicillamine (48) or gold salts (49) develop a membranous glomerulopathy as Wistar rats injected with $HgCl_2$ (37). LEW rats are resistant to the three toxin-induced autoimmune diseases.

D. D-Penicillamine- and Gold Salt–Induced Autoimmunity in Mice

Mice bearing the H-2^s haplotype, susceptible to $HgCl_2$-induced autoimmunity, also produce antinuclear antibodies when treated with either gold sodium thiomalate or D-penicillamine (50). An increase in total serum IgG, IgE, and IgM concentrations is detected in A-SW mice injected with gold salts (43).

E. Gold Salt–Induced Autoimmune Nephritis in Guinea Pigs

Hartley guinea pigs injected with gold sodium aurothiomalate developed an autoimmune tubulointerstitial nephritis and an immune complex glomerulopathy (51). Anti–tubular basement membrane (TBM) antibodies were found linearly deposited along the TBM. Anti–brush border antibodies have been considered to be involved in the pathogenesis of the glomerular disease.

F. Cadmium-Induced Autoimmunity

Cadmium can induce in ICR but not in BALB/c mice antinuclear antibodies (52). Cadmium has been reported to induce an immune complex type glomerulonephritis in rats (53). Autoantibodies such as antilaminin and anti–type IV collagen antibodies are found in cadmium-injected Sprague-Dawley rats.

G. Propylthiouracil-Induced SLE in Cats

Fifty to 70% of mongrel cats receiving propylthiouracil (PTU) develop an autoimmune disease marked by lymphadenopathies, autoimmune hemolytic anemia, and autoantibodies such as anti–native DNA antibodies (54). The presence of a free sulfhydryl group on PTU is required for autoimmunity to occur (55).

H. L-Caravanine–Induced SLE

In monkeys, alfalfa sprouts can induce anemia, low serum complement, antibodies to DNA, and deposition of immunoglobulins in skin and kidneys (56). This autoimmunity is attributed to the nonprotein amino acid constituent, L-canavanine (57). It has been suggested that this disease could be due to the abrogation of suppressor functions (57).

I. Hydralazine- and Procainamide-Induced Autoimmunity

Though mice are poor acetylators, hydralazine does not induce a clear autoimmunity in this species. Hydralazine, given orally at the dose of 0.5–1 mg/day for 6–8 months increases the incidence of antinuclear antibodies in A/J and C57BL/6 mice (58–59). In one report, procainamide given orally at the dose of 20 mg/day for 8 months has the same effect in these two strains (59).

J. Cyclosporin A–Induced Autoimmunity

Cyclosporin A (CsA) is an immunosuppressive drug used to prevent allograft rejection and graft-versus-host disease in allogeneic bone marrow transplantation (reviewed in Ref. 60). This drug acts by inhibiting lymphokine production by T-helper cells as shown in vitro. Surprisingly, irradiated host transplanted with syngeneic or even autologous bone marrow cells and treated with CsA develop a lupus-like disease after the drug has been withdrawn (61–63). This phenomenon was described in humans, rats, and mice. This autoimmune disease is transferable by T cells from diseased animals (64), whereas removal of the thymus in transplanted recipients prevents the autoimmune disease (65). Recently, it was shown that engrafting from the thymus of CsA-treated mice into a T-cell–depleted congeneic mouse leads to an autoimmune disease avoided by the cotransplantation of a normal thymus (66). Thus the thymus is required for the appearance of CsA-induced autoreactive T cells in periphery. CsA interferes with the thymic maturation of T cells bearing $\alpha\beta$ receptor since single positive T cells are greatly reduced in the thymus of CsA-treated mice (67). The lineage of $\gamma\delta$ $CD4^-CD8^-$ T cells seems not to be altered by CsA treatment (67). When inoculated to newborn mice, even for a short time, CsA can also trigger autoimmunity (68). Interestingly, autoreactive T cells are found at the periphery at this early time of life. Cyclophosphamide, another immunosuppressive drug, can trigger the transient occurrence of autoreactive cells in the spleen of normal mice, but mechanisms are not yet elucidated (69).

III. MECHANISMS OF DRUG-INDUCED IMMUNE RESPONSE TOWARDS AN AUTOANTIGEN

There are several possible mechanisms for this response. The immune response can be directed against the drug or its metabolites, and in this case it does not correspond stricto sensu to an autoimmune response. A toxin can be stuck onto an autoantigen which becomes an "innocent victim" of antidrug immune responses. This mechanism was suggested to occur during hemolytic anemia mediated by penicillin covalently bound to red blood cells (3). Hemagglutination by serum or eluate from patient red blood cells is only observed in the presence of the drug or its metabolites (3).

An autoantigen can adsorb a drug–antidrug complex. Quinidin–antiquinidin antibodies bind to the major glycoprotein complex of platelets and lead to thrombopenia (3). Drug–antidrug antibody complexes could be passively trapped in the glomeruli and could be responsible for some drug-induced membranous glomerulopathies. However, in human mercurial- and gold-induced glomerulopathies, the drugs were not found in the glomerular deposits.

Following alteration by a toxic agent, an autoantigen can become immunogenic. This mechanism presumably is inferred in several methicillin or diphenylhydantoin interstitial nephritides (9). In patients injected with methicillin, dimethoxyphenylpenicilloyl, a metabolite of methicillin, has been found along the tubular basement membrane (TBM) together with IgG linearly deposited (5). Whether these IgG recognize the TBM or the hapten bound to the TBM is unknown. However, circulating anti-TBM antibodies are detected in several patients, which argues for the former hypothesis. The relevance of these antibodies in the pathogeny of the disease remains to be determined.

A drug could modify a glomerular structure; specific antibodies would be generated and bind the renal autoantigen. Alternatively circulating immune complexes consisting of "modified autoantigen" antibodies could be trapped passively in the glomeruli (5,9). Hepatitis induced by halothane or tienilic acid are characterized by antifluoroacetylated carboxylesterase and anti–cytochrome P-450 antibodies, respectively. It is likely that these diseases are a consequence of a modification of the autoantigen (70,71).

Several agents such as mercurials and gold salts are toxic towards proximal convoluted tubules. As a result of the toxic alteration, some tubular autoantigens could be released and an immune response towards these autoantigens initiated. Antigens such as glycoprotein 330 are expressed both on brush border of convoluted tubules and glomerular epithelial cells. This explains how the autoantibodies to such antigens also cause a membranous glomerulopathy. This mechanism was proposed by Ueda et al. (51) in a model of gold-induced glomerulopathy.

IV. MECHANISMS OF DRUG-INDUCED SYSTEMIC AUTOIMMUNITY

Several mechanisms may explain the appearance of systemic autoimmune manifestations following drug exposure.

A. Defect of Clearance of the Immune Complexes

The elevated concentration of immune complexes (IC) and the deposition of the IC in the tissues such as in $HgCl_2$-treated mice (40) led to the proposal that toxins as $HgCl_2$ might depress the clearance of IC by the reticuloendothelial system; this is unlikely since this toxin does not modify the clearance of preformed IC (40). This mechanism was also evoked for drugs that interact with complement components (72). Hydralazine, procainamide, and D-penicillamine inactivate the C4 complement component in vitro. Inactivation of the early complement components could lead in vivo to decreased solubilization and removal of immune complexes. Such a mechanism could be at play in systemic lupus erythematosus but does not explain the increased production of autoantibodies.

B. Action of a Drug on B Cells

There are no experimental arguments that a drug can induce an autoimmune disease by directly stimulating B cells to proliferate/differentiate. However, in vitro, lithium salts increase the lipopolysaccharide (LPS)-mediated polyclonal activation of B cells from responder mice (73). Lithium also allows B cells from nonresponder mice to proliferate in the presence of LPS. Lithium alone is able to promote RNA synthesis in B cells from these mice, while LPS alone is not.

C. Drug-Induced Autoreactive T Cells

T cells specific for class II molecules are responsible for the occurrence of autoimmunity during the allogeneic responses in the chronic graft-versus-host reaction (74,75) as well as in the host-versus-graft disease (76,77). We will detail the former disease, which led Gleichmann et al. to propose similar mechanisms in some drug-induced autoimmune disorders (78).

1. *Chronic Graft-Versus-Host Disease*

The graft-versus-host (GVH) reaction happens when T cells from a parent X are injected into a (X × Y) F_1 hybrid. The parental T cells are not rejected and react with the recipient cells expressing alloantigens inherited from the parent Y (74,75). In most cases, when F_1 hybrid and parent X differ at both class I and class II molecules, the GVH is deeply immunosuppressive and lethal. However, in genetic combinations in which parents X and Y are only class II incompatible, donor X's $CD4^+$ T cells specific for Y class II alloantigens are stimulated, In turn, these allo-class II T cells polyclonally activate B cells expressing Y class II molecules (Fig. 1). It is noteworthy that several but not all B-cell clones are triggered by anti–class II T cells (79–80); this suggests that B cells should be preactivated as demonstrated for several antiself class II T-cell clones (81–82). A lupus-like autoimmune disease arises consequently to the polyclonal B-cell activation.

2. *Anti-"Modified" Class II T Cells*

Gleichmann has suggested that a virus or a toxin could bind class II molecules and modify them in such a way that they mimic allogeneic class II antigens and stimulate specific autologous T-cell clones, as depicted in Figure 2 (78). These clones could activate B cells expressing the "modified" class II molecules. This hypothesis is in agreement with the results of Nagata et al. (83), who showed that spleen cells from BALB/c mice exposed to D-penicillamine elicited the proliferation of syngeneic T cells. However, it is not clear whether these cells are relevant to autoimmunity since BALB/c mice do not produce antinuclear antibodies (50). Although lead and zinc are not known to be responsible for autoimmunity, they can promote in vitro the proliferation of autologous $CD4^+$ and $CD8^+$ T cells. Anti–class II or an anti-CD4 monoclonal antibodies block the proliferation of the two T-cell populations, which emphasizes the requirement of both class II^+ cells and $CD4^+$ T cells for the occurrence of the proliferations (84,85). Interactions between class II molecules and nickel are more interesting. From patients with nickel-induced contact dermatitis, Kapsenberg et al. (86) cloned T cells originated either from skin lesions or from the circulating blood lymphocytes. In both cases, the authors demonstrated that the majority of the clones are stimulated by autologous class II^+ cells and nickel. All these clones are $CD4^+$, and their proliferation is abolished in the presence of an anti–class II monoclonal antibody. Sinigaglia et al. (87) obtained similar results and showed in addition

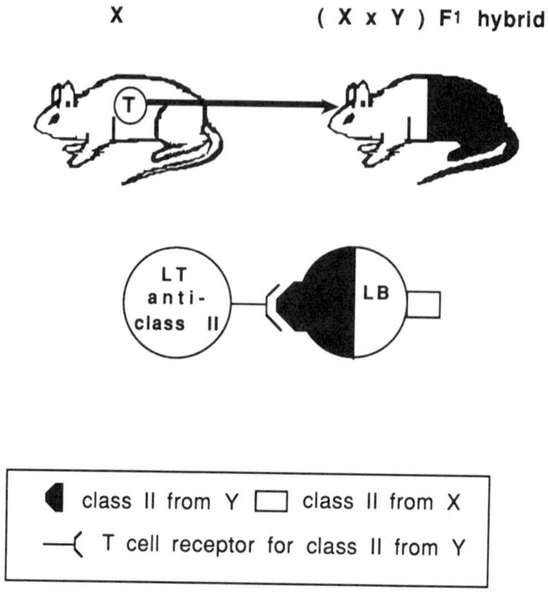

FIGURE 1 Chronic graft-versus-host reaction can occur when parental X T cells are injected into a class II incompatible (X × Y) F_1 hybrid. Donor anti-Y class II are stimulated and polyclonally activate host B lymphocytes.

that the T cells stimulated by class II^+ cells in the presence of nickel are able to polyclonally activate autologous B cells. Interestingly, patients suffering from nickel-induced contact dermatitis do not exhibit systemic manifestations. This could be due to the exclusive presence of nickel in the skin, to a differential ability of class II positive cells to trigger T cells, or to the fact that these T cells are preferentially triggered by class II molecules presenting a skin-specific antigen.

3. Antinative Class II T Cells

Anti–Class II T Cells in the Normal Immune System and Their Physiology. T cells specific for self class II molecules are generated during the autologous mixed lymphocyte reaction defined as the ability of T cells to proliferate in the presence of autologous class II^+ non-T cells (88–91). Anti–class II T cells have been shown to originate from antigen-stimulated precursors and clones of autoreactive antiself class II T cells are produced from immunized animals or humans

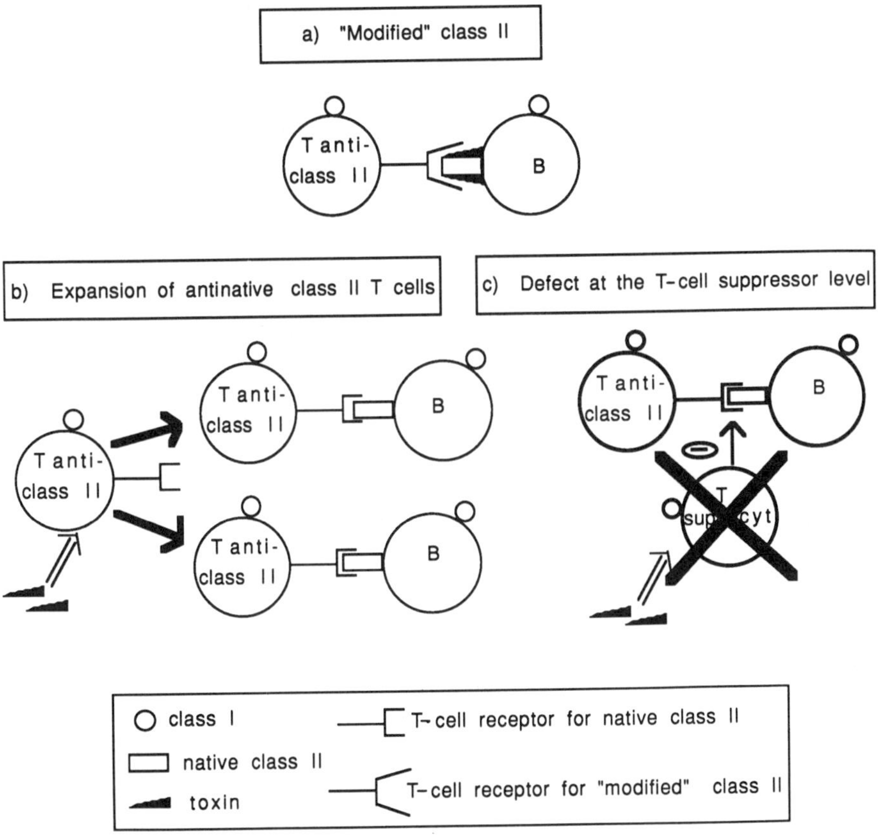

FIGURE 2 Three possible pathways of polyclonal B-cell activation by anti–class II T cells. Class II molecules could be modified by a toxin and then mimic allogeneic molecules; the specific antiallogeneic clones are activated (a). A toxin could induce expansion of potential autoreactive antinative class II cells (b). A toxin-induced defect at the suppressor level could also lead to the expansion of antinative class II T cells (c).

(92,93). Such clones were also obtained from nonmanipulated animals (94). Their roles were investigated in many laboratories (as reviewed in Refs. 88–97) and both interferon-γ and IL-2–producing T_H1 and IL-4–secreting T_H2 anti–class II T cells have been reported. Recently, Nagarkatti (98) has described an autoreactive clone able to secrete both IL-2 and IL-4. Anti–class II T-cell clones have essentially regulatory functions (81,82,94,95,97–101). They can provide helper signals that enhance MHC-restricted B-cell proliferation and maturation

(81,82,92–101). But they can also have suppressor (81,82,100) and even contrasuppressor activities (82). Bocchieri et al. (102) showed that anti–class II T cells obtained from normal mice secrete interferon-γ, whereas those produced from lupus-prone mice do not. It is of note that some autoreactive T-cell clones did not stimulate all B cells; Saito et al. (101) demonstrated by limiting dilution analysis that an autoreactive T-cell clone stimulated only 1 in 100 B cells, hence suggesting that other signals are required for the B-cell activation to occur.

Fine specificity of autoreactive T cells remains to be elucidated; they could recognize either empty class II molecules or a peptide in the peptide groove associated or not to class II molecules. Coeshott et al. (96) reported that an autoreactive T-cell hybridoma secretes IL-2 after stimulation by liposomes containing affinity-purified class II molecules; that this hybridoma recognizes class II alone is assumed. However, one has to keep in mind that processed peptides remain associated with MHC molecule as supported for crystalline class I molecule (103). Whether or not autoreactive T cells are present in normal individuals is controversial. There are lines of evidence that T cells specific for empty self class II molecules are deleted in the thymus. Kourilsky and Claverie (104) suggested that T cells recognizing self peptides presented by self-MHC with a high affinity are silenced in the thymus. Several hypotheses can be proposed to take into account the positive selection in the thymus. One is that T cells with weak affinity for self antigens presented by the MHC could escape inactivation and grow. The foreign epitopes would be recognized since they cross-react with self epitopes (105–107). In any case, thymus deletion of potentially autoreactive T cells is incomplete. Peripheral autoreactive T cells are found at a low frequency in normal individuals (108) and are controlled by T-cell circuits involving suppressor cells as shown by many authors (108–112).

b. How Could a Drug Induce Anti–Class II T Cells? A toxin could lead to polyclonal B-cell activation by expanding antinative class II T cells (Fig. 2). Several nonexclusive mechanisms can be proposed to explain this phenomenon.

Under certain circumstances, a drug may allow anti–class II T cells to escape thymic deletion as suggested to explain cyclosporine-induced autoimmunity (67,113).

A drug may induce the expansion of anti-class II T cells by increasing class II expression (114). Indeed, mercurials, zinc, lead, and nickel enhance in vitro class II expression, and this effect is antagonized by anti–interferon-γ antibodies (84,85,115). The increase of class II expression could stimulate autoreactive T cells as suggested in lupus-prone mice (116).

Antiself class II T cells can be induced following a disturbance of the T-cell network as suggested for mercury-induced autoimmunity in BN rats (117,118). Thus, in BN rats mercury promotes autoreactive cells, the frequency of which was calculated by limiting dilution analysis at different times of the disease (118).

Two different autoreactive cells were defined: One recognizes native class II on syngeneic B cells and is probably responsible for the B-cell polyclonal activation found in this model, and the other is triggered by T cells exposed to mercury. The former interaction is blocked by an anti–class II monoclonal antibody and the second by an anti-CD4 monoclonal antibody. In this case, it is proposed that mercury acts on the CD4 molecule, which normally interacts with class II molecules (Fig. 3). Since "class II-like" structures can be present on T-cell receptors, a CD4 "modified" T cell could stimulate T cells expressing "class II-like" determinants, which in turn induce antiself class II T cells.

A drug could generate anti–class II T cells by modifying T lymphocytes specific for an exogenous antigen in such a way that they become exclusively specific for self class II. As shown by Richardson et al. (119), a tetanus toxoid–specific $CD4^+$ T-cell clone is stimulated by autologous class II^+ cells only in the presence of 5-azacytidine. This agent, known to inhibit DNA methylation, could in this way derepress gene expression that would allow the expression of normally silent genes and then generate autoreactivity. Hydralazine and procainamide could cause autoimmunity in the same manner (120).

Double-negative T cells are present in the pool of normal spleen cells (121,122). When cultured in the presence of ionomycin + phorbol myristate acetate, 30% of these cells become $CD4^+$ self-reactive (122). However, CD4 expression is not an absolute requirement for self-reactivity (123). A toxin might directly generate proliferation and differentiation of such cells.

A defect at the T-suppressor level was evoked during responses to nickel, lead, zinc, and mercury that could also favor the emergence of anti–class II T cells (Fig. 2).

c. *Could a Drug Interact with T Cells Specific for Self Peptides?* Another interesting hypothesis concerns the ability of a drug to expand T cells specific for "self peptide/class II molecule." Assuming that only T cells with high affinity for self peptides presented by self MHC are deleted in the thymus (104), a drug could enhance the low affinity between the self peptide and a T-cell receptor. Such a T cell could be able to stimulate the corresponding B cell. A drug might act either by binding the T-cell receptor or the class II molecules, as outlined in Figure 4. Thus nickel interacting with a defined peptidic sequence could bind some T-cell receptor determinants (86) and then promote autoreactivity as well as gold-binding class II molecules. Such a concept could explain why drug-induced anti–class II T cells triggered preferentially some B-cell clones. It could also explain (1) that the differences in the third hypervariable region of DRβ gene that may contain the α helix of the peptide groove, govern the susceptibility to the autoimmune rheumatoid arthritis in humans (124,125), and (2) that the H2-^{bm12} mice differing from the wild type by only three amino acids in the third hypervariable region of one class II β chain molecule (126), mount an immune response

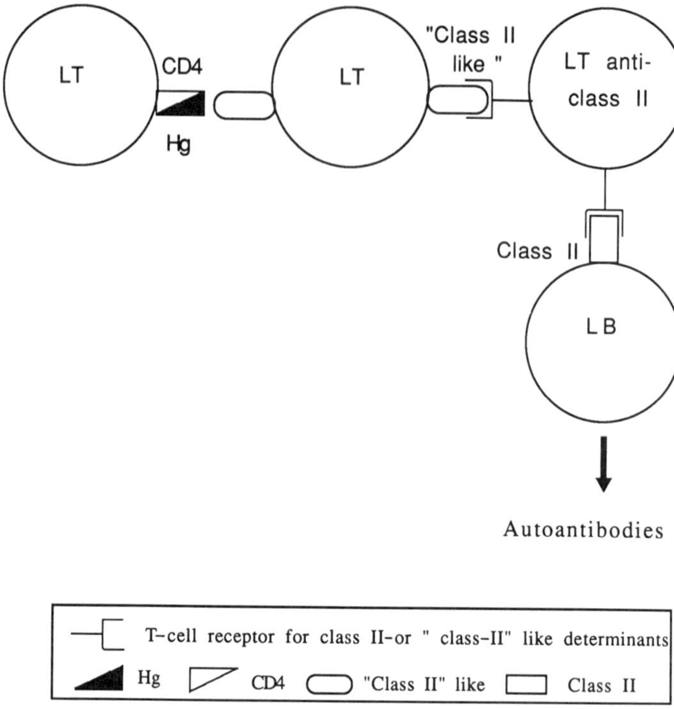

FIGURE 3 How could $HgCl_2$ induce autoreactive T cells in BN rats? Possible interactions between CD4 and Hg could activate T cells that recognize both class II molecules on B cells and "class II-like" determinants on T cells.

pattern very different from that of the wild type (127). More interestingly, $H2^{-bm12}$ mice are resistant to experimentally induced autoimmune myasthenia gravis, while the wild type is susceptible (128).

V. IgE RESPONSES AND INVOLVEMENT OF THE DIFFERENT CYTOKINES IN DRUG-INDUCED AUTOIMMUNITY

The IgE class poses a particular dilemma. On one hand, IgE arises as a defense against parasitic infections and is of benefit to the host. On the other hand, IgE inextricably linked in the sequence of atopic reactions against harmless antigens represents an undesirable side effect and is detrimental. Involved in many immediate hypersensitivity reactions against industrial chemicals and medicines, IgE

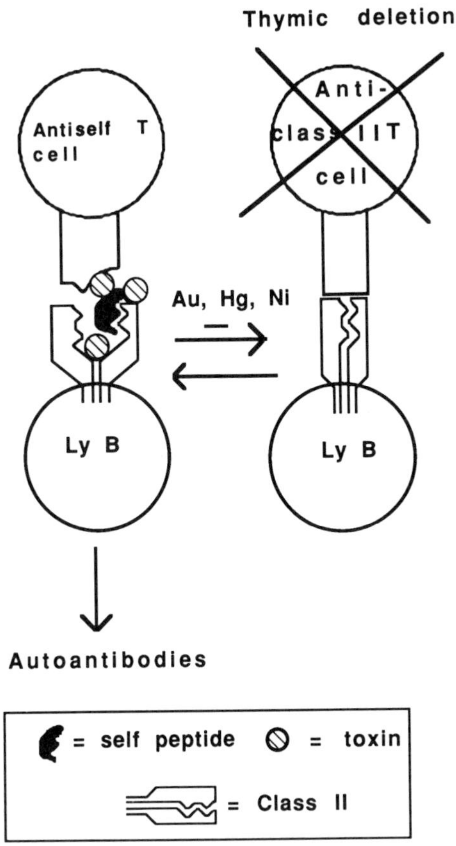

FIGURE 4 Binding of a toxin to either class II molecules or a self peptide presented by class II molecules or the specific T-cell receptor could enhance the affinity of the T-cell receptor for the self peptide and lead to autoreactivity.

is seldom implicated in human toxin-induced immune disorders. In BN rats, mercurials, D-penicillamine, and gold salts induce autoimmune diseases characterized by high concentrations of circulating IgE without any signs of immediate hypersensitivity. In these diseases, IgE might be neither beneficial nor detrimental but might be rather a marker of immune dysregulation.

Many heavy metal transition salts involved in atopic reactions have an effect on lymphocytes. Nickel, cadmium, cobalt, zinc, and mercury all produce nonspecific stimulatory effects on unsensitized human and animal blood lymphocytes. Furthermore, in rats, $HgCl_2$ and several platinum group metal salts exhibit an enhancing effect on specific IgE antibody response to ovalbumin (31,129). Experimental data concerning platinum salts suggest that in both sensitized and nonsensitized workers, this enhancing effect is obtained when there are already stimulated and multiplying B cells. This is likely to be true in $HgCl_2$-injected BN rats since $HgCl_2$ was proven to act as a T-dependent polyclonal B-cell activator. Further in-depth studies showed that $HgCl_2$ induces anti–class II autoreactive $CD4^+$ T cells (118) contributing to the polyclonal activation of B cells (23). In human, interactions of autoreactive T-helper clones derived from nonatopic subjects, with autologous B cells led to B-cell proliferation and IgE secretion (130). Regarding the considerable increase of circulating IgE level during mercury-induced autoimmune disease in BN rats, the aformentioned mechanism should be taken in account. For IgE synthesis to occur, a cognitive T_H–B-cell interaction is necessary together with another signal involving IL-4 (131). Not all T_H cells can infer IgE synthesis. In human, data from Quint et al. (132) suggest that $CD4^+$ T cells secreting predominantly IL-4 and belonging to the memory $CD45R^-$ subset are involved. Because they express surface antigen of the integrin family of adhesion proteins, these cells could possibly enhance T–B interactions and thus provide more efficient transfer of IL-4.

Little information is available that characterize the IgE committed B cell sublineage. Recently, MacKenzie and Dosch (133) demonstrated that IgE-committed B cells represent a unique B-cell subset where coexpression of IgE plus IgM and plus IgD is the rule. In mouse, IgE-secreting clones have been shown to produce IgM and IgE in the same proportion as human IgE-secreting clones, consistent with the view that IgE expression may follow similar pathways in either species. In BN rats, a toxic agent could stimulate, directly or not, such a B-cell subset. Moreover, a toxin could prevent downregulation of $sIgE^+$ B cells by altering Peyer's patches (PP), anatomic sites in which this modulation occurs. In the patients with the hyper IgE syndrome (HIES), PP are not detectable. It is tempting to speculate that the abnormalities of IgE regulation observed in HIES are due to the absence of PP or to an altered lymphoid traffic in these organs (134).

Like monocytes, platelets, and T lymphocytes, B cells express low affinity receptors for $Fc\epsilon$ ($Fc\epsilon RII$) that play a major role in the regulation of IgE production. The interaction between IgE and its receptor initiates a cascade of events that increases $Fc\epsilon RII$ expression and ultimately controls IgE synthesis. Recent studies by Richards et al. (135) showed that IgE–antigen complexes provide a stronger signal for inducing new $Fc\epsilon$ RII than monomeric IgE and, very excitingly, that these IgE–antigen complexes increase in parallel class II expression on B cells. Binding of IgE to $Fc\epsilon RII$ could decrease the turnover of the receptor and then enhance its expression on B cells. A similar mechanism might explain the increased expression of class II antigen since Bonnefoy et al. (136) reported that the FcϵRII and HLA-DR are spatially associated on human B-cell membranes. Other experimental data agree with a transmembrane communication for FcϵRII-mediated control of class II antigen expression. In $HgCl_2$-injected BN rats developing mercury-induced autoimmune disease, increase of class II expression may lead to an enhancement of FcϵRII expression on B cells. Such a mechanism might account for the hyperproduction of IgE.

In mouse as in human, involvement of IL-4 in IgE synthesis is well documented (137–140). Because of the impressive increase of IgE production during mercury-induced autoimmunity in BN rats (31), it was tempting to look for other effects of IL-4 during the course of the disease. C. Dubey et al. (unpublished) demonstrated a transient enhancement of class II expression by B cells that paralleled the kinetics of total serum IgE level. These results strongly suggest a role for IL-4. An increase of class II expression was observed on lymph node B cells as soon as the third day of $HgCl_2$ injections, and so far this is the earliest marker of immunotoxic effects of $HgCl_2$. Rat recombinant IL-4 is not yet available, and it is difficult to definitively relate increase of class II expression on B cells and IgE hyperproduction to IL-4 activity. Gleichmann et al. developed in the mouse a mercury-induced autoimmune disease similar to mercury-induced autoimmune disease in BN rats (43) and showed that anti-mouse IL-4 monoclonal antibody (11 B11) inhibited IgE synthesis in vivo (personal communication).

IL-4 produced by activated T_H cells enhances class II expression on B cells, which in turn stimulates anti–class II autoreactive T_H cells to proliferate and to release lymphokines. In the mouse, T_H1 and T_H2, two T_H cell subsets, have been defined according to their specific secretion of cytokines (141). Recently Mosmann and Coffman (142) proposed a model to predict which immune response should be expected depending upon the T_H1 and/or the T_H2 contributions. If the isotype produced may predict which of the two T_H subsets is implicated, high levels of IgE and IgG1 in the mercury model would predict a strong preferential T_H2 response with minimal T_H1 activation (if any). This overwhelming T_H2 response would lead to high production of IL-4 and IL-5 and low secretion (or absence) of interferon-γ and IL-2. A previous study by Baran et al. (143) showed that injections of $HgCl_2$ in BN rats for 7, 14, or 28 days resulted in a significant decrease of IL-2 production following Con A stimulation in vitro. These data are consistent with the poor IL-2 production by lymphoid cells from animals or humans with autoimmune diseases (144,145). It is likely that in BN rats, $HgCl_2$ induces anti–class II autoreactive T_H cells of the T_H2 subset preferentially. Consequently, IgE and IgG1 anti-GBM antibody production are enhanced while IL-2 secretion is decreased. Profound defects of IL-2 demonstrated as early as the 7th day of $HgCl_2$ injections suggests a strong inhibitory effect of the T_H2 subset towards the T_H1 subset.

V. REGULATORY MECHANISMS OF DRUG-INDUCED AUTOIMMUNITY

Autoregulation is the hallmark of drug-induced autoimmunity in BN rats. Mechanisms that could be at play will be discussed in this section.

A. Suppressor Mechanisms

The spontaneous resolution of drug-induced autoimmunity described in BN rats treated with $HgCl_2$, D-pencillamine, or gold salts while the drug was still inoculated led the authors to suspect the emergence of suppressor cells. This was supported by (1) the detection of elevated numbers of $CD8^+$ T-suppressor cells in blood lymphocytes during downregulation of autoimmunity (146), (2) the in vitro demonstration of $CD8^+$ T cells able to inhibit the proliferation of autoreactive T cells from the end of the second week (this was associated to a decrease in the frequency of anti–class II $CD4^+$ cells (118)), and (3) the attenuation of mercury-induced disease by transfer of $CD8^+$ T cells from healing rats into syngeneic $HgCl_2$-injected rats (35). However, in vivo $CD8^+$ cell depletion of BN rats treated with $HgCl_2$, gold salts, or D-penicillamine does not rule out the spontaneous regulation of the disease, evoking other regulatory mechanisms (47).

B. IgE Regulation

During the course of D-penicillamine, gold, and mercury autoimmune disease in BN rats, IgE synthesis is enhanced and then autoregulated. Alternative and non exclusive suppressive mechanisms can be proposed.

$CD8^+$ T cells have been involved in the regulation of IgE synthesis. Geha et al. (147) demonstrated that addition of normal $CD8^+$ T cells markedly decrease IgE secretion of B lymphocytes from patients with HIES. Lanzavecchia and Parodi (148) suggested that a possible mechanism for the inhibition of IgE production is the induction of specific cytotoxic cells. In contrast, $CD8^+$ T-cell depletion was ineffective on the course of mercury-induced disease, clearly demonstrating that lack of suppressor T cells does not modify IgE kinetics.

Production of anti-IgE isotype autoantibodies could participate to IgE regulation in drug-induced autoimmunity. In rats inoculated with autologous IgE, autoanti-IgE antibodies selectively suppress IgE responsiveness of neonates and adults (149,150). In human, IgG anti-IgE antibodies have been described in allergic and autoimmune disorders, as a part of circulating immune complexes (151). Another study demonstrated that Ig batches contain both IgE and IgG anti-IgE antibodies that inhibit spontaneous IgE production in vitro, such inhibition being correlated with IgE and IgG anti-IgE antibody concentrations (152). This latter finding led to the suggestion that IgG anti-IgE antibodies mimic an IgE-binding factor suppressor of IgE synthesis. It cannot be ruled out that circulating immune complexes found in mercury-induced autoimmune disease are partly IgG–anti-IgE immune complexes.

Finally, IgE production might be regulated by idiotypic–anti-idiotypic interactions that can involve both B and T lymphocytes (153). In BALB/c mice primary IgE response against benzylpenicilloyl (BPO) group (responsible for human allergic disease) was suppressed following immunization with purified anti-BPO antibodies (154). Such a suppression was also observed after injections of syngeneic spleen cells chemically coupled with idiotype-expressing antibodies or with cells natively bearing the relevant idiotype. Furthermore, an established IgE response against the same BPO hapten was specifically suppressed for 2 or 3 weeks by a single intravenous injection of autologous anti-BPO anti-idiotype antibodies. The suppressive effect could be due to direct inactivation or depletion of B cells expressing idiotypes and later by specific T-suppressor cells. So far, during mercury-induced autoimmune disease in BN rats, idiotypic regulation of IgE synthesis has not been proven to occur. However, there are lines of evidence that idiotypic interactions are at play to regulate the production of the numerous anti-nonself and antiself antibodies induced by $HgCl_2$-mediated polyclonal B-cell activation.

IgE could downregulate its production. Regulation of IgE antibody production starting the third week of $HgCl_2$ injections is consistent with an antibody effect that counteracts the bias imposed by cytokines. The regulatory effect of IgE on the T_H2 subset would lead to the inhibition of antibody synthesis (142). In addition, IgE can favor activation of the T_H1 subset and, consequently, production of interferon-γ. This latter interleukin antagonizes IL-4 and therefore depresses IgE synthesis (155). Such a mechanism might explain the return of the immune system to a state of balance; it is unlikely to explain the unresponsiveness of the immune system to $HgCl_2$.

C. Idiotypic Regulations

In mercury-induced autoimmune disease of BN rats, autoanti-GBM antibodies share cross-idiotypic determinants (CRid Hg) borne by kidney-eluted, kidney-bound, and circulating anti-GBM antibodies. The kinetics of Ig-bearing CRid Hg paralleled that of anti-GBM antibody activity (156). Like mercury-induced autoimmune disease, gold and D-penicillamine autoimmune diseases are considered a consequence of a T-dependent polyclonal B-cell activation probably mediated by anti–class II T cells and responsible for the production of circulating and kidney-bound autoanti-GBM antibodies. The demonstration that the CRid Hg expressed in the mercury model are also borne by kidney-eluted Ig in gold- and D-penicillamine-treated BN rats suggests that anti–class II T cells activate the same B-cell clones (46). Moreover, in $HgCl_2$- and D-penicillamine–induced autoimmune diseases in BN rats, circulating IgE has been shown to bear CRid Hg, the kinetics of CRid Hg expression paralleling that of serum IgE during the course of the diseases (B. Bellon, unpublished). Since no IgE has ever been found that exhibits anti-GBM specificity, it is likely that IgE CRid$^+$ anti-GBM$^-$ represent the idiotypic parallel set described by Oudin and Cazenave. These results are in agreement with the emphasis on public idiotype in autoimmunity (157). In active systemic lupus erythematosus (SLE) common idiotypes of anti-DNA antibodies (16/6 and 32/15 idiotypes) have been described and were also detected on anti-DNA antibodies from patients with procainamide-induced lupus (158). Moreover, serum concentrations of 16/6 public idiotype have been proven better markers of disease activity in SLE than concentrations of anti-DNA antibodies (158). These latter antibodies could be tied up in immune complexes and therefore not easily detectable by conventional tests, whereas they could be identified by a public idiotype. Thus, T-dependent polyclonal B-cell activation can be considered to have CRid Hg as markers, and according to the prediction of Jerne's network theory its regulation could involve autoanti-CRid Hg antibodies. In mercury-induced autoimmune disease, Chalopin and Lockwood gave evidence of humoral factors behaving as auto-andi-Id antibodies able to block GBM specific cells (36). Recently Guéry obtained an autoanti-idiotypic monoclonal antibody that recognizes a V_K-associated idiotype expressed on two anti-GBM monoclonal antibodies, one of them produced in the same fusion, thus demonstrating that anti-GBM antibodies and their corresponding autoanti-idiotypic antibodies are simultaneously produced during the disease (159). Indeed such autoanti-idiotype antibodies may have a regulatory role, but they may also exert a pathogenic effect. Idiotype–anti-idiotype immune complexes were found in glomeruli from LPS-injected mice exhibiting polyclonal activation (160). Such idiotype–anti-idiotype immune complexes could be responsible in part for the granular IgG deposits observed in the mercury model. Although not investigated in drug-induced autoimmune diseases, a possible role for T cells in idiotypic regulation should not be ruled out (161). It is well documented that B and T cells share idiotypic determinants (162–164). There are examples of idiotype-specific T cells characteristically MHC restricted (165), the Ig idiotype being probably recognized as a peptide in association with class II antigen. Alternatively, direct interaction between Ig idiotype and T-cell receptor may occur independently of MHC (166). This latter process may lead to pathological conditions and autoimmune diseases (167).

VII. HOW CAN A TOXIN LEAD TO LYMPHOCYTE ACTIVATION?

The intracellular mechanisms of activation have been primarily studied by physiologists or biochemists. Thus little is known about the effects of drugs on the activation of lymphocyte. Multiple intracellular targets have been demonstrated for metals and particularly for cationic ones (114) (Table 6). It is noteworthy that metals are frequently responsible for immunotoxic manifestations presumably

TABLE 6 Possible Mechanisms of Drug-Induced Cellular Activation

Ligand mimicry
Modification of the membrane lipid bilayer
Modification of the ligand–receptor interaction
Modification of activation via T-cell receptor–class II-peptide interaction
Activation via accessory molecules (CD4, CD2)
Modulation of transducers
Modification of the metabolism of second messengers
Modulation of enzymatic functions (kinases, phosphodiesterases)
Modifications of the oxidative metabolism of the cell
Modulation of intracellular ionic activities
Interactions with nucleoproteins

due to their ability to interact with many compounds involved in cellular activation. Cationic metals may bind to sulfhydryl, phosphoryl, carboxyl, or nitryl groups. For example, Hg and Au bind sulfhydryl groups with a 10^{15}–10^{20} and 10^5 affinity constant, respectively (168,169); Hg also has a substantial affinity constant for hydroxyl, carboxyl, or phosphoryl groups (constant of affinity of 10^{15}), (170,171). To understand how a metal can lead to cellular activation or inhibition of activation is of great interest.

Figure 5 summarizes the three pathways leading to the activation of a cell (114,172–174). Recognition and transduction are always required; sometimes second messengers are generated, but in any case the biological effects are mediated by phosphorylated proteins. Current models of T-cell activation involve hydrolysis of phosphoinositol, activation of protein kinase C (PKC), and increase in intracellular $Ca2^+$ concentration (Figs. 5,6a), (174); the latter can be affected by cationic metals as shown in Figure 6a (84,85,115,175–177). However, it is not excluded that toxins such as Pb, Cd, and Zn can enhance cAMP and activate T cells via the PKC pathway (178) (Fig. 6). Indeed, PKC could be a target for protein kinase A (PKA) as shown in B cells (178); cAMP-elevating agents stimulate nuclear translocation of PKC—this nuclear PKC could upregulate its gene expression. Finally, some membrane receptors that possess a tyrosine kinase activity are involved in the regulation of cellular growth (173,179). Initially, they were defined as numerous retroviral oncogenes involved in cellular transformation, but they also include receptors for growth factors (e.g., EGF) (179). These receptors have a capacity for autophosphorylation. Murine T cells have a high level of protein kinase activity, and it was recently shown that murine leukocytes and particularly T cells express a gene encoding for a transmembrane protein-kinase belonging to this family (180). The corresponding protein is an integral membrane protein of 56 kD. The $p56^{lck}$ is physically associated to CD4 and CD8

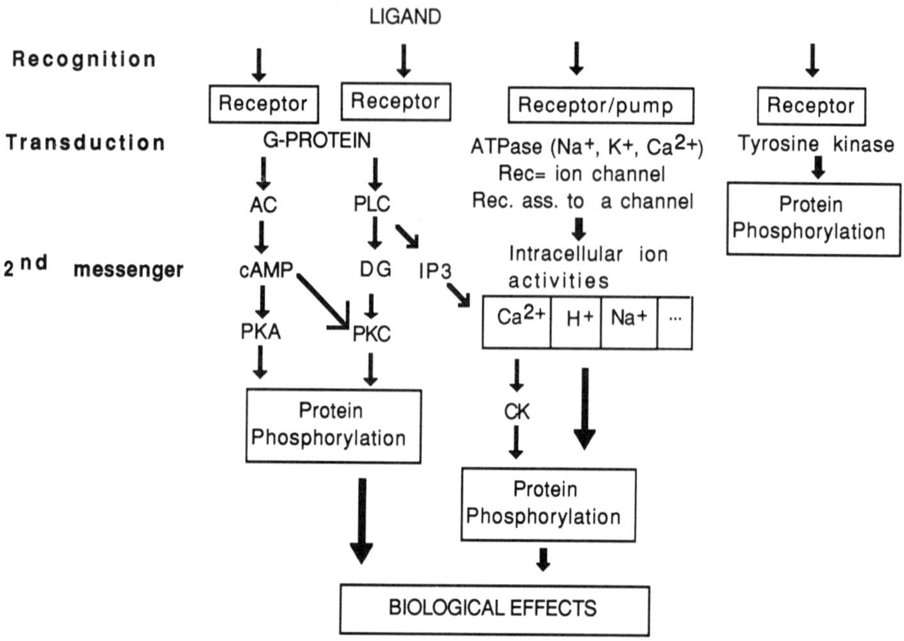

FIGURE 5 One ligand–receptor interaction can lead to cellular activation via either the protein kinase A (PKA)– or the protein kinase C (PKC)–mediated pathways. Growth factors can bind a receptor with a tyrosine kinase activity. Receptors (Rec) can be either pumps or ion channels or can be associated to these (Rec ass. to a channel). Interaction of a ligand with such a receptor can modify ion intracellular activities and cell activation status. AC = adenylate cyclase; cAMP = cyclic adenosine 5′ monophosphate; PLC = phospholipase C; DG = diacylglycerol; IP3 = insitol-1,4,5-triphosphate; CK = calmodulin kinase.

molecules by a possible binding sequence Lys-Arg-Lys-Arg-X-Cys-X-Cys-Pro-X-X-X-X-Lys-Thr/Ser. The cysteine residues, targets for Hg, Au, Zn, and Pb, are crucial in this interaction. CD4 and CD8 antigens modulate the T-cell response depending upon the proximity of these accessory molecules to the Ti/CD3 receptor (179,181,182); $p56^{lck}$ associated to CD4/CD8 might phosphorylate the ζ chain of the CD3 molecule and perhaps other chains of the CD3 molecule or other substrates (Fig. 7) (179). The toxins could bind molecules such as CD4 and CD2 molecules and deliver a positive signal to the cell as can some specific antibodies (181–184). Metals such as mercurials are known to modify the membrane lipid bilayer (185); since the proximity of CD4 and Ti/CD3 or the proximity of CD4 and other molecules such as CD45 play a crucial role in

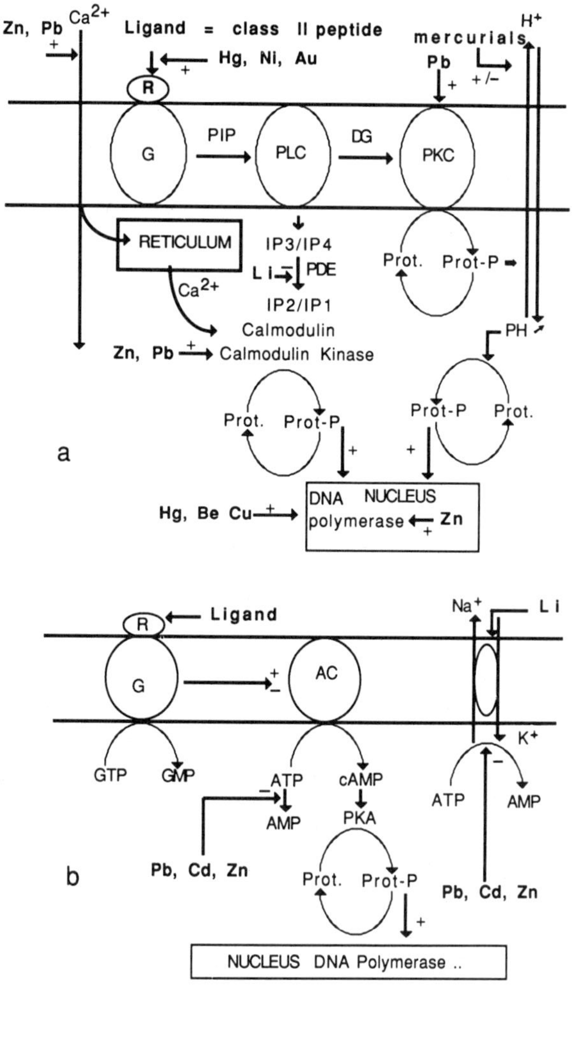

FIGURE 6 Interactions of cationic metals with the protein kinase A (PKA)–mediated (a) or protein kinase C (PKC)–mediated (b) pathways. R = receptor; G = GTP binding protein; PIP = phosphatidyl inositol-4,5-biphosphate, PLC = phospholipase C; DG = diacylglycerol; Prot = protein; Prot-P = phosphorylated protein; IP3 = inositol-1,4,5-triphosphate; IP4 = inositol-1,3,4,5-tetraphosphate; IP2 = inositol-3,4-bisphosphate; IP1 = inositol-4-monophosphate; PDE = phosphodiesterase; AC = adenylate cyclase GTP = guanosine triphosphate; GDP = guanosine diphosphate; ATP = adenosine triphosphate; AMP = adenosine monophosphate; cAMP = cyclic adenosine 5′ monophosphate.

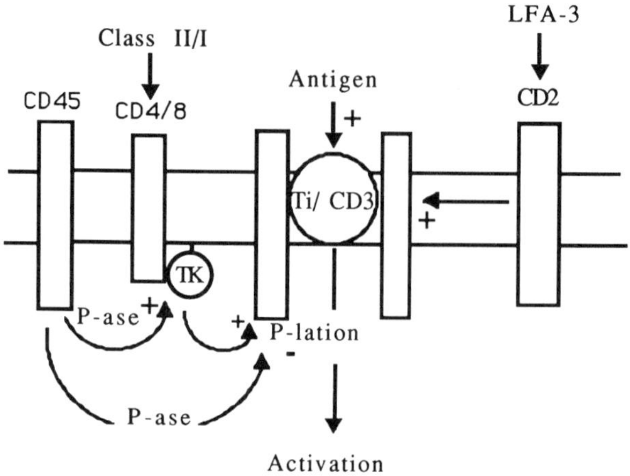

FIGURE 7 Cooperative regulatory interactions between CD4/8$^-$ tyrosine kinase (p56^{lck}), CD45, CD2, and the CD3-receptor complex (Ti/CD3). CD45 could dephosphorylate p56^{lck}, which would increase p56^{lck} activity and indirectly activate the CD3 complex. Alternatively, CD45 could directly interact with CD3 and counteract p56^{lck} effects. P-ase = phosphatase; P-lation = phosphorylation.

activation (179) (Fig. 7), physical modifications of the membrane fluidity could be sufficient to up- or downregulate cellular activation.

A toxin could also act directly at every level involved in the protein phosphorylation, as shown in Figure 6 (reviewed in Ref. 114). In summary, lead, zinc, and lithium can act on the $Ca2^+$-dependent pathway of activation, whereas mercurials that affect the regulation of proton intracellular activities could modify pH-dependent protein phosphorylation. Little is known about interactions between toxin and nucleoproteins involved in the regulation of gene expression except for the copper able to activate metallothionein gene by altering the conformation of a specific DNA-binding protein (186). However, nuclear receptors were evoked for Hg and beryllium (187,188). Zinc is a normal cofactor of DNA polymerase and acts by binding nuclear proteins through a Cys-Cys loop (189). Exogenous zinc is able to increase the activity of this enzyme and promote DNA synthesis; other metals could have the same effects.

The results obtained from experimental models should make it possible to dissect molecular aspects of drug-induced activation or inhibition of the lymphocytes involved in the immune response. Such studies, however, require T-cell clones. It is noteworthy that such T-cell clones are already available in some human situations.

REFERENCES

1. Hahn, L. J., Kloiber, R., Vimy, M. J., Takahashi, Y., and Lorscheider, F. L. 1989. Dental "silver" tooth fillings: A source of mercury exposure revealed by whole-body image scan and tissue analysis. *FASEB J.*, *3*: 2641-2646.
2. Bigazzi, P. E. 1988. Autoimmunity induced by chemicals. *Clin. Toxicol.*, *26*: 125–156.
3. Habibi, B. 1987. Drug-induced immune haemolytic animals. *Clin. Immunol. Allerg.*, *1*: 343–356.
4. Charpentier, B., Moullot, P., Faux, N., Manigand, G., and Fries, D. 1981. Fonctions lymphocytaires T au cours d'une glomerulonephrite extramembraneuse induite par une intoxication chronique au mercure. Arguments pour un defaut lymphocytaire de presentation des molecules de classe II d'histocompatibilite. *Nephrologie*, *2*: 153–157.
5. Fillastre, J. P., Druet, P., and Mery, J. P. 1988. Proteinuria associated with drugs and substances of abuse. In *The Nephrotic Syndrome* (J. S. Cameron and Glassock, eds.). Marcel Dekker, New York, pp. 697–744.
6. Kammüller, M. E., Bloksma, N., and Seinen, W. 1989. Autoimmunity and toxicology. Immune disregulation induced by drugs and chemicals. In *Autoimmunity and Toxicology* (M. E. Kammüller, N. Bloksma, and W. Seinen, eds.). Elsevier, New York, pp. 3-35.
7. Tournade, H., Pelletier, L., Glotz, D., and Druet, P. 1989. Toxiques et autoimmunité. *Med. Sci.*, *5*: 303–310.
8. Davies, D. M. 1977. *Textbook of Adverse Drug Reactions*. Oxford University Press.
9. Wilson, C. B. 1982. Drug- and toxin-induced nephritis. Anti-kidney antibody and immune complex mediation. In *Nephrotoxic Mechanisms of Drugs and Environmental Toxins* (G. A. Porter, eds.). Plenum, pp. 389-392.
10. Hall, C. 1982. Gold and D-penicillamine induced renal disease. In *The Kidney and Rheumatic Disease* (P. A. Bacon and N. M. Hadler, eds.). Butterworth, London, pp. 246-266.
11. Ainsworth, Swain, R. P., Watabe, N., Brackett, N. C., Pilia, P., and Henniger, G. R. 1981. Gold nephropathy. *Arch. Pathol. Lab. Med.*, *105*: 371–378.
12. Shaloub, R. J. 1974. Pathogenesis of lipoid nephrosis: A disorder of T-cell function. *Lancet*, *ii*: 556–559.
13. Alder, R., Boxstein, D., Schaff, P., and Kelly, D. 1982. Metallic mercury vapor poisoning simulating mucocutaneous lymph node syndrome. *J. Pediatrics*, *101*: 967–968.
14. Wooley, P. H., Griffin, J., Panayi, G. S., Batchelor, J. R., Welsh, K. I., and Gibson, T. J. 1980. HLA-DR antigens and toxic reaction to sodium aurothiomalate and D-penicillamine in patients with rheumatoid arthritis. *N. Engl. J. Med.*, *303*: 300–302.
15. Emery, P., Panayi, G. S., Huston, G., Welsh, K. L., Mitschell, S. C., Shah, R. R., Idle, J. R., Smith, R. L., and Waring, R. H. 1984. D-penicillamine induced toxicity in rheumatoid arthritis: the role of sulphoxidation status and HLA-DR3. *J. Rheum.*, *11*: 626–632.

16. Woosley, R. L., Drayer, D. E., Reidenberg, M. M., Nies, A. S., Carr, K., and Oates, J. A. 1978. Effect of acetylator phenotype on the rate at which procainamide induces antinuclear antibodies and the lupus syndrome. *N. Engl. J. Med., 298*: 1157–1159.
17. Batchelor, J. R., Welsh, K. L., Tinoco, R. M., Dollery, C. T., Hugues, G. R. V., Bernstein, R., Ryan, P., Naish, P. F., Aber, G. M., Bing, R. F., and Russell, G. I. 1980. Hydralazine-induced systemic lupus erythematosus: Influence of HLA-DR and sex on susceptibility. *Lancet, i*: 1107–1109.
18. Polak, L., Barnes, J. M., and Turk, J. L. 1968. The genetic control of contact sensitization to inorganic metal compounds in guinea pigs. *Immunol., 14*: 707–711.
19. Weening, J. J., Fleuren, G. J., and Hoedemaeker, P. J. 1978. I Demonstration of anti-nuclear antibodies in mercury-induced glomerulopathy in the rat. *Lab. Invest., 39*: 405–411.
20. Weening, J. J., Hoedemaeker, P. J., and Bakker, W. W. 1981. Immunoregulation and anti-nuclear antibodies in mercury-induced glomerulopathy in the rat. *Clin. Exp. Immunol., 45*: 64–71.
21. Sapin, C., Druet, E., and Druet, P. 1977. Induction of anti-glomerular basement membrane antibodies in the Brown-Norway rat by mercuric chloride. *Clin. Exp. Immunol., 28*: 173–178.
22. Druet, P., Druet, E., Potdevin, F., and Sapin, C. 1978. Immune type glomerulonephritis induced by $HgCl_2$ in the Brown Norway rat. *Ann. Immunol. (Inst. Pasteur), 129C*: 777–792.
23. Hirsch, F., Couderc, J., Sapin, C., Fournie, G., and Druet, P. 1982. Polyclonal effect of $HgCl_2$ in the rat, its possible role in an experimental autoimmune disease. *Eur. J. Immunol., 12*: 620–625.
24. Bellon, B., Capron, M., Druet, E., Verroust, P., Vial, M. C., Sapin, C., Girard, J. F., Foidart, J. M., Mahieu, P., and Druet, P. 1982. Mercuric chloride-induced autoimmunity in Brown Norway rats: Sequential search for anti-basement membrane antibodies. *Eur. J. Clin. Invest., 12*: 127–133.
25. Burres, S. A., Kanter, M. E., Richman, D. P., and Arnason, B. G. W. 1981. Studies on the pathophysiology of chronic D-penicillamine-induced myasthenia. *Ann. N. Y. Acad. Sci., 377*: 640–650.
26. McVicker, J. H., Lava, N. S., Mittag, T. W., and Ringel, S. P. 1982. D-penicillamine-induced neuromuscular disease in guinea pigs. *Exper. Neurol., 76*: 46–57.
27. Donker, A. J., Rocco, C. V., Vladutiu, A. O., Brentjens, J. R., and Andres, G. A. 1984. Effects of prolonged administration of D-penicillamine or captopril in various strains of rats. Brown-Norway rats treated with D-penicillamine develop autoantibodies, circulating immune complexes and disseminated intravascular coagulation. *Clin. Immunol. Immunopathol., 30*: 142–155.
28. Tournade, H., Pelletier, L., Pasquier, R., Vial, M. C., Mandet, C., and Druet, P. 1990. D-penicillamine-induced autoimmunity in Brown-Norway rats: Similarities with $HgCl_2$-induced autoimmunity. *J. Immunol., 144*: 2985–2991.
29. Pelletier, L., Pasquier, R., Guettier, C., Vial, M. C., Mandet, C., Nochy, D., Bazin, H., and Druet, P. 1988. $HgCl_2$ induces T and B cells to proliferate and differentiate in BN rats. *Clin. Exp. Immunol., 71*: 336–342.

30. Pusey, C. D., Bowman, C., Morgan, A., Weetman, A. P., Hartley, B., Lockwood, C. M. 1990. Kinetics and pathogenicity of autoantibodies induced by mercuric chloride in the Brown Norway rat. *Clin. Exp. Immunol., 81*: 76–82.
31. Prouvost-Danon, A., Abadie, A., Sapin, C., Bazin, H., and Druet, P. 1981. Induction of IgE synthesis and potentiation of anti-ovalbumin IgE response by $HgCl_2$ in the rat. *J. Immunol., 126*: 699–702.
32. Sten, J., Bosman, C. B., Rosing, J., Stjnen, T., Hoedemaeker, P. J., and Weening, J. J. 1988. Mercuric chloride-induced autoimmunity in the Brown Norway rat. Cellular kinetics and major histocompatibility complex antigen expression. *Am. J. Pathol., 133*: 127–138.
33. Pelletier, L., Pasquier, R., Vial, M. C., Mandet, C., Moutier, R., Salomon, J. C., and Druet, P. 1987. Mercury-induced autoimmune glomerulonephritis: Requirement for T cells. *Nephrol. Dial. Transplant., 1*: 211–218.
34. Pelletier, L., Pasquier, R., Rossert, J., Vial, M. C., Mandet, C., and Druet, P. 1988. Autoreactive T cells in mercury disease. Ability to induce the autoimmune disease. *J. Immunol., 140*: 750–754.
35. Bowman, C., Mason, D. W., Pusey, C. D., and Lockwood, C. M. 1984. Autoregulation of antibody synthesis in mercuric chloride nephritis in the Brown Norway rat. I. A role for T suppressor cells. *Eur. J. Immunol., 14*: 464–470.
36. Chalopin, J. M., and Lockwood, C. M. 1984. Autoregulation of antibody synthesis in mercuric chloride nephritis in the Brown Norway rat. II. Presence of antigen augmentable plaque forming cells in the spleen is associated with humoral factors behaving as auto-antiidiotypic antibodies. *Eur. J. Immunol., 14*: 470–475.
37. Druet, E., Sapin, C., Günther, E., Feingold, N., and Druet, P. 1977. Mercuric chloride induced anti-glomerular basement membrane antibodies in the rat. Genetic control. *Eur. J. Immunol., 7*: 348–351.
38. Aten, J., Bruijn, J. A., Veringa, A., de Heer, E., and Weening, J. J. 1988. Anti-laminin autoantibodies and mercury-induced membranous glomerulopathy. *Kidney Int., 33*: 309.
39. Roman-Franco, A., Turiello, A., Albini, M., Ossi, E., Milgrom, F., and Andres, G. A. 1978. Anti-basement membrane antibodies and antigen-antibody complexes in rabbits injected with mercuric chloride. *Clin. Immunol. Immunopathol., 9*: 464–481.
40. Eneström, S., and Hultman, P. 1984. Immune-related glomerulonephritis induced by mercuric chloride in mice. *Experientia, 40*: 1234–1240.
41. Hultman, P., and Eneström, S. 1987. The induction of immune complex deposits in mice by peroral and parenteral administration of mercuric chloride: Strain dependent susceptibility. *Clin. Exp. Immunol., 67*: 283–292.
42. Hultman, P., and Eneström, S. 1988. Mercury-induced antinuclear antibodies in mice: Characterization and correlation with renal immune complex deposits. *Clin. Exp. Immunol., 71*: 269–274.
43. Pietsch, P., Vohr, H. W., Degitz, K., and Gleichmann, E. 1989. Immunopathological signs inducible by mercury compounds. II. $HgCl_2$ and gold sodium thiomalate enhance serum IgE and IgG concentrations in susceptible mouse strains. *Int. Arch. Allergy. Appl. Immun., 90*: 47–53.
44. Robinson, C. J. G., Abraham, A. A., and Balazs, T. 1984. Induction of anti-nuclear antibodies by mercuric chloride in mice. *Clin. Exp. Immunol., 58*: 300–306.

45. Balazs, T., Robinson, C. J. G., and Abramam, A. A. 1984. Drug-induced autoimmunity in rats (abstract). Sixth Int. Congress of Immunology, Toronto, Canada.
46. Guery, J. C., Tournade, H., Pelletier, L., Druet, E., and Druet, P. 1990. Rat anti-glomerular basement membrane antibodies in toxin-induced autoimmunity and in chronic graft-versus-host reaction share recurrent idiotypes. *Eur. J. Immunol., 20*: 101–105.
47. Pelletier, L., Rossert, J., Pasquier, P., Vial, M. C., and Druet, P. 1990. Role of $CD8^+$ T cells in mercury-induced autoimmunity or immunosuppression in the rat. *Scand. J. Immunol., 31*: 65–74.
48. Batsford, S. R., Rohrbach, Reide, U. N., Sandritter, and Kluthe, R. 1976. Effects of D-penicillamine administration to rats, induction of renal changes: preliminary communication. *Clin. Nephrol., 6*: 394–397.
49. Nagi, A. H., Alexander, F., and Barabas, A. Z. 1971. Gold nephropathy in rats. Light and electron microscopic studies. *Exp. Mol. Pathol., 15*: 354–362.
50. Robinson, C. J. G., Balazs, T., and Egorov, I. K. 1986. Mercuric chloride, gold sodium thiomalate, and D-penicillamine-induced anti-nuclear antibodies in mice. *Clin. Exp. Immunol., 58*: 300–306.
51. Ueda, S., Wakashin, M., Wakashin, Y., Yoshida, H., Iesato, K., Mori, T., Mori, Y., Akikusa, B., and Okuda, K. 1986. Experimental gold nephropathy in guinea pigs: Detection of autoantibodies to renal tubular antigens. *Kidney Int., 29*: 539–548.
52. Ohsawa, M., Takahashi, K., and Otsuka, F. 1988. Induction of anti-nuclear antibodies in mice orally exposed to cadmium at low concentrations. *Clin. Exp. Immunol., 73*: 98–102.
53. Johsi, B. C., Dwivedi, C., Powell, A., and Holscher, M. 1981. Immune complex nephritis in rats induced by long-term exposure to cadmium. *J. Comp. Path., 91*: 11–15.
54. Aucoin, D. P. 1989. Propylthiouracil-induced immune-mediated disease syndrome in the cat: A novel model for a drug-induced lupus-like disease. In *Autoimmunity and Toxicology* (M. E. Kammüller, N. Bloksma, and W. Seinen, eds.). Elsevier, New York, pp. 309–323.
55. Aucoin, D. P., Rubin, R. L., Peterson, M. E., Reidenberg, M. M., Drayer, D. D., Hurvitz, A. I., and Lahita, R. G. 1988. Dose-dependent induction of anti-native DNA antibodies in cats by propylthiouracil. *Arthritis Rheum., 31*: 688–693.
56. Malinow, M. R., Bardana, E. J., Pirofsky, B., and Craig, S. 1982. Systemic lupus erythematosus-like syndrome in monkeys fed alfalfa sprouts: Role of a nonprotein ammino acid. *Science, 216*: 415–417.
57. Alcocer-Varela, J., Iglesias, A., Lorente, L., and Alarcon-Segovia, D. 1985. Effects of L-canavanine on T cells may explain the induction of systemic lupus erythematosus by alfalfa. *Arthritis. Rheum., 28*: 52–57.
58. Cannat, A., and Seligmann, M. 1968. Induction by isoniazid and hydralazine of antinuclear factors in mice. *Clin. Exp. Immunol., 3*: 99–105.
59. Ten Venn, J. H., and Feltkamp, T. E. W. 1972. Studies on drug induced lupus erythematosus. I. Drug induced antinuclear antibodies (ANA). *Clin. Exp. Immunol., 11*: 265–276.
60. Thomson, A. W., and Webster, L. M. 1988. The influence of cyclosporin A on cell mediated immunity. *Clin. Exp. Immunol., 71*: 369–376.

61. Santos, G. W., Hess, A. D., and Vogelsang, G. B. 1984. Graft-versus-host reactions. *Immunol. Rev., 88*: 169-192.
62. Glazier, A., Tustschka, P. J., Farmer, E. R., and Santos, G. W. 1985. Graft-versus host disease in cyclosporin A-treated rats after syngeneic and autologous bone marrow reconstitution. *J. Exp. Med., 158*: 1-8.
63. Hess, A. D., Horwitz, L., Beschorner, W. E., and Santos, G. W. 1985. Development of graft-vs.-host disease-like syndrome in cyclosporine-treated rats after syngeneic bone marrow transplantation. I. Development of cytotoxic T lymphocytes with apparent polyclonal anti-Ia specificity, including autoreactivity. *J. Exp. Med., 161*: 718-730.
64. Fischer, A. C., Beschorner, W. E., and Hess, A. D. 1989. Requirements for the induction and adoptive transfer of cyclosporin-induced syngeneic graft-versus host disease. *J. Exp. Med., 169*: 1031-1041.
65. Sorokin, R., Kimura, H., Schroder, K., Wilson, D. H., and Wilson, D. B. 1986. Cyclosporin-induced autoimmunity: Conditions for expressing, requirement for intact thymus, and potency estimates of autoimmune lymphocytes in drug-treated rats. *J. Exp. Med., 164*: 1615-1625.
66. Sakaguchi, S., and Sakaguchi, N. 1988. Thymus and autoimmunity. Transplantation of the thymus from cyclosporin A-treated mice cause organ-specific autoimmune disease in athymic nude mice. *J. Exp. Med., 167*: 1479-1485.
67. Jenkins, M. K., Schwartz, R. H., and Pardoll, D. M. 1988. Effects of cyclosporin A on T cell development and clonal deletion. *Science, 241*: 1655-1657.
68. Sakaguchi, S., and Sakaguchi, N. 1989. Organ-specific autoimmune disease induced by elimination of T cell subsets. V. Neonatal administration of cyclosporin A causes autoimmune disease. *J. Immunol., 142*: 471-480.
69. L'age-Stehr, J., and Diamantstein, T. 1978. Studies on induction and control of cell-mediated-autoimmunity. I. Induction of "autoreactive" T lymphocytes in mice by cyclophosphamide. *Eur. J. Immunol., 8*: 620-624.
70. Satoh, H., Martin, B. M., Schulick, A. H., Christ, D. D., Kenna, J. G., and Phol, L. R. 1989. Human anti-endosplamic reticulum antibodies in sera of patients with halothane-induced hepatitis are directed against a trifluoroacetylated carboxylesterase. *Proc. Natl. Sci., 86*: 322-326.
71. Beaune, P., Dansette, P. M., Mansuy, D., Kiffel, L., Finck, M., Leroux, J. P., and Homberg, J. C. 1987. Human anti-endoplasmic reticulum autoantibodies appearing in a drug-induced hepatitis are directed against a human liver cytochrome P-450 that hydroxylates the drug. *Proc. Natl. Acad. Sci. USA, 84*: 551-555.
72. Sim, E. 1989. Drug interactions with complement components in relation to the induction of auto-immune-like interactions. In *Autoimmunity and Toxicology* (M. E. Kammüller, N. Bloksma, and W. Seinen, eds.). Elsevier, New York, pp. 3-35.
73. Ishizaka, S., and Moller, G. 1982. Lithium chloride induces partial responsiveness to LPS in nonresponder B cells. *Nature, 299*: 363-365.
74. Rolink, A. G., Pals, S. T., and Gleichmann, E. 1983. Allosuppressor and allohelper T cells in acute and chronic graft-versus-host disease. II. F1 recipients carrying mutations at H-2k and/or I-A. *J. Exp. Med., 157*: 755-771.
75. Rolink, A. G., Pals, S. T., and Gleichmann, E. 1983. Allosuppressor and allohelper

T cells in acute and chronic graft-versus-host disease. III Different Lyt subsets of donor T cells induce different pathological syndromes. *J. Exp. Med.*, *158*: 546–558.

76. Abramowicz, D., Goldman, M., Bruyins, C., Lambert, P. H., Thoua, Y., and Toussaint, C. 1987. Autoimmune disease after neonatal injection of semi-allogeneic spleen cells in mice; involvement of donor B and T cells and characterization of glomerular deposits. *Clin. Exp. Immunol.*, *70*: 61–67.
77. Abramowicz, D., Vandervost, P., Bruyins, C., and Goldman, M. 1987. In vitro demonstration of alloreactive T cells involved in anti-DNA antibody production after neonatal induction of transplantation tolerance in mice (abstract). *Int. Arch. Allergy Appl. Immunol.*, *83*: 821.
78. Gleichman, E., Pals, S. T., Rolink, A. G., Radaszkiewicz, T., and Gleichmann, H. 1984. Graft-versus host reactions: Clues to the etiopathology of a spectrum of immunological diseases. *Immunol. Today*, *5*: 324–332.
79. Gleichman, E., van Elven, E. H., and van der Veen, J. P. W. 1982. Systemic lupus erythematosus (SLE)-like disease in mice induced by abnormal T-B cell cooperation. Preferential formation of autoantibodies characteristic of SLE. *Eur. J. Immunol.*, *12*: 152–159.
80. Van der Veen, J. P. W., Kiesel, F. M., Poels, L., Schuler, W., Melief, C. J. M., Landegent, J., and Gleichmann, E. 1984. Further evidence against random polyclonal antibody formation in mice with lupus-like graft-versus-host disease. *J. Immunol.*, *132*: 1814–1820.
81. Clayberger, C., DeKruyff, R. H., and Cantor, H. 1984. Immunoregulatory activities of autoreactive-T cells: An Ia-specific T cell clone mediates both help and suppression of antibody responses. *J. Immunol.*, *132*: 2237–2243.
82. Quintans, J., Suzuki, H., Sosman, J. A., and Shah, P. D. 1986. Immunoregulation by T cells. I. Characterization of the IEk-specific Lbd self reactive T cell clone that helps, suppresses and contrasuppresses B cell responses. *J. Immunol.*, *136*: 1974–1981.
83. Nagata, N., Hurtenbach, U., and Gleichmann, E. 1986. Specific sensitization of Lyt-1+2− T cells to spleen cells modified by the drug D-penicillamine or a stereoisomer. *J. Immunol.*, *136*: 136–142.
84. Warner, G. L., and Lawrence, D. A. 1986. Stimulation of murine lymphocyte responses by cations. *Cell. Immunol.*, *101*: 425–439.
85. Warner, G. L., and Lawrence, D. A. 1986. Cell surface and cell cycle analysis of metal-induced murine T cell proliferation. *Eur. J. Immunol.*, *16*: 1337–1342.
86. Kapsenberg, M. L., van der Pouw-Kraan, T., Stiekema, F. E., Schootemeijer, A., and Bos, J. D. 1988. Direct and indirect nickel specific stimulation of T lymphocytes from patients with allergic contact dermatitis to nickel. *Eur. J. Immunol.*, *18*: 977–982.
87. Sinigaglia, F., Scheidegger, D., Garotta, G., Scheper, R., Pletscher, M., and Lanzavecchia, A. 1985. Isolation and characterization of Ni-specific T cell clones from patients with Ni-contact dermatitis. *J. Immunol.*, *135*: 3929–3932.
88. Yamashita, U., and Shevach, E. M. 1980. The syngeneic mixed lymphocyte culture: The genetic requirements of self resembles the requirements for the recognition of antigens in association with self. *J. Immunol.*, *124*: 1773–1778.
89. Glimcher, L. H., Longo, D. L., Green, I., and Schwartz, R. H. 1981. Murine

syngeneic mixed lymphocyte response. I. Target antigens are self Ia molecules. *J. Exp. Med., 154*: 1652–1670.
90. Weksler, M. E., Moody, C. E., Jr., and Kozak, R. W. 1981. The autologous mixed-lymphocyte reaction. *Adv. Immunol., 31*: 271–312.
91. Zauderer, M., Campbell, H., Johnson, D. R., and Seman, M. 1984. Helper functions of antigen-induced specific and autoreactive T-cell colonies. *J. Mol. Cell. Immunol., 1*: 65–72.
92. Tilkin, A. F., Michon, J., Juy, D., Kayibanda, M., Henin, Y., Sterkers, G., Betuel, H., and Levy, J. P. 1987. Autoreactive T cell clones of MHC class II specificities are produced during responses against foreign antigens in man. *J. Immunol., 138*: 674–679.
93. Faherty, D. A., Johnson, D. R., and Zauderer, M. 1985. Origin and specificity of autoreactive T cells in antigen-induced populations. *J. Exp. Med., 161*: 1293–1301.
94. Nagarkatti, P. S., Snow, C., and Kaplan, A. M. 1985. Characterization and function of autoreactive T-lymphocyte clones isolated from normal unprimed mice. *Cell. Immunol., 94*: 32–48.
95. Finnegan, A., Needleman, B., and Hodes, R. J. 1984. Activation of B cells by autoreactive T cells: Cloned-autoreactive T cells activate B cells by two distinct pathways. *J. Immunol., 133*: 78–85.
96. Coeshott, C. M., Chesnut, R. W., Kubo, R. T., Grammer, S. F., Jenis, D. M., and Grey, H. M. 1986. Ia-specific mixed leukocyte reactive T cell hybridomas: analysis of their specificity by using purified class II MHC molecules in a synthetic membrane system. *J. Immunol., 136*: 2832–2838.
97. Zauderer, M. 1989. Origin and significance of autoreactive T cells. *Adv. Immunol., 45*: 417–437.
98. Nagarkatti, P. S., Seth, A., Kakkanaiah, V. N., and Nagarkatti, M. 1989. $CD4^+$ autoreactive T cell clones having the properties of both T_H1 and T_H2 type of T helper cells (abstract). 7th International Congress of Immunology (Berlin). Gustav Fischer Verlag; Stuttgart, New York, p. 434.
99. Bensussan, A., Meuier, M. C., Schlossman, S. F., and Reinherz, E. L. 1984. Delineation of an immunoregulatory amplifier population recognizing autologous Ia molecules: Analysis with human T cell clones. *J. Exp. Med., 159*: 559–576.
100. Kotani, H., Mitsuya, H., Jarret, R. F., Yenokida, G. G., James, S. P., and Strober, W. 1986. An autoreactive T cell clone which can be activated to provide both helper and suppressor functions. *J. Immunol., 136*: 1951–1959.
101. Saito, T., and Rajewsky, K. 1985. A self-Ia reactive T cell clone directly stimulates every hundredth B cell and helps antigen-specific B cell responses. *Eur. J. Immunol., 15*: 927–934.
102. Bocchieri, M. H. 1989. Immunoregulatory effects of cloned T cells on B-cell responses: Comparison of autoimmune and non-autoimmune derived clones. *Immunology, 66*: 526–531.
103. Bjorkman, P. J., Saper, M. A., Samraoui, B., Bennett, W. S., Strominger, J. L., and Wiley, D. C. 1987. The foreign antigen binding site and T cell recognition regions of class I histocompatibility regions. *Nature, 329*: 512–518.
104. Kourilsky, P., and Claverie, J. M. 1989. MHC-antigen interactions: What does the T cell receptor see? *Adv. Immunol., 45*: 107–193.

105. Singer, A., Munitz, T. I., Golding, H., Rosenberg, A., and Mizuochi, T. 1987. Recognition requirements for the activation differentiation and function of T-helper cells specific for class I MHC alloantigens. *Immunol. Rev.*, *98*: 145–170.
106. Sprent, J., and Webb, S. R. 1987. Function and specificity of T cell subsets in the mouse. *Adv. Immunol.*, *41*: 39–133.
107. Sprent, J., Lo, D., Gao, E. K., and Ron, Y. 1988. T cell selection in the thymus. *Immunol. Rev.*, *101*: 172–189.
108. Nagarkatti, P. S., Nagarkatti, M., Mann, L. W., Jones, L. A., and Kaplan, A. M. 1988. Characterization of an endogenous Lyt 2+ T-suppressor-population regulating autoreactive T cells in vitro and in vivo. *Cell. Immunol.*, *112*: 64–77.
109. Romain, P. L., Morimoto, C., Daley, J. F., Palley, L. S., Reinherz, E. L., and Schlossman, S. F. 1984. Reactivity of inducer cell subsets and T8-cell activation during the human autologous mixed lymphocyte reaction. *Clin. Immunol. Immunopathol.*, *30*: 117–128.
110. Rosenkrantz, K., Dupont, B., and Flomenberg, N. 1985. Generation and regulation of autocytotoxicity in mixed lymphocyte cultures: evidence for active suppression of autocytotoxic cells. *Proc. Natl. Acad. Sci.*, *82*: 4508–4512.
111. Deusch, K., Moebius, U., Meyer zum Büschenfelde, K-H., and Meuer, S. C. 1986. T lymphocyte control of autoreactivity: Analysis with human T cell clones and limiting dilution culture. *Eur. J. Immunol.*, *16*: 1433–1438.
112. Sano, K., Fujisawa, I., Abe, R., Asano, Y., and Tada, T. 1987. MHC-restricted minimal regulatory circuit initiated by a class II-autoreactive T cell clone. *J. Exp. Med.*, *165*: 1284–1295.
113. Gao, E-K., Cheney, R., Kanagawa, O., and Sprent, J. 1988. Abnormal differentiation of thymocytes in mice treated with cyclosporine A. *Nature, 336*: 176–179.
114. Pelletier, L., Tournade, H., and Druet, P. *Immunologically-Mediated Manifestations Induced by Metals*. Plenum Press (in press).
115. Warner, G. L., and Lawrence, D. A. 1988. The effects of metals on IL-2 related lymphocyte proliferation. *Int. J. Pharmacol.*, *10*: 629–637.
116. Weston, K. M., Yeh, E. T. H., and Sy, M. S. 1987. Autoreactivity accelerates the development of autoimmunity and lymphoproliferation in MRL/Mp-lpr/lpr mice. *J. Immunol.*, *139*: 734–742.
117. Pelletier, L., Pasquier, R., Hirsch, F., Sapin, C., and Druet, P. 1986. Autoreactive T cells in mercury-induced autoimmune disease: In vitro demonstration. *J. Immunol.*, *137*: 2548–2554.
118. Rossert, J., Pelletier, L., Pasquier, R., and Druet, P. 1988. Autoreactive T cells in mercury-induced autoimmune disease. Demonstration by limiting dilution analysis. *Eur. J. Immunol.*, *18*: 1761–1766.
119. Richardson, B. 1986. Effect of an inhibitor of DNA methylation on T cells. II. 5-azacytidine induces self reactivity in antigen-specific T4+ cells. *Human Immunol.*, *17*: 456–470.
120. Cornacchia, E., Golbus, J., Maybaum, J., Strahler, J., Hanash, S., and Richardson, B. 1988. Hydralazine and procainamide inhibit T cell DNA methylation and induce autoreactivity. *J. Immunol.*, *140*: 2197–2200.
121. de Talance, A., Regnier, D., Spinella, S., Morisset, J., and Seman, M. 1986.

Origin of autoreactive T helper cells. I. Characterization of Thy-1^+, Lyt^-, $L3T4^-$ precursors in the spleen of normal mice. *J. Immunol., 137*: 1101–1108.
122. Reimann, J., Bellan, A., and Conradt, P. 1988. Development of autoreactive $L3T4^+$ T cells from double-negative ($L2T4^-$/Ly-2^-) Thy-1^+ spleen cells of normal mice. *Eur. J. Immunol., 18*: 989–999.
123. Sainis, K., and Datta, S. K. 1988. CD4+ T cell lines with selective patterns of autoreactivity as well as CD4-CD8- T helper cell lines augment the production of idiotypes shared by pathogenic anti-DNA autoantibodies in the NZB × SWR model of lupus nephritis. *J. Immunol., 140*: 2215–2224.
124. Gregersen, P. K., Silver, J., and Winchester, R. J. 1987. The shared hypothesis. An approach to understanding the molecular genetics of susceptibility to rheumatoid arthritis. *Arthritis Rheum., 30*: 1205–1213.
125. Mackay, I. R., Rowley, M. J., and Tait, B. D. 1989. The relationship of "shared epitopes" of major histocompatibility complex molecules to autoimmune disease. *Arthritis Rheum., 32*: 509.
126. Mengle-Gaw, L., Conner, S., McDevitt, H. O., and Fathman, C. G. 1984. Gene conversion between murine class II major histocompatibility complex loci: functional and molecular evidence from the bm12 mutant. *J. Exp. Med., 160*: 1184–1194.
127. Hochman, P. S., and Huber, B. T. 1984. A class II gene conversion event defines an antigen specific Ir gene epitope. *J. Exp. Med., 160*: 1925–1930.
128. Christadoss, P., Lindstrom, J. M., Melvoid, R. W., and Talal, N. 1985. Mutation of I-A beta chain prevents experimental autoimmune myasthenia gravis. *Immunogenetics, 21*: 33–38.
129. Murdoch, R. D., and Pepys, J. 1984. Immunological responses to complex salts of platinium. II. Enhanced IgE antibody responses to ovalbumin with concurrent administration of platinium salts in the rat. *Clin. Exp. Immunol., 58*: 478–485.
130. Leung, D. Y. M., Young, M. C., and Geha, R. S. 1986. Induction of IgG and IgE synthesis in normal B cells by autoreactive T cell clones. *J. Immunol., 136*: 2851–2855.
131. Umetsu, D. T., Leung, D. Y. M., Siraganian, R., Jabara, H. H., and Geha, R. S. 1985. Differential requirements of B cells from normal and allergic subjects for the induction of IgE synthesis by an alloreactive T cell clone. *J. Exp. Med., 162*: 202–214.
132. Quint, D. J., Bolton, E., Solari, R., McNamee, A., Hissey, P., Champion, R., and Zanders, E. D. 1989. Functional and phenotypic properties of T-cell clones which regulate IgE synthesis. *J. Autoimmunity, 2* (Suppl): 131–140.
133. MacKenzie, T., and Dosch, H. M. 1989. Clonal and molecular characteristics of the human IgE-committed B cell subset. *J. Exp. Med., 169*: 407–430.
134. Durkin, H. G., Auci, D. L., Chice, S. M., Smith, M. C., Murali, M. R., Bazin, H., Tarcsay, L., and Dukor, P. 1989. Control of IgE responses. *Clin. Immunol. Immunopathol., 50*: 852–872.
135. Richards, M. L., Marceletti, J. F., and Katz, D. H. 1988. IgE-antigen complexes enhance Fcϵ R and Ia expression by murine B lymphocytes. *J. Exp. Med., 168*: 571–587.

136. Bonnefoy, J. Y., Guillot, O., Spits, H., Blanchard, D., Ishizaka, K., and Banchereau, J. 1988. The low affinity receptor for IgE (CD23) on B lymphocytes is spatially associated with HLA-DR antigens. *J. Exp. Med., 167*: 57–72.
137. Coffman, R. L., Ohara, J., Bond, M. W., Carty, J., Zlotnik, A., and Paul, W. E. 1986. B cell stimulatory factor-1 enhances the IgE response of lipopolysaccharide-activated B cells. *J. Immunol., 136*: 4538–4541.
138. Finkelman, F. D., Katona, I. M., Urban, J. F., Snapper, C. M., Ohara, J., and Paul, W. E. 1986. Suppression of in vivo polyclonal IgE responses by monoclonal antibody to the lymphokine B-cell stimulatory factor-1. *Proc. Natl. Acad. Sci. USA, 83*: 9675–9678.
139. Del Prete, G. F., Maggi, E., Paronci, P., Chretien, I., Tiri, A., Macchia, D., Ricci, M., Banchereau, J., de Vries, J. E., and Romagnani, S. 1988. IL4 is an essential factor for the IgE synthesis induced in vitro by human T cell clones and their supernatants. *J. Immunol., 140*: 4193–4198.
140. Pene, J., Rousset, F., Briere, F., Chretien, I., Paliard, X., Banchereau, J., Spits, H., and de Vries, J. E. 1988. IgE production by normal human B cells induced by alloreactive T cell clones is mediated by Il-4 and suppressed by IFN-γ. *J. Immunol., 141*: 1218–1224.
141. Mosmann, T. R., Cherwinski, H., Bond, M. W., Giedlin, M. A., and Coffman, R. L. 1986. Two types of murine helper T cell clones I. Definition according to profiles of lymphokines activities and secreted proteins. *J. Immunol., 136*: 2348–2357.
142. Mosmann, T. R., and Coffman, R. L. 1989. Heterogeneity of cytokine suppression patterns and functions of helper T cells. *Adv. Immunol., 46*: 111–147.
143. Baran, D., Lantz, O., Dosquet, P., Sfaksi, A., and Druet, P. 1988. Interleukin-2 production in Brown-Norway rats with $HgCl_2$-induced autoimmune disease: Paradoxical in vivo versus in vitro findings. *Clin. Exp. Immunol., 73*: 401–405.
144. Altmann, A., Theofilopoulos, A. N., Weiner, R., Katz, D. H., and Dixon, F. J. 1981. Analysis of T cell function in autoimmune murine strains. Defects in production of and unresponsiveness to interleukin-2. *J. Exp. Med., 154*: 791–808.
145. Linker-Israeli, M., Bakke, A. C., Kitridou, R. C., Gendler, S., Gillis, S., and Horwitz, D. A. 1983. Defective production of interleukin 1 and interleukin 2 in patients with systemic lupus erythematosus (SLE). *J. Immunol., 130*: 2651–2655.
146. Bowman, C., Green, C., Borysiewicz, L., and Lockwood, C. M. 1987. Circulating T-cell populations during mercuric chloride-induced nephritis in the Brown Norway rat. *Immunology, 61*: 515–520.
147. Geha, R. S., Reinherz, E., Leung, D., McKee, K. T., Schlossman, S., and Rosen, F. S. 1981. Deficiency of suppressor T cells in the hyperimmunoglobulin E syndrome. *J. Clin. Invest., 68*: 783–790.
148. Lanzavecchia, A., and Parodi, B. 1983. In vitro stimulation of IgE production at a single precursor level by human alloreactive T helper clones. *Clin. Exp. Immunol., 55*: 197–203.
149. Hall, E. P., and Gault, E. A. 1986. Suppression of IgE responses by hyperimmune serum in rats. *Immunology, 59*: 577–581.
150. Marshall, J. S., and Bell, E. B. 1985. Induction of an auto-anti-IgE response in rats. I. Effects on serum IgE concentrations. *Eur. J. Immunol., 15*: 272–277.

151. Magnusson, C. G. M., and Johansonn, S. G. O. 1989. Clinical significance of anti-IgE autoantibodies and immune complexes containing IgE. *Clin. Rev. Allergy, 7*: 73–103.
152. Rigal, D., Baboin-Jaubert, M., Rousset, F., El Habib, R., and Monier, J. C. 1988. Immunodulation induced by immunoglobulins I. Action of placental immunoglobulin on in vitro spontaneous synthesis of IgE in man. *Clin. Immunol. Immunopathol., 49*: 1–5.
153. Geha, R. S., and Comunale, M. 1983. Regulation of immunoglobulin E antibody synthesis in man by antiidiotypic antibodies. *J. Clin. Invest., 71*: 46–54.
154. Blaser, K., Wetterwald, A., Weber, A., Gerber, V. E., and de Weck, A. L. 1983. Immune networks in immediate type allergic disease. *Ann. NY Acad. Sci., 418*: 330–345.
155. Coffman, R. L., Carty, J. 1986. A T cell activity that enhances polyclonal IgE production and its inhibition by interferon γ. *J. Immunol., 136*: 949–954.
156. Guery, J. C., Druet, E., Glotz, D., Hirsch, F., Mandet, C., De Heer, E., and Druet, P. 1990. Specificity and cross-reactive idiotypes of antiglomerular basement membrane antibodies in $HgCl_2$-induced autoimmune glomerulonephritis. *Eur. J. Immunol., 20*: 93–100.
157. Burdette, S., and Schwartz, R. S. 1987. Current concepts in immunology. Idiotypes and idiotypic networks. *N. Engl. J. Med., 317*: 219–224.
158. Shoenfeld, Y., Teplizki, H. A., Mendlovic, S., Blank, M., Mozes, E., and Eisenberg, D. A. 1989. The role of the human anti-DNA anti-idiotype 16/6 in autoimmunity. *Clin. Immunol. Immunopathol., 51*: 313–253.
159. Guery, J. C., and Druet, P. 1990. A spontaneous hybridoma producing auto anti-idiotypic antibodies that recognize a Vk-associated idiotope in mercury-induced autoimmunity. *Eur. J. Immunol., 20*: 1027–1031.
160. Goldman, M., Rose, L. M., Hochmann, A., and Lambert, P. H. 1982. Deposition of idiotype-antiidiotype complexes in renal glomeruli after polyclonal B cell activation. *J. Exp. Med., 155*: 1385–1399.
161. Kearney, J. F. 1989. Idiotypic networks. In *Fundamental Immunology*, 2nd ed. (W. E. Paul, ed.). Raven Press, New York, pp. 663–676.
162. Binz, H., and Wigzell, H. 1975. Shared idiotypic determinants on B and T lymphocytes reactive against the same antigenic determinants. I. Demonstration of similar or identical idiotypes on IgG and T cell receptors with specificity for some alloantigens. *J. Exp. Med., 142*: 197–211.
163. Cazenave, P. A., Cavaillon, J. M., and Bona, C. 1977. Idiotypic determinants on rabbit B and T derived lymphocytes. *Immunol. Rev., 34*: 34–49.
164. Eichman, K., and Rajewsky, K. 1975. Induction of T and B cell immunity by antiidiotypic antibody. *Eur. J. Immunol., 5*: 661–666.
165. Bogen, B., Malissen, B., and Haas, W. 1986. Idiotope specific T cell clones that recognize syngeneic immunoglobulin fragment in the context of class II molecules. *Eur. J. Immunol., 16*: 1373–1378.
166. Bottomly, K. 1988. The idiotype-specific repertoire is determined by idiotype prevalence. In *Biological Applications of Anti-idiotypes* (C. Bona, ed.). CRC Press, Boca Raton, FL, pp. 153–163.
167. Marcos, M. A. R., de la Hera, A., Gaspar, M. L., Marques, C., Bellas, C.,

Mampaso, F., Toribio, M. L., and Martinez, C. 1986. Modification of emerging repertoires by immunosuppression in immunodeficient mice results in autoimmunity. *Immunol. Rev.*, *90*: 51–74.

168. Simpson, R. B. 1961. Association constants of methylmercury with sulphydryl and other bases. *J. Am. Chem. Soc.*, *83*: 4711–4717.

169. Shaw, C. B. 1980. The biochemistry and subcellular distribution of gold in kidney tissue: Implication for chrysotherapy and nephrotoxicity. *Agent Actions*, *8*: 509–528.

170. Passow, H. 1970. The red blood cell: Penetration, distribution, and toxic actions of heavy metals. In *Effects of Metals on Cells, Subcellular and Macromolecules* (J. Maniloff, J. R. Coleman, and M. Miller, eds.). Charles C. Thomas, Springfield, IL, pp. 291–340.

171. Clarkson, T. W. 1972. The pharmacology of mercury compounds. *Ann. Rev. Pharmacol.*, *19*: 375–406.

172. Enjalbert, A. 1988. Recepteurs membranaires et mecanismes de transduction. *Med. Sci.*, n° special: 40–48.

173. Evans, W. H., and Graham, J. M. 1989. Membrane receptors. In *Membrane Structure and Function* (D. Rickwood and D. Male, eds.). Oxford University Press, pp. 31–51.

174. Isakov, N., Scholtz, W., and Altman, A. 1986. Signal transduction and intracellular events in T-lymphocyte activation. *Immunol. Today*, *7*: 271–277.

175. Lawrence, D. A. 1981. Heavy metal modulation of lymphocyte activities. *Toxicol. Appl. Pharmacol.*, *57*: 439–451.

176. Noelle, R. J., and Lawrence, D. A. 1981. Modulation of T-cell functions. II. Chemical basis for the involvement of cell surface thiol-reactive sites in control of T-cell proliferation. *Cell. Immunol.*, *60*: 453–469.

177. Lawrence, D., Mudzinsky, S., Rudofsky, U., and Warner, G. 1984. Mechanisms of metal-induced immunotoxicity. In *International Seminar on the Immunological System as a Target for Toxic Damage.* Luxemburg, November 6–9.

178. Li, Y. S., Kouassi, E., and Revillard, J. P. 1989. Cyclic AMP can enhance mouse B cell activation by regulating progression into the late G1/S phase. *Eur. J. Immunol.*, *19*: 1721–1725.

179. Rudd, C. E., Anderson, P., Morimoto, C., Streuli, M., and Schlossman, S. F. 1989. Molecular interactions, T-cell subsets and a role of the CD4/CD8:p56lck complex in human T-cell activation. *Immunol. Rev.*, *111*: 225–267.

180. Ben-Neriah, Y., and Bauskin, A. R. 1988. Leukocytes express a novel gene encoding a putative transmembrane protein-kinase devoid of an extracellular domain. *Nature*, *333*: 672–676.

181. Ledbetter, J. A., June, C. H., Rabinovitch, P. S., Grossmann, A., Tsu, T. T., and Imboden, J. B. 1988. Signal transduction through CD4 receptors: Stimulatory vs inhibitory activity is regulated by CD4 proximity to the CD3/T cell receptor. *Eur. J. Immunol.*, *18*: 525–532.

182. Mittler, R. S., Goldman, S. J., Spitalny, G. L., and Burakoff, S. J. 1989. T-cell receptor-CD4 physical association in a murine T-cell hybridoma: Induction by antigen receptor ligation. *Proc. Natl. Sci.*, *86*: 8331–8335.

183. Owens, T., and Fazekas de St. Groth. 1987. Participation of L3T4 in T cell activation in the absence of class II major histocompatibility complex antigens. Inhibition by anti-L3T4 antibodies is a function both of epitope density and mode of presentation of anti-receptor antibody. *J. Immunol.*, *132*: 2402–2409.

184. Meuer, S. C., Hussey, R. E., Fabbi, M., Fox, D., Acuto, O., Fitzgerald, A., Hodgdon, S. C., Protentis, J. P., Schlossman, S., and Reinherz, E. 1984. An alternative pathway to T cell activation: A functional role for the 50Kd T11 sheep erythrocyte receptor protein. *Cell, 36*: 897–906.

185. Boudou, A., Desmazes, J. P., and Georgescauld, D. 1982. Fluorescence quenching study of mercury compounds and liposome interactions: Effect of charged lipid and pH. *Ecotox. Environment. Safety, 6*: 379–382.

186. Fürst, P., Hu, S., Hackett, R., and Hammer, D. 1988. Copper activates metallothionein gene transcription by altering the conformation of a specific DNA binding protein. *Cell, 55*: 705–717.

187. Nordlind, K. 1984. Binding and uptake of mercuric chloride in human lymphoid cells. *Int. Archs. Allergy. Appl. Immun.*, *77*: 405–408.

188. Skilleter, D. N., and Price, R. J. 1984. Lymphocyte beryllium binding: Relationship to development of delayed beryllium hypersensitivity. *Int. Archs. Allergy. Appl. Immun.*, *73*: 181–183.

189. Berg, J. M. 1988. Proposed structure for the zinc-binding domains from transcription factor IIIa and related proteins. *Proc. Natl. Acad. Sci. USA, 85*: 99–102.

17

The Natural Anti-Gal Antibody: Evolution and Autoimmunity in Man

Uri Galili
Medical College of Pennsylvania, Philadelphia, Pennsylvania

I. NATURAL ANTIBODIES, EVOLUTION, AND AUTOIMMUNITY

Autoimmune diseases are pathologic states in which the immune system acts against seemingly normal autologous tissues. Diagnosis of autoimmune diseases is usually based on demonstration of humoral or cellular immune components within the damaged tissue and, on the in vitro demonstration of antibody or lymphoid reactivity with tissues, cells, or specific organelles. It is well accepted that the immune system in man contains a large number of lymphoid clones capable of reacting with self antigens and which are nonreactive in healthy individuals. As reflected in the various chapters of this book, the in vivo initiation of lymphoid reactivity against self antigens is attributed to multiple factors, part of which includes regulatory defects in suppressive mechanisms, breakdown of tolerance because of antigenic mimicry by infectious agents and of abnormal expression of HLA antigens. The present chapter describes yet another mechanism which may explain the initiation of autoimmune processes as a result of the interaction between natural antibodies and autologous antigens. In addition to the theoretical considerations discussed below, an example of such an antigen/antibody system is presented. The antigen discussed is the carbohydrate epitope Galα1→3Galβ1→4ClcNAc-R (α-galactosyl epitope) and the corresponding natural antibody is the natural "anti-Gal" antibody that constitutes 1% of circulating IgG in man.

The majority of the circulating 10 mg/ml of immunoglobulins in healthy individuals seem to be natural antibodies (i.e., antibodies made without active preimmunization by the corresponding antigen) which are produced as a result of constant stimulation by various environmental antigens such as gastrointestinal bacteria. It is conceivable that many of the natural antibodies within the serum of a given species are the result of a dynamic evolutionary process selecting for individuals capable of producing protective antibodies against environmental pathogens. Thus natural antibodies greatly contribute to the *modus vivendi* between different species and their environmental pathogens. The excessive sensitivity of agammaglobulinemic patients to various infections (1) is but one example of the importance of natural antibodies in protection against infections by bacteria which are nonpathogenic in healthy individuals. Natural antibodies may differ in related species or in members of the same species separated by geographic barriers, as a result of selective exposure to endemic pathogens. One distinct example is that of natural antibodies of primates to Epstein–Barr virus (EBV). This virus evolved in the Old World (i.e., Africa, Asia, and Europe) from the herpesvirus family after the separation of South America from Africa. As a result of continuous exposure to EBV, Old World monkeys, apes, and, ultimately, humans have evolved with the capacity to produce natural antibodies against the virus, whereas New World monkeys are incapable of producing such antibodies (2). It has therefore been suggested that these natural anti-EBV antibodies participate in limiting the effect of EBV infection in man to a transient infection (i.e., infectious mononucleosis (2,3). In contrast, EBV-infected New World monkeys develop polyclonal lymphomas consisting of the EBV-transformed B-lymphoid cells (2). The observations that immunosuppressed individuals would occasionally develop EBV-induced polyclonal lymphomas homologous to those observed in New World monkeys (4,5) further indicate the role of natural immunity in protection against EBV.

In an attempt to evade effective immune response, many infectious agents express surface antigens which mimic host antigens (6). When such pathogens become detrimental to the survival of a given species, a selective pressure is exerted for the evolution of subspecies which do not express the mimicked antigen and can thus produce protective antibodies against the pathogen. This process, which alters the repertoire of natural antibodies, can be a surprisingly rapid one. Natural antibodies to blood group antigens in man are an example of such a process. The natural antibodies to blood groups A and B are produced in humans as a result of constant immunization by gastrointestinal bacteria (7,8). Because of immune tolerance, individuals with blood group A produce anti-B antibodies and those with blood group B produce anti-A antibodies, whereas individuals with blood group O produce both anti-A and anti-B antibodies. Most human populations are polymorphic and include variable proportions of blood groups O, A, B, and AB phenotypes (9). However, the Indians of the Amazon basin all have blood group O (10). These Indians, who migrated to South America some 10,000–20,000 years ago, are believed to share common ancestors with North American Indians, many of whom have blood group A. Furthermore, blood group A antigens have been identified in human bones from 1500-year-old Amazonian burial sites (11). The diminished expression of blood group A among Amazonian Indians may be attributed to the ineffective immune response of individuals with blood group A against bacteria expressing a similar antigen. Therefore, within a span of less than 20,000 years, this Indian population seems to have been selected for individuals with only blood group O who could produce both anti-A and anti-B antibodies (11).

Blood group antigens have a polymorphic expression in man; therefore, selection may occur by elimination of the disadvantageous alleles from the gene pool. However, when the antigen subjected to the selective pressure is expressed by all members of the affected species, one may speculate that this process would result in selection for diminished expression of the antigen, loss of immune tolerance against it, and subsequent production of protective antibodies toward the similar epitope on the pathogen(s). These changes in autologous antigenic expression can occur as a result of regulatory mutations which affect the biosynthetic rate of the antigen (12), structural mutations which alter the antigenicity of the epitope selected against, or deletion of the antigen-encoding gene. These evolutionarily suppressed antigens become "forbidden antigens" since, upon reexpression, they would interact with the natural antibody, which is continuously produced. Reexpression of such forbidden antigens may occur because of either reversion of structural mutations or impairment of the regulatory mechanisms which prevent the expression of these antigens. The interaction of the de novo synthesized forbidden antigen and the natural antibody recognizing it is likely to result in an autoimmune process in the tissue expressing such antigens.

The hypothetical considerations discussed above are reflected in the evolutionary relationship between the natural anti-Gal antibody and the carbohydrate epitope, with the structure Galα1→3Galβ1→4GlcNAc-R (the α-galactosyl epitope).

II. THE NATURAL ANTI-Gal ANTIBODY

Anti-Gal is a natural antibody which is produced in all humans and constitutes 1% of circulating IgG (13). This antibody can be readily isolated from normal serum by affinity chromatography on melibiose (Galα1→6Gal)-Sepharose (Sigma Chemicals, St. Louis, MO) (14,15) or a synthetic Galα1→3Galβ1→4GlcNAc adsorbent column (16) (Synsorb # 115 column, Chemibiomed, Edmonton, Alberta, Canada). Subsequent extensive washing of such immunoadsorbents and elution with either low pH or with α-methylgalactoside results in the isolation of an IgG preparation that corresponds to 50–100 μg IgG per ml serum. The eluted antibody is designated anti-Gal or anti-α-galactosyl IgG (13) and, although it is a polyclonal antibody (13), anti-Gal interacts with high specificity with mammalian glycoconjugates (glycolipids and glycoproteins) which have the terinal carbohydrate structure Galα1→3Galβ1→4GlcNAc-R (14,16,18–20). One way of demonstrating the specificity of this antibody is by the immunostaining of glycolipids with chemically defined carbohydrate structures and which are chromatographed on thin-layer chromatography (TLC) plates (14,16). An example of such analysis is shown in Figure 1, where rabbit red cell neutral glycolipids were separated on a TLC plate. The two major neutral glycolipids (i.e., glycolipids lacking sialic acid) in rabbit red cell membrane are ceramide trihexoside (CTH) with the terminal residue Galα1→4Galβ1→4Glc-R and ceramide pentahexoside (CPH) with the terminal residue Galα1→3Galβ1→4GlcNAc-R (Fig. 1, lane 1) (21,22). Immunostaining of the TLC plate with anti-Gal revealed specific binding of the antibody to CPH and to glycolipids with longer carbohydrate chains (Fig. 1, lane 2) which were previously reported to have 15–25 carbohydrate units with terminal Galα1→3Galβ1→4GlcNAc residues (23). Immunostaining of other glycolipids with anti-Gal demonstrated interaction with Galα1→3Galβ1→4GlcNAc residues and not

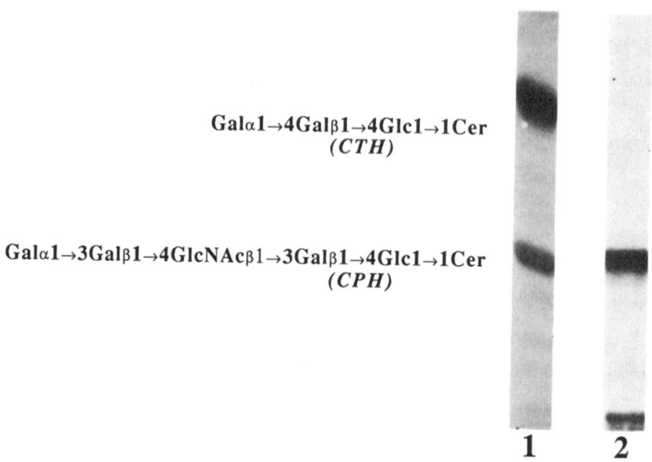

FIGURE 1 Thin-layer chromatogram of rabbit red cell neutral glycolipids immunostained with anti-Gal. Nonspecific staining with orcinol in lane 1 demonstrates the two major glycolipid molecules: CTH (ceramide trihexoside) and CPH (ceramide pentahexoside (21,22). Immunostaining with anti-Gal shows the specific binding of anti-Gal to CPH and to glycolipid molecules with longer carbohydrate chains, found near the origin of the chromatogram. The extraction of glycolipids and immunostaining procedures are described in detail elsewhere (14,16).

with Galα1→4Galβ1→4GlcNAc, sialyl, fucosyl, or other carbohydrate residues described in Table 1 (16). A similar specificity was observed when glycoproteins or synthetic oligosaccharides were assayed for interaction with anti-Gal [14,18,20). It should be stressed that anti-Gal can interact with Galα1→6 residues as in melibiose (Galα1→6Glc) (13,14) and hypothetically may bind to Galα1→2 residues, however, no such residues have been found on mammalian glycoconjugates.

The specificity of anti-Gal antibody clones in individuals with blood group B or AB is restricted to the Galα1→3Galβ1→4GlcNAc structures. However, in individuals with blood group A or O, a substantial proportion of anti-Gal clones also can interact with the blood group B antigen. Blood group B antigen has, in addition to the structure described above, a fucosyl residue which is linked α1-2 to the penultimate glucose, i.e., Galα1→3(Fucα1→2)Galβ1→4GlcNAc. Most (>85%) of the so-called anti-blood group B antibodies in A and O individuals are in fact anti-Gal antibodies which can bind to the Galα1→3Galβ1→4GlcNAc residue, regardless of fucosyl binding to the penultimate galactose (for detailed discussion, see Refs. 16,24).

The high concentration of anti-Gal in human serum throughout life suggested constant antigenic stimulation for the production of this antibody. Indeed, we could isolate a number of gastrointestinal bacteria strains which readily interacted with anti-Gal (25). Furthermore, anti-Gal staining of Western blots of bacterial lipopolysaccharides (LPS) demonstrated the occurrence of α-galactosyl residues in LPS of a number of *E. coli*, *Klebsiella*, and *Serratia* strains (25). Biochemically characterized Galα1→3Gal residues on bacterial LPS were previously reported (26,27). These findings support the assumption that anti-Gal is continuously synthesized in man as a result of immunologic stimulation by bacterial antigens.

III. EVOLUTION OF THE Galα1→3Galβ1→4GLCNAC-R (α-GALACTOSYL) EPITOPE

The abundant synthesis of anti-Gal in man implied that the Galα1→3Galβ1→4GlcNAc epitope it recognizes (for convenience, hereafter referred to as the α-galactosyl epitope) is absent from human cells. This epitope was, however, reported to be abundantly expressed on murine Ehrlich ascites cells (28), lymphoma cells (29) and 3T3 fibroblasts (30), rat carcinoma cells (31), bovine red cells and thyroid cells (32–34), and rabbit red cells (21–23,35). In addition, the α-galactosyl epitope was found on murine and bovine laminin (36,37) and on bovine thyroglobulin (38). In view of the widespread distribution of the α-galactosyl epitope in nonprimate mammals, it was reasonable to assume that its suppression and subsequent anti-Gal production might have been initiated at a certain stage of primate or human evolution. In order to determine the evolutionary stage at which suppression of the α-galactosyl epitope occurred, we studied

TABLE 1 Glycolipids Tested for Anti-Gal Binding

Name	Source	Structure	Anti-Gal binding
CPH (ceramide pentahexoside)	Rabbit	Galα1→3Galβ1→4GlcNAcβ1→3Galβ1→4Glc1→3Cer	+
CHH (ceramide heptahexoside)	Cow	Galα1→3(Galβ1→4GlcNAcβ1→3)$_2$Galβ1→4Glc1→1Cer	+
Glucosyl ceramide	Human	Glc1→1Cer	–
Lactosyl ceramide	Human	Galβ1→4Glc1→1Cer	–
CTH (ceramide trihexoside)	Rabbit	Galα1→4Galβ1→4Glc1→1Cer	–
Globoside	Human/Pig	GalNAcβ1→3Galα1→4Galβ1→4Glc1→1Cer	–
Paragloboside	Human	Galβ1→4GlcNAcβ1→3Galβ1→4Glc1→1Cer	–
Forsman	Sheep	GalNAcα1→3GalNAcβ1→3Galα1→4Galβ1→4Glc1→1Cer	–
P_1	Human	Galα1→4Galβ1→4GlcNAcβ1→3Galβ1→4Glc1→1Cer	–
B_I	Human	Galα1→3(Fucα1→2)Galβ1→4GlcNAcβ1→3Galβ1→4Glc1→1Cer	–
GM_3	Human	NeuAcα2→3Galβ1→4Glc1→1Cer	–
Sialylparagloboside	Human	NeuAcα2→3Galβ1→4GlcNAcβ1→3Galβ1→4Glc1→1Cer	–

the expression of this structure on nucleated cells of a large number of species (17). No such epitopes were detected on fish-, amphibian-, reptile-, or bird-derived fibroblasts. A distinct pattern of α-galactosyl epitope distribution was observed in mammals (Table 2). The α-galactosyl epitope was found to be abundantly expressed (1×10^6–35×10^6 epitopes per cell) on fibroblasts from marsupials such as opossum and kangaroo, as well as placentals such as mouse, rabbit, pig, cow, horse, sheep, dog, cat, bat, and dolphin. Among primates, the α-galactosyl epitope is abundant on cells of lemurs (prosimians living in Madagascar) and New World monkeys (primates of South American and Central America) but is undetectable on cells of Old World monkeys (primates of Asia and Africa), apes, and humans. Analysis of red cells revealed a similar pattern of α-galactosyl epitope expression (24,39,40). Furthermore, the CPH molecule initially found in rabbit red cells (Fig. 1) was identified in cow and New World monkey red cells, but not in Old World monkey or human red cells (39,40). In contrast to the α-galactosyl epitope distribution, anti-Gal was found to be present in large amounts in the serum of Old World monkeys and apes, as in man, and not detectable in serum of New World monkeys, lemurs, or nonprimate mammals as mouse and rabbit (24,39). These data imply that the α-galactosyl epitope appeared early in the evolution of mammals, before the divergence of marsupial and placental mammals, i.e., more than 120 million years ago (MYA). This carbohydrate structure has since been conserved in many mammalian species, including ancestral primates. It is presently expressed in lemurs, a prosimian group which diverged from primates approximately 65 MYA, and is found in New World monkeys, which diverged from Old World monkeys approximately 35 MYA (41). The α-galactosyl epitope expression was suppressed, however, in ancestral Old World monkeys, probably before the divergence between monkeys and apes (i.e., more than 23 MYA) (41).

The distribution pattern of the α-galactosyl epitope in primates may suggest

TABLE 2 Distribution of the α-Galactosyl Epitope and of the Natural Anti-Gal Antibody in Mammals

Species group	α-Galactosyl epitope	Anti-Gal antibody
Nonprimate mammals (marsupial and placental)	+	−
Prosimians (lemurs)	+	−
New World monkeys	+	−
Old World monkeys	−	+
Apes	−	+
Humans	−	+

Source: Adapted from Refs. 17,20,24,38,39,40.

that, subsequent to the divergence between New World monkeys and Old World monkeys, ancestral primates in the Old World were exposed to an endemic detrimental infectious agent which expressed carbohydrate antigenic epitopes with a structure similar to the α-galactosyl epitope. Such a pathogen could have exerted a selective pressure for the evolution of primates, which produced anti-Gal antibodies as a protective response, with concomitant suppression of autologous α-galactosyl epitope expression, thus avoiding autoimmunity. It is impossible at present to determine the identity of such a hypothetical agent. Nevertheless, a whole variety of infectious agents expressing α-galactosyl or α-galactosyl-like epitopes has been identified. These include murine Friend leukemia virus (42), bacteria such as *Salmonella* (26), *Klebsiella*, and *E. coli* (25), and parasites such as *Trypanosoma cruzi* and *Leishmania mexicana* (43). Furthermore, anti-Gal was found to induce complement-mediated lysis of *Trypanosoma cruzi* (44), implying the abundant expression of α-galactosyl epitopes on these infectious agents. An alternative scenario might have been the evolution of ancestral Old World primates suppressing α-galactosyl epitope expression as a result of exposure to a pathogen that exerted its detrimental efffect via receptors containing the α-galactosyl epitope. Such a possibility has been studied by Krivan et al. (45), who have shown that the binding sites for *Clostridium difficile* enterotoxin-A on intestinal epithelial cells is the α-galactosyl epitope. A pathogen producing a detrimental toxin with similar specificity in ancentral Old World primates could exert a selective pressure for the suppression of α-galactosyl epitopes, the subsequent loss of immune tolerance toward this carbohydrate structure, and the resulting production of anti-Gal response to gastrointestinal bacterial antigens.

Although the evolutionary events leading to the suppression of the α-galactosyl epitope expression in ancestral Old World primates may only be a subject of speculation, the biosynthetic aspects underlying this phenomenon are better understood. The lack of α-galactosyl epitopes in man and in Old World primates is the result of diminished activity of one enzyme, the α1-3 galactosyltransferse (17). This is a Golgi membrane-bound enzyme that catalyzes the reaction:

$$\underset{\text{(N-acetyllactosamine)}}{\text{Gal}\beta 1\rightarrow 4\text{GlcNAc-R}} + \text{UDP-Gal} \xrightarrow{\text{Mn}^{2+}} \underset{(\alpha\text{-galactosyl epitope})}{\text{Gal}\alpha 1\rightarrow 3\text{Gal}\beta 1\rightarrow 4\text{GlcNAc-R}} + \text{UDP}$$

The activity of this enzyme has been demonstrated in microsomal fractions obtained from mouse Ehrlich ascites cells and teratocarcinoma cells (46,47), rabbit bone marrow and stomach mucosa (48,49), and cow thymus cells (50). In addition, it has been purified to homogeneity from mouse Ehrlich ascites cells (51) and cow thymus (50). We could demonstrate the reactivity of this enzyme in mouse, rat, cow, rabbit, guinea pig, and New World monkey cells, but not in Old World monkey or human cells (17,52). Thus the diminished expression of

α-galactosyl epitopes in ancestral Old World primates is the result of the specific suppression of α1-3 galactosyltransferase.

The molecular basis for the suppression of α1-3 galactosyltransferase activity in Old World primates and humans has not been elucidated as yet. Recent studies have indicated that the α1-3 galactosyltransferase gene is present within the human genome but is not expressed. Joziasse et al. (53) have cloned α1-3 galactosyltransferase cDNA from a bovine cDNA library and could demonstrate, by Northern blot analysis, the presence of transcripts for the α1-3 galactosyltransferase gene in various nonprimate species and New World monkeys, but not in Old World monkeys and human cells. Southern blot analysis, however, clearly identified homologous sequences for α1-3 galactosyltransferase in human genomic DNA. Similarly, Lowe and colleagues (54,55) have cloned the α1-3 galactosyltransferase cDNA from a mouse cDNA library, and have found homologous sequences in man. Furthermore, they have found 81% homology between the human genomic DNA sequence and the mouse cDNA sequence. These studies strongly imply that the gene encoding for α1-3 galactosyltransferase is indeed present in the human genome, but that its expression is suppressed on the transcriptional level. Hypothetically, a structural mutation in the α1-3 galactosyltransferase gene resulting in an unstable transcript, stop codon or frame shift, or a regulatory mutation(s) impairing the capacity of the promoter region to facilitate effective initiation of transcription by RNA polymerase II, could have caused the suppression of α-galactosyl epitope expression in ancestral primates. Such a mutation(s) would have been fixed in the progeny of Old World monkeys, apes and, ultimately, humans. Individuals expressing de novo the α-galactosyl epitopes would have been eliminated from the population as a result of autoimmune processes mediated by the natural anti-Gal antibody. The mechanism suppressing the α1-3 galactosyltransferase gene expression may be elucidated by cloning and sequencing of the human α1-3 galactosyltransferase gene and its flanking regions, and subsequently by studying the activity of the structural and regulatory regions of the gene in cell transfection experiments.

IV. α1-3 GALACTOSYLTRANSFERASE AND AUTOIMMUNITY IN MAN

The finding of the α1-3 galactosyltransferase gene within the human genome in a suppressed form has raised the possibility that, under certain conditions that are not yet understood, this gene may undergo deregulation resulting in the synthesis of the enzyme and subsequent de novo expression of α-galactosyl epitopes. Reports on the expression of this epitope by some human malignant cells suggest the possible occurrence of this process. Kagawa et al. (56) analyzed the carbohydrate residues of recombinant DNA interferon-β molecules produced by a *human* lung carcinoma cell line. These investigators have found that, while the majority of the N-linked carbohydrate residues have the structure SA-Galβ1→4GlcNAc-R (SA, sialic acid), one-tenth of the residues is the α-galactosyl epitope with the structure Galα1→3Galβ1→4GlcNAc-R. Castronovo et al. (57) have reported the expression of α-galactosyl epitopes on the surface of mammary carcinoma cell lines and on malignant cells obtained by aspiration biopsy from primary lesions of 50% of patients with mammary carcinoma. These studies on human malignant cells suggest that the mechanism which causes the suppression of α1-3 galactosyltransferase expression in man can be overridden under certain circumstances.

The potential of α1-3 galactosyltransferase to be aberrantly expressed and to synthesize the α-galactosyl epitope in human cells is of substantial pathologic significance, for the following reason: In the Golgi apparatus of human cells, the N-acetyllactosamine residues (Galβ1-4GlcNAc-R) of human cell membrane glycoproteins are usually sialylated by sialyltransferases which catalyze the synthesis of SAα2→3Galβ1⁄4GlcNAc residues or SAα2→6Galβ1→4GlcNAc residues (58). Aberrant activity of α1-3 galactosyltransferase in vivo would result in the synthesis of a number of Galα1→3Galβ1→4GlcNAc residues on membrane glycoproteins. The binding of anti-Gal to these de novo-produced α-galactosyl epitopes, as demonstrated in Figure 2, would lead to a local inflammatory reaction mediated by granulocytes, macrophages, and killer lymphoid cells interacting with the Fc portion of the bound anti-Gal. These cytotoxic cells would subsequently exert their lytic activity toward the cells producing the α-galactosyl epitope in an antibody-dependent, cell-mediated cytolysis (ADCC) process. A relatively low number of α-galactosyl epitopes per cell would be sufficient to bind the threshold amount of anti-Gal IgG molecules required to induce ADCC. Thus, a human mammary carcinoma cell line expressing $\sim 10^5$ epitopes per cell is readily killed in an ADCC reaction in the presence of anti-Gal, whereas human fibroblasts, which do not express this epitope, are completely resistant to lysis (59).

Studies on the expression of α-galactosyl epitopes and α1-3 galactosyltransferase in mammalian thyroid glands may illustrate this point. The α-galactosyl epitope is expressed in variable amounts on thyroglobulin molecules and thyrocyte membrane of species such as rat, guinea pig, rabbit, pig, cow, and squirrel monkey (New World monkey) but not in rhesus monkey (Old World monkey) and man (20,34,38,52). These findings correlated with the activity of α1-3 galactosyltransferase which was found to be high in microsomal preparations of nonprimate mammalian and New World monkey thyroids, but diminished in Old World monkey and human thyroid (52). Aberrant expression of the α1-3 galactosyltransferase gene in human thyroid cells could induce an ADCC reaction toward the thyrocytes. This process would, in turn, damage physiologic barriers, increase exposure of the immune system to other thyroid antigens, and ultimately lead to expansion of B- and T-lymphoid clones that react with thyroid-specific antigens. Eventually, an antoimmune inflammatory reaction initiated by anti-Gal would be perpetuated.

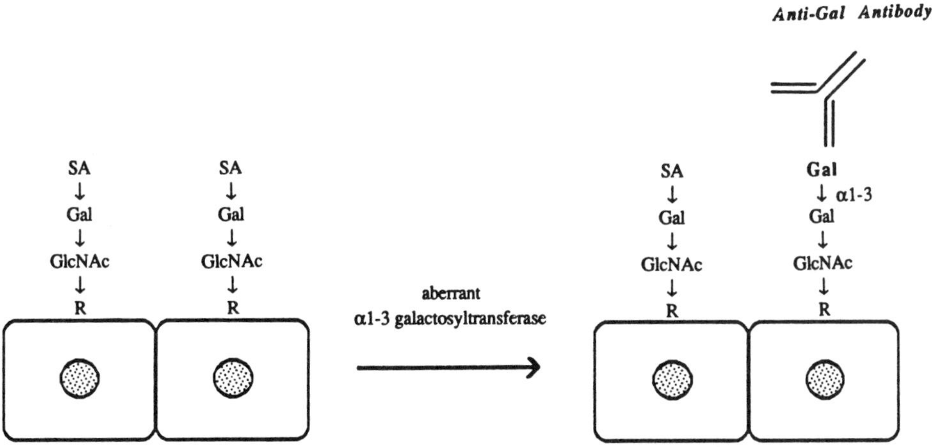

FIGURE 2 Human cells normally synthesize glycoconjugates in which the carbohydrate chains are mostly sialylated. Aberrant activity of α1-3 galactosyltransferase in human cells would result in the synthesis of α-galactosyl epitopes. Binding of anti-Gal to these epitopes may initiate an autoimmune process. Gal, galactose; GlcNAc, N-acetylgalactosamine; SA, sialic acid.

This hypothetical scenario is supported by findings in healthy individuals of B-lymphoid clones that can produced antibodies to human thyroglobulin (60). Such clones may be expanded upon chronic exposure to thyroglobulin. Abnormal expression of α-galactosyl epitopes in patients with autoimmune disorders of the thyroid has been suggested by Winand et al. (61,62). These investigators observed a marked elevation in anti-Gal titer in patients with Graves' disease (possibly a result of overimmunization by α-galactosyl epitopes on thyrocytes) and reported on the expression of α-galactosyl epitopes in the thyroid of a patient with Graves' disease. In a recent study, we have found a significant elevation in α1-3 galactosyltransferase activity in thyroid microsomal fractions of two out of three patients with Graves' disease, and no increase in this enzyme activity in patients with nontoxic goiter or adenoma of the thyroid. Hypothetically, activation of the α1-3 galactosyltransferase in vivo may occur as a result of viral infection or mutations induced by chemicals or irradiation. Such factors may impair the suppressive mechanism normally preventing expression of the α1-3 galactosyltransferase gene, thus leading to the pathologic synthesis of glucoconjugates with α-galactosyl epitopes. Although such preliminary studies suggest the involvement of αgalactosyl epitopes and anti-Gal in the pathologic process within the thyroid, a more detailed study is needed to better assess the contribution of α1-3 galactosyltransferase to the etiology of autoimmune disorders of the thyroid. Such a study should combine measurement of α1-3 galactosyltransferase gene transcription, activity of this enzyme in microsomal fractions, and the expression of α-galactosyl epitopes on thyroid cell membranes in pathologic specimens.

It is theoretically possible that a similar mechanism exists for other autoimmune disorders where α-galactosyl epitopes might be synthesized de novo. Thus abnormal expression of the α1-3 galactosyltransferase gene in synovial cells may result in rheumatoid arthritis, whereas a similar event in Langerhans islet cells in the pancreas may initiate diabetes.

An alternative source for α1-3 galactosyltransferase synthesizing pathologic α-galactosyl epitopes on human normal cells may be an exogenous one, i.e., bacterial, α1-3 galactosyltransferase. The activity of such an enzyme has been demonstrated in *Salmonella* (63). Since α-galactosyl residues are common in bacteria of the human flora, it is possible that some "promiscuous" bacterial α-galactosyltransferases can use human N-acetyllactosamine residues as acceptors for de novo synthesis of α-galactosyl epitopes on human cell membranes. The interaction of anti-Gal with such epitopes would result in an inflammatory process causing the destruction of autologous tissues and propagation of autoimmune reactions as discussed above. We are currently studying the capacity of bacterial galactosyltransferases to synthesize the α-galactosyl epitope in vitro.

V. ANTI-Gal AND HUMAN RED CELL AGING

Our studies on the immunoglobulin molecules involved in the removal of human senescent red cells suggest that there is a residual synthesis of a cryptic α-galactosyl epitope in human erythropoietic cells. Studies by Kay (64) have suggested that as red cells age in the circulation, cryptic antigens are exposed, binding a few hundred molecules of natural antibodies. The bound IgG molecules label the aging red cells for phagocytosis by the macrophages of the reticuloendothelial system. Senescent red cells could be obtained by centrifugation of red cells on a density gradient and isolation of the 1% of cells with the highest density (>1.11 g/ml) (65). Elution experiments with various free carbohydrates revealed that a large proportion of the IgG molecules on normal human aging red cells (i.e., high-density red cells) display anti-Gal specificity (66,67). Incubation of high-density red cells (>1.11 g/ml) with melibiose or α-methylgalactose resulted in extensive elution of the bound antibodies, whereas lactose and β-methylgalactose did not elute the bound antibodies from the senescent red cells. Incubation of IgG-depleted senescent red cells with anti-Gal resulted in binding of the natural antibody to these cells, whereas no anti-Gal binding was observed with young red cells (66,67). Furthermore, senescent red cells were readily phagocytized in vitro by macrophages, but following elution of the IgG antibodies with α-methylgalactose, phagocytosis was diminished. Rebinding of anti-Gal resulted in reinduction of the in vitro phagocytosis of the senescent red cells by macrophages (66,67).

It is of interest to note that, while anti-Gal binds in vivo to the senescent red cells which in healthy individuals comprise less than 1% of the red cells, in patients with β-thalassemia or sickle cell anemia where red cells are destroyed prematurely, the same antibody is detectable on 30–40% of the red cells (13,66–69). In addition, proteolytic treatment of normal young red cells can result in the exposure of cryptic binding sites for anti-Gal on the red cell membrane (13). All of these studies suggest that human red cells have a low number of cryptic α-galactosyl epitopes, which are exposed upon the aging of red cells, possibly by removal of surface glycoproteins in the course of red cell aging. Scatchard plotting analysis of the binding of labeled *Bandeirea simplicifolia* IB_4 lectin (which interacts with the α-galactosyl epitope) revealed the occurrence of 1000–2000 such epitopes per red cell (67). In order to identify such putative α-galactosyl epitopes as cryptic structures on human red cell glycolipids, we produced a monoclonal antibody, designated Gal-13, which is highly specific for this epitope on glycolipids (40). By using this monoclonal antibody, we could identify a small population of glycolipids with α-galactosyl epitopes in human red cells (40). These findings implied that the α1-3 galactosyltransferase gene may be marginally expressed in human erythropoietic cells, resulting in residual synthesis of a few cryptic α-galactosyl epitopes on the red cell membrane. It is suggested that, because of gradual removal of surface glycoproteins, possibly by proteases on the surface of reticuloendothelial macrophages (70), cryptic α-galactosyl epitopes are exposed and subsequently bind the natural anti-Gal antibody. After approximately 120 days in circulation, a sufficient number of anti-Gal IgG molecules are attached to the aging red cells, labeling them for phagocytosis by the reticuloendothelial macrophages. In patients ith β-thalassemia and sickle cell anemia, the red cells are trapped in the reticuloendothelial system in an early stage in the circulation because of intrinsic structural defects, and are subjected to accelerated exposure of the α-galactosyl epitope and thus premature destruction mediated by anti-Gal. It should be stressed that anti-Gal is not viewed as an antibody present in the circulation to probe for senescent red cells. Rather, it is primarily produced as a result of antigenic stimulation by environmental antigens. Hypothetically, if anti-Gal would not have been produced in man, red cells might circulate for more than 120 days, and eventually would have been removed by other mechanisms related to the "wear and tear" processes occurring on the circulating red cell membrane. In species that lack anti-Gal and synthesize an abundance of α-galactosyl epitopes, removal of red cells from the circulation involves other mechanisms in which natural antibodies may or may not participate. The large variation in the lifespan of red cells in different mammalian species may be attributed to the variety of mechanisms participating in the removal of senescent red cells, and may imply that there is no "unified theory" for explaining destruction of aging red cells in mammals.

VI. CONCLUDING REMARKS

Autoimmune diseases are defined as diseases in which the immune system, for some unknown reason, recognizes autologous tissue and cell components as foreign. Thus many of the characteristics observed in the immunization response to foreign antigens are attributed to the autoimmune process. The studies presented in this chapter offer an additional aspect to this complex issue: The interaction between natural antibodies and de novo synthesized "forbidden antigens." The information for biosynthesis of such antigens has been conserved within the human genome in a suppressed form as a result of particular events which occurred in the course of evolution. Theoretically, carbohydrate structures may comprise a considerable proportion of such "forbidden antigens," since these structures are among the main components of bacterial antigenicity. Evolutionarily, production of antibodies against such carbohydrates coupled with the suppression of the autologous antigenic structures could have been an effective way of coping with new pathogens. The anti-Gal antibody and the α-galactosyl epitope offer one example of such a relationship. The suppression of the glycosyltransferase synthesizing the α-galactosyl epitope, whether the result of a structural mutation or regulatory mechanism, may represent a more general mechanism for evolutionary suppression of carbohydrate antigens. Aberrant synthesis of such structures may result in autoimmune processes mediated by natural antibodies, which are primarily directed against environmental pathogens.

Most of the current information on autoimmune diseases has been derived from animal models, many of which have evolved along pathways different from that of humans, for more than 70 million years. The study of autoimmune diseases in animal models such as rodents may thus not provide insight on forbidden antigens in man. The identification of antigens recognized by natural human antibodies in such animals may, however, provide preliminary clues as to which antigens have been evolutionarily suppressed in man and, if reexpressed, would contribute to autoimmune processes.

ACKNOWLEDGMENTS

Dr. Galili's work has been supported by NIH grants AG-06299 and GM-40205.

REFERENCES

1. Douglas, S. D., Goldberg, L. S., and Fudenberg, H. H. 1970. Clinical serological and leukocyte function studies on patients with idiopathic "acquired" agammaglobulinemia and their families. *Am. J. Med.*, *48*: 48–53.

2. Frank, A., Andeman, W. A., and Miller, G. 1976. Epstein-Barr virus and nonhuman primates. Natural and experimental infection. *Adv. Cancer Res.*, *23*: 171–201.
3. DeThe, G. 1980. Role of Epstein-Barr virus in human diseases: Infectious mononucleosis, Burkitt's lymphoma and nasopharyngeal carcinoma. In *Viral Oncology* (G. Klein, ed.). Raven Press, New York, pp. 169–197.
4. Hanto, D. W., Frizzera, G., Gajl-Plczalska, K. J., Sakamoto, K., Purtilo, D. T., Balfour, H. H., Simmons, R. L., and Najarian, J. S. 1982. Epstein-Barr virus induced B-cell lymphoma after renal transplantation. *N. Engl. J. Med.*, *306*: 913–918.
5. Cleary, N. L., and Sklar, J. 1984. Lymphoproliferative disorders in cardiac transplant recipients are multiclonal lymphoma. *Lancet*, *i*: 489–493.
6. DeVay, J. E., and Adle, H. E. 1976. Antigens common to host and parasites. *Ann. Rev. Microbiol.*, *30*: 147–168.
7. Wiener, A. S. 1951. Origin of naturally occurring hemagglutinins and hemolysins: A review. *J. Immunol.*, *66*: 287–295.
8. Springer, G. F., and Horton, R. F. 1969. Blood group isoantibody stimulation in man by feeding blood group-active bacteria. *J. Clin. Invest.*, *48*: 1280–1291.
9. Mourant, A. E., Kopéc, A. C., and Domaniewska-Sobczak, O. 1976. *The Distribution of Blood Groups and Other Polymorphisms*, Vol. 1, 2nd ed. Oxford Press, p. 1050.
10. Salzano, F. M. 1957. The blood groups of South American Indians. *Am. J. Phys. Anthropol.*, 555–579.
11. Pereira, M., Rohr, P. J. A., Langyel, I., and Barretto, O. C. O. P. 1984. Os grupos sanguineos ABO em esqueletos pré-históricos de aborigines de Ilha de Santa Catarina, Brasil. *Cienca e Cultura*, *36*: 1597–1599 (in Portuguese, abstract in English).
12. Wilson, A. C. 1985. The molecular basis of evolution. *Sci. Am.*, (Oct): 164–173.
13. Galili, U., Rachmilewitz, E. A., Peleg, A., and Flechner, I. 1984. A unique natural human IgG antibody with anti-α-galactosyl specificity. *J. Exp. Med.*, *160*: 1519–1531.
14. Galili, U., Macher, B. A., Buehler, J., and Shoet, S. B. 1985. Human natural anti-α-galactosyl IgG. II. The specific recognition of α(1-3)-linked galactose residues. *J. Exp. Med.*, *162*: 573–582.
15. Davin, J. C., Malaise, M., Foidart, J. M., and Mahieu, P. 1987. Anti-α-galactosyl antibodies and immune complexes in children with Henoch-Schönlein purpura or IgA nephropathy. *Kidney Res.*, *31*: 1132–1139.
16. Galili, U., Buehler, J., Shohet, S. B., and Macher, B. A. 1987. The human natural anti-Gal IgG. III. The subtlety of immune tolerance in man as demonstrated by crossreactivity between natural ati-Gal and anti-B antibodies. *J. Exp. Med.*, *165*: 693–704.
17. Galili, U., Shohet, S. B., Kobrin, E., Stults, C. L. M., and Macher, B. A. 1988. Man, apes, and Old World monkeys differ from other mammals in the expression of α-galactosyl epitopes on nucleated cells. *J. Biol. Chem.*, *263*: 17755–17762.
18. Towbin, H., Rosenfelder, G., Wieslander, J., Avila, J. L., Rojas, M., Szarfman, A., Esser, K., Nowack, H., and Timple, R. 1987. Circulating antibodies to mouse laminin in Chagas disease, American cutaneous Leishmaniasis and normal individuals recognize terminal galactosyl (α1-3) galactose epitopes. *J. Exp. Med.*, *166*: 419–432.

19. Suzuki, E., and Naiki, M. 1984. Heterophile antibodies to rabbit erythrocytes in human sera and identification of the antigen as a glycolipid. *J. Biochem.* (Tokyo), *83*: 103–108.
20. Thall, A., and Galili, U. Distribution of Galα1→3Galβ1→4GlcNAc residues on secreted mammalian glycoproteins (thyroglobulin, fibrinogen and immunoglobulin G) as measured by a sensitive solid-phase radioimmunoassay. *Biochemistry* (in press).
21. Eto, T., Iichikawa, Y., Nishimura, K., Ando, S., and Yamakawa, T. 1968. Chemistry of lipids of the posthemolytic residue or stroma of erythrocytes. XVI. Occurrence of ceramide pentasaccharide in the membrane of erythrocytes and reticulocytes in rabbit. *J. Biochem.* (Tokyo), *64*: 205–213.
22. Stellner, K., Saito, H., and Hakomori, S. 1973. Determination of aminosugar linkage in glycolipids by methylation. Aminosugar linkage of ceramide pentasaccharides of rabbit erythrocytes and of Forssman antigen. *Arch. Biochem. Biophys.*, *133*: 464–472.
23. Egge, H., Kordowicz, M., Peter-Katalinic, J., and Hanfland, P. 1985. Immunochemistry of I/i-active oligo- and polyglycosylceramides from rabbit erythrocyte membranes. *J. Biol. Chem.*, *260*: 4927–4935.
24. Galili, U. 1988. The two antibody specificities within human anti-blood group B antibodies. *Tarnsfus. Med. Rev.*, *2*: 112–121.
25. Galili, U., Mandrell, R. E., Hamadeh, R. M., Shohet, S. B., and Griffiss, J. M. 1988. The interaction between the human natural anti-α-galactosyl IgG (anti-Gal) and bacteria of the human flora. *Infect. Immun.*, *57*: 1730–1737.
26. Lüderitz, O., Simmons, D. A. R., and Westphal, O. 1965. The immunochemistry of *Salmonella* chemotype VI O-antigen. The structure of oligosaccharides from *Salmonella* group U 043 lipopolysaccharides. *Biochem. J.*, *97*: 820–826.
27. Jansson, P. E., Linberg, A. A., Lindberg, B., and Walling, R. 1981. Structural studies on the hexose region of the core lipopolysaccharide from enterobacteriaceae. *Eur. J. Biochem.*, *115*: 571–577.
28. Eckhardt, A. E., and Goldstein, I. J. 1983. Isolation and characterization of a family of α-D-galactosyl-containing glycopeptides from Ehrlich ascites tumor cells. *Biochemistry*, *22*: 5290–5297.
29. Cummings, R. D., and Kornfeld, S. 1984. The distribution of separating [Galβ1,4GlcNAcβ1,3] sequences in asparagine-linked oligosaccharides of the mouse lymphoma cell lines BW 5147 and PHA 2.1. *J. Biol. Chem.*, *259*: 6253–6260.
30. Santer, U. V., DeSantis, R., Hård, K. J., van Kuik, J. A., Vliegenthart, J. F. G., Won, B., and Glock, M. C. 1989. N-linked oligosaccharide changes with oncogenic transformation require sialylation of multiantennae. *Eur. J. Biochem.*, *181*: 249–260.
31. Hull, S. R., Laine, R. A., Kaizu, T., Rodriguez, I., and Carraway, K. L. 1984. Structures of O-linked oligosaccharides of the major cell surface sialoglycoprotein of MAT-B and MAH-C, ascites sublines of the 13762 rat mammary adenocarcinoma. *J. Biol. Chem.*, *259*: 4866–4877.
32. Uemura, K., Yuzawa, M., and Taketomi, T. 1978. Characterization of major glycolipids in bovine erythrocyte membrane. *J. Biochem.* (Tokyo), *83*: 463–471.
33. Chien, J. L., Li, S. C., and Li, Y. T. 1979. Isolation and characterization of a heptaglycosylceramide from bovine erythrocyte membrane. *J. Lipid Res.*, *20*: 669–673.

34. Edge, A. S. B., and Spiro, R. G. 1985. Thyroid cell surface glycoproteins. Nature and disposition of carbohydrate units and evaluation of their blood group I activity. *J. Biol. Chem.*, *260*: 15332–15338.
35. Honma, K., Manabe, H., Tomita, M., and Hamada, A. 1981. Isolation and partial structure characterization of macroglycolipids from rabbit red cell membrane. *J. Biochem.* (Tokyo), *90*: 1187–1196.
36. Arumugham, R. G., Hsieh, T. C. Y., Tanzer, M. L., and Laine, R. A. 1986. Structures of the asparagine-linked sugar chains of laminin. *Biochim. Biophys. Acta, 883*: 112–126.
37. Mohan, P. S., and Spiro, R. G. 1985. Macromolecular organization of basement membranes. Characterization and comparison of glomerular basement membrane and lens capsule components by immunochemical and lectin affinity procedures. *J. Biol. Chem.*, *261*: 4328–4336.
38. Spiro, R. G., and Bhoyroo, V. D. 1984. Occurrence of α-D-galactosyl residues in the thyroglobulin from several species. Localization in the saccharide chains of the complex carbohydrate units. *J. Biol. Chem.*, *259*: 9858–9866.
39. Galili, U., Clark, M. R., Shohet, S. B., Buehler, J., Macher, B. A. 1987. Evolutionary relationship between the anti-Gal antibody and the Galα1→3Gal epitope in primates. *Proc. Natl. Acad. Sci. USA, 84*: 1369–1373.
40. Galili, U., Basbaum, C. B., Shohet, S. B., Buehler, J., and Macher, B. A. 1987. Identification of erythrocyte Galα1→3Gal glycosphingolipids with a mouse monoclonal antibody, Gal-13. *J. Biol. Chem.*, *262*: 4683–4688.
41. Napier, J. R., and Napier, P. H. 1985. *The Natural History of Primates*. MIT Press, Cambridge, MA.
42. Geyer, R., Geyer, H., Strim, S., Hunsmann, G., Schneider, J. Dabrowski, U., and Dabrowski, J. 1984. Major oligosaccharides in the glycoprotein of Friend murine leukemia virus: Structure elucidation by one- and two-dimensional proton nuclear magnetic resonance and methylation analysis. *Biochemistry, 23*: 5628–5634.
43. Avila, J. L., Rojas, M., and Galili, U. 1989. Immunogenic Galα1→3Gal carbohydrate epitopes are present on pathogenic American. *Trypanosoma* and *Leishmania*. *J. Immunol.*, *142*: 2828–2834.
44. Milani, S. R., and Travassos, L. R. 1988. Anti-α-galactosyl antibodies in chagasic patients. Possible biological significance. *Braz. J. Med. Biol. Res.*, *21*: 1275–1286.
45. Krivan, H. C., Clark, G. F., Smith, D. F., and Wilkins, D. T. 1986. Cell surface binding site for *Clostridium difficile* enterotoxin: Evidence of a glycoconjugate containing the sequence Galα1→3Galβ1→4GlcNAc. *Infect. Immun.*, *53*: 573–581.
46. Blake, D. D., and Goldstein, I. J. 1981. An α-D-galactosyltransferase in Ehrlich ascites tumor cells. Biosynthesis and characterization of a trisaccharide (α-D-galactose (1-3)-N-acetylgalatosamine). *J. Biol. Chem.*, *256*: 5387–5393.
47. Cummings, R. D., and Mattox, S. A. 1988. Retinoic acid-induced differentiation of the mouse teratocarcinoma cell line F9 is accompanied by an increase in the activity of UDP-galactose: β-D-galactosyl-α1,3-galactosyltransferase. *J. Biol. Chem.*, *263*: 511–519.
48. Basu, M., and Basu, S. 1973. Enzymatic synthesis of a blood group-related pentaglycosyl ceramide by an α-galactosyltransferase from rabbit bone marrow. *J. Biol. Chem.*, *248*: 12700–12706.

49. Betteridge, A., and Watkins, W. M. 1983. Two α-2-D-galactosyltransferases in rabbit stomach mucosa with different acceptor substrate specificities. *Eur. J. Biochem., 132*: 29–35.
50. Blanken, W. M., and Van den Eijnden, D. H. 1985. Biosynthesis of terminal Galα1→3Galβ1→4GlcNAc-R oligosaccharide sequence on glycoconjugates: Purification and acceptor specificity of a UDP-Gal: N-acetyllactosaminide α1-3 galactosyltransferase. *J. Biol. Chem., 260*: 12927–12934.
51. Elices, M. J., Blake, D. D., and Goldstein, I. J. 1986. Purification and characterization of a UDP-Gal: β-D-Gal(1,4)-D-GlcNAc α(1-3) galactosyltransferase from Ehrlich ascites tumor cells. *J. Biol. Chem., 261*: 6064–6072.
52. Thall, A., Etienne-Decerf, J., Winand, R., and Galili, U. α1-3 Galactosyltransferase in mammalian thyroid cells. (submitted).
53. Joziasse, D. H., Shaper, J. H., Van den Eijnden, D. H., Van Tunen, A. H., and Shaper, N. L. 1989. Bovine α1-3 galactosyltransferase: Isolation and characterization of a cDNA clone. Identification of homologous sequences in human genomic DNA. *J. Biol. Chem., 264*: 14290–14297.
54. Lowe, J. B., Larsen, R. D., Ruff, M. M., and Cummings, R. D. 1989. Isolation of cloned cDNAs that direct expression of oligosaccharides recognized by *Griffonia simplicifolia* isolectin B_4. *J. Cell Biochem., 13*A (Suppl): 129.
55. Larsen, R. D., Rajan, V. P., Ruff, M., Jukowska-Latialle, J., Cummings, R. D., and Lowe, J. B. 1989. Isolation of a cDNA encoding murine UDP galactose: βD-galactosyl-1,4-N-acetyl-D-glycosaminide α1,3-galactosyltransferase: Expression cloning by gene transfer. *Proc. Natl. Acad. Sci. USA, 86*: 8227–8231.
56. Kagawa, Y., Takasaki, S., Utsumi, J., Hasoi, K., Shimizu, H., Kochibe, N., and Kobata, A. 1988. Comparative study of the asparagine-linked sugar chains of natural human interferon-β1 and recombinant human interferon-β1 produced by three different mammalian cells. *J. Biol. Chem., 263*: 17508–17515.
57. Casronovo, V., Parent, B., Steeg, P. S., Colin, C., Foidart, J. M., Lambotte, R., and Mahieu, F. 1989. Human natural anti-Gal antibodies may play a role in the natural anti-tumor defense system. *J. Natl. Cancer Inst., 81*: 212–216.
58. Kornfeld, R., and Kornfled, S. 1985. Assembly of asparagine-linked oligosaccharides. *Ann. Rev. Biochem., 54*: 631–634.
59. Galili, U. 1989. Abnormal expression of α-galactosyl epitopes in man: A trigger for autoimmune processes? *Lancet, ii*: 358–361.
60. Casali, P., Inghirami, G., Nakamura, M., Davis, T. F.,a nd Notkins, A. L. 1986. Human monoclonals from antigen-specific selection of B lymphocytes and transformation by EBV. *Science, 234*: 476–479.
61. Etienne-Decerf, J., Mahieu, P., Malaise, M., and Winand, R. 1987. Measurement of anti-α-galactosyl antibodies in the course of various thyroid disorders and isolation of an antigenic glycopeptide fraction. In (Pinchera, A., Ingbar, S. H., McKenzie, J. M., and Fenzi, G. F., eds.). Plenum Press, pp. 297–301.
62. Etienne-Decerf, J., Malaise, M., Mahieu, P., and Winand, R. 1987. Elevated anti-α-galactosyl antibody titers. A marker of progression in autoimmune thyroid disorders and in endocrine ophthalmology. *Acta Endocrinol., 115*: 67–74.
63. Endo, A., and Rothfield, L. 1969. Studies on phospholipid-requiring bacteria enzymes.

I. Purification and properties of uridine diphosphate galactose: lipopolysaccharide α-3 galactosyltransferase. *Biochemistry, 8*: 3500–3507.

64. Kay, M. M. B. 1975. Mechanism of removal of red cells by macrophages in situ. *Proc. Natl. Acad. Sci. USA, 72*: 3521–3525.
65. Piomelli, S., Lurinsky, G., and Wasserman, R. L. 1967. The mechanism of red cell aging. I. Relationship between cell age and specific gravity evaluated by centrifugation in a discontinuous density gradient. *J. Lab. Clin. Med., 69*: 659–674.
66. Galili, U., Flechner, I., Kniszinski, A., Danon, D., and Rachmilewitz, E. A. 1986. The natural anti-α-galactosyl IgG on human normal senescent red blood cells. *Br. J. Haematol., 62*: 317–326.
67. Galili, U., Clark, M. R., and Shohet, S. B. 1986. Excessive binding of the natural anti-α-galactosyl IgG to sickle red cells may contribute to extravascular cell destruction. *J. Clin. Invest., 77*: 27–33.
68. Galili, U., Korkesh, A., Kahane, I., and Rachmilewitz, E. A. 1983. Demonstration of a natural anti-galactosyl IgG antibody on thalasseic red blood cells. *Blood, 61*: 1258–1264.
69. Galili, U. 1988. The natural anti-Gal antibody, the B-like antigen and human red cell aging. *Blood Cells, 14*: 205–220.
70. Galili, U., Kobrin, E., Macher, B. A., and Shohet, S. B. 1989. Anti-Gal and human red cell aging. In *The Red Cell: 7th Ann Arbor Conference* (G. J. Brewer, ed.). A. R. Liss Publications, pp. 225–245.

Index